日英対訳

日本における医薬品のリスクマネジメント 第3版

－新たな改正 GPSP 省令への対応と
　医薬品医療機器等法の改正に向けて－

企画・編集

一般財団法人 医薬品医療機器レギュラトリーサイエンス財団

Drug Risk Management in Japan 3rd ed.

- compatible with Newly revised GPSP
  Ordinance and including expectations for the
  forthcoming revision of the PMD Act -
  (in Japanese and English)

Edited by　Pharmaceutical and Medical Device
　　　　　　Regulatory Science Society of Japan

じほう

Drug Risk Management in Japan 3rd ed.
-compatible with Newly revised GPSP Ordinance
and including expectations for the forthcoming revision of the PMD Act-
(in Japanese and English)

ISBN: 978-4-8407-5170-4

Edited and planned by
Pharmaceutical and Medical Device Regulatory Science Society of Japan (PMRJ).

First published 2019

©Copyright 2019 by Jiho, Inc.
Published in Japan by Jiho, Inc.,
1-5-15, Kandasarugakucho, Chiyoda-ku, Tokyo, 101-8421, Japan,
phone: +81-3-3233-6361, fax: +81-3-3233-6369

None of the contents of this publication may be reproduced by any means without
the prior written permission of the publisher, Jiho, Inc.

Notice

　発行者等は，本書の記載内容について，正確かつ最新（2019 年 3 月現在）の情報であるよう細心の注意を払って編集作業を行っております。しかし，本書の主たる情報源である法令，厚生労働省および独立行政法人 医薬品医療機器総合機構（PMDA）等による運用・行政執行の方針は常に改正，更新されております。実際の薬事行政や企業における薬事業務実施にあたりましては，ご自身で必ず最新の関連法令等を参照の上，適宜，厚生労働省および独立行政法人 医薬品医療機器総合機構（PMDA）等に直接確認していただきますようお願い申し上げます。

　本書の内容に関連して生じたいかなる損害等について，一般財団法人 医薬品医療機器レギュラトリーサイエンス財団，本書の執筆者，英文監修者，および株式会社 じほうは一切の責任を負いません。

The issuer, etc. have performed the editing work with great attention so that the descriptions in this book are accurate and latest (as of March 2019) information. However, the main information sources for this book, such as laws/regulations and the guidelines on operations or administrative executions provided by the Ministry of Health, Labour and Welfare (MHLW), the Pharmaceuticals and Medical Devices Agency (PMDA), etc. are always being revised or updated. When implementing actual pharmaceutical regulations or pharmaceutical affairs-related duties in your company, please directly check with the MHLW, the PMDA, etc. in an appropriate manner after referring to latest related laws/regulations.

The Pharmaceutical and Medical Device Regulatory Science Society of Japan, the authors and English editorial supervisor of this book, and Jiho, Inc. assume no responsibility whatsoever for any damages, etc. occurring in relation to the contents of the book.

序

　医薬品による最適な治療効果を引き出すためには，有効かつ安全で，品質の確保された医薬品が，必要かつ十分な情報とともに医療の場に提供され，適正に使用され，さらには，医療の場からの情報が迅速かつ正確にフィードバックされ，より有効で安全な使用へと生かされることが重要である。そのためには，開発・審査段階から製造販売後までの，医薬品のライフサイクル全般にわたり，一貫したリスクマネジメントが必要である。

　本書は，2010年に初版が発行され，2014年の改訂を経て，医薬品の製造販売後安全管理や製造販売後調査担当の方々などに幅広く活用されてきた「日本における医薬品のリスクマネジメント」を，国際的な変化などに対応した，わが国の薬事規制などの見直しの内容などを取り入れるため，今回，新たに大改訂を行ったものである。

　医薬品を巡る国際的な環境は，ICHが始まった1990年当時に比べると，21世紀に入り，急速に変化してきている。米国における製造販売後安全対策の強化などの動きにもみられるように，従来，開発・審査段階に重点が置かれていた医薬品のリスク管理が，開発・審査から製造販売後までの一貫したものとして捉える方向に大きく動き出している。

　さらには，医薬品規制の在り方も，単に規制を厳しくすることにより医薬品の品質や有効性・安全性を確保するという考え方から，医薬品製造販売業者の自主性を重視し，無駄な規制はできるだけ廃止し，より合理的かつ効率的な規制とすることによって，ICHの目標でもある，「より良い医薬品をより早く患者さんのもとに届ける」ことを重視する規制へと，国際的にも大きく変化しつつある。

　わが国においては，ICHの一員として，欧米との調和が重視されつつも，なお，わが国の長い歴史を背景とした，独特の薬事規制が存在している。そのため，欧米との共通化が難しく，効率的な医薬品のリスクマネジメントを行うための障害となっているといわれている。わが国固有の習慣や考え方は，欧米からは，わが国の規制が理解しにくい，規制の理由がわかりにくいなどといわれる原因ともなっている。

　本書が，わが国の医薬品リスクマネジメントに関する歴史や仕組みを，国内だけではなく，外国の方々にも理解していただくための一助となり，将来的には，わが国を含む3極の医薬品のリスクマネジメントに関する規制がよりグローバルなものに統一されることを期待している。

2019年4月

　　　　　　　　一般財団法人　医薬品医療機器レギュラトリーサイエンス財団

　　　　　　　　　　　　理事長　　土　井　　脩

Preface

To achieve the optimum therapeutic effects of drugs, it is of utmost importance to provide drugs with assured efficacy, safety and quality to medical practices hand in hand with sufficient and necessary information so that proper use can be achieved. Moreover, feedbacks from medical practices must be obtained promptly and accurately and utilized for ever more effective and safer use. For this purpose, consistent risk management must be employed throughout the lifecycle of drugs from the stage of development and review to post-marketing stage.

This document was first published in 2010 and revised in 2014. "Drug Risk Management in Japan" extensively utilized by those involved in post-marketing safety control and investigation of drugs has now been substantially revised to incorporate results of review of pharmaceutical regulations in Japan, taking account of global changes, etc.

The global environment surrounding drugs has been changing rapidly in the 21st century, compared to 1990 when the ICH was started. As seen by the strengthening of post-marketing risk management in the United States, major steps have been taken to expand drug risk management from its previous emphasis on the development and review stages to a consistent approach covering not only clinical development and review but also post-marketing.

Furthermore, the purpose of pharmaceutical regulations has also been changing globally, from the assurance of quality, efficacy and safety of drugs by simply strengthening the regulations to the one which places importance on "Faster delivery of better drugs to patients", which is also the goal of the ICH, by honoring the independence of marketing authorization holders, abolishing unnecessary regulations as much as possible, and making regulations more rational and efficient.

In Japan, although it is considered important to harmonize with the US and Europe as a member of the ICH, we have distinctive pharmaceutical regulations based on the long history of our country. As such, it can be difficult to standardize regulations with the US and Europe, and it is considered that these regulations may hinder efficient drug risk management. Also, the habits and concepts unique to Japan may be the reasons why it is difficult for the US and Europe to understand Japanese regulations and reasons behind them.

I hope that this book helps not only Japanese people but also people overseas understand the history and structure of drug risk management in Japan, and expect that regulations on drug risk management in three major regions including Japan would be globally unified in the future.

April 2019
Pharmaceutical and Medical Device Regulatory Science Society of Japan
Osamu Doi, Ph.D., Chief Executive

今回の改訂にあたって

　2010年4月に公表された「薬害肝炎事件の検証及び再発防止のための医薬品行政のあり方検討会」の最終提言,並びに2010年8月に公表された「医薬品の安全対策における医療関係データベースの活用方策に関する懇談会」の提言を受けて,PMDAでは以下の2つのプロジェクトが進行していました。

　MIHARI（Medical Information for Risk Assessment Initiative）projectは電子診療情報等を安全対策へ活用する体制を構築することを目的として,安全対策業務の強化・充実策の一環として2009年4月に発足し,2014年4月以降の5年間で実際の安全対策措置に活用するとしています。また,並行して新規データソースや,新規手法については引き続き各種試行調査を通じて,その利用可能性について検討を重ねています。

　MID-NET（Medical Information Database Network）のprojectは医療ビッグデータの活用により現在の副作用報告制度の限界を補い,薬剤疫学的手法による医薬品等の安全対策を推進することを目的として2011年4月からそのシステム構築が開始され,2015年4月からの行政,協力医療機関によるシ

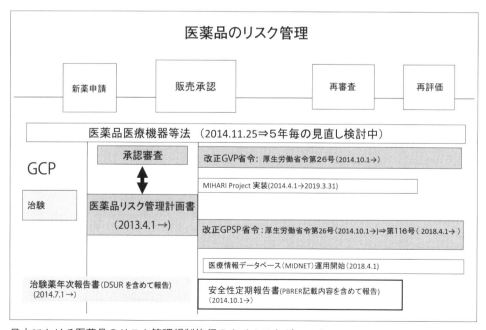

日本における医薬品のリスク管理規制施行のタイムスケジュール

About the Present Revision

In response to the final recommendations of the "Review Committee on Drug Administration for Investigation and Prevention of Recurrence of Drug-induced Hepatitis Cases" released in April 2010 and the recommendations of the "Informal Conference on Measures for Utilization of Medical Databases in Safety Measures for Drugs" released in August 2010, the following 2 projects were promoted by the PMDA.

Medical Information for Risk Assessment Initiative (MIHARI) project was started in April 2009 to construct a structure for utilization of electronic medical information, etc. in safety measures as a part of the measures for strengthening and enriching safety measure operations. It is planned to utilize such information in the actual safety measures and actions in 5 years from April 2014. At the same time, repeated investigations are conducted on usability of new data sources and new approaches through various experimental surveys.

For Medical Information Database Network (MID-NET) project, the construction of the system was started in April 2011 to compensate for limitations of present ADR reporting system by utilizing medical big data and to promote safety measures for drugs, etc. by pharmacoepidemiologic approach. After the trial operation of the system by the government and cooperative medical institutions since April 2015, full-scale operation has been carried out since April 2018 and it has been available for utilization by pharmaceutical companies and researchers.

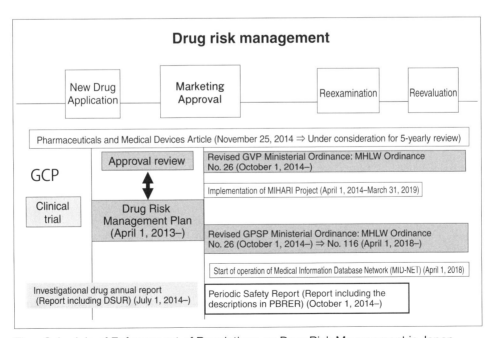

Time Schedule of Enforcement of Regulations on Drug Risk Management in Japan

ステムの試行運用を経て，2018 年 4 月からシステムを本格運用，製薬企業や研究者等による利活用も可能となっています。

　一方，2014 年 11 月に施行された「医薬品，医療機器等の品質，有効性及び安全性の確保等に関する法律（略称：医薬品医療機器等法）により，「医薬品リスク管理計画書」の作成は承認条件となり，結果として「安全性監視計画」の作成について欧米との調和の面から，官民合同の勉強会を通じて検討されていました。

　「改正 GPSP 省令：医薬品の製造販売後の調査及び試験の実施の基準に関する省令等の一部を改正する省令（平成 29 年厚生労働省令第 116 号）」が 2017 年 10 月 26 日に公布され，2018 年 4 月 1 日から施行されています。この省令により，医療情報データベースを用いて実施する調査として「製造販売後データベース調査」が新たに定義され，平成 29 年 12 月 5 日付薬生薬審発 1205 第 1 号，薬生安発 1205 第 1 号厚生労働省医薬・生活衛生 局医薬品審査管理課長，医薬安全対策課長連名通知「「医薬品リスク管理計画の策定について」の一部改正について」が発出されました。

　そこで，本改訂版では第 4 章「わが国の市販後の医薬品リスクマネジメント」，第 7 章「市販後安全対策」の大幅な見直しを行い，第 8 章「製品基本情報と適正使用情報」を新設し，併せて，2014 年 11 月に施行された医薬品医療機器等法の 5 年毎の見直し（2019 年中に公布予定）について検討された医薬品医療機器制度部会での「薬機法改正の取りまとめ案」から「日本の医薬品リスクマネジメント」に関連する内容についても第 1 章で紹介しています。

On the other hand, "Act on Securing Quality, Efficacy and Safety of Pharmaceuticals, Medical Devices, Regenerative and Cellular Therapy Products, Gene Therapy Products, and Cosmetics (Abbreviated name: PMD Act)" enacted in November 2014 made the preparation of "Drug Risk Management Plan" a condition for approval. Consequently, investigations were conducted for preparation of "Pharmacovigilance Plan" through study meetings co-held by public and private sectors, in relation to harmonization with the US and Europe.

"Revised GPSP Ministerial Ordinance: Ministerial Ordinance for Partial Revision of the Ministerial Ordinance on Good Post-marketing Study Practice (MHLW Ordinance No. 116, 2017) was promulgated on October 26, 2017 and enacted on April 1, 2018. This ministerial ordinance newly defined "Post-marketing database survey" as the study conducted using medical information databases. Also, Joint PSEHB/PED Notification No. 1205-1 and PSEHB/PSD Notification No. 1205-1, "Partial Revision of 'Establishment of Risk Management Plan'" was issued by the Directors of Pharmaceutical Evaluation Division and Pharmaceutical Safety Division, Pharmaceutical Safety and Environmental Health Bureau, MHLW on December 5, 2017.

Therefore, Chapter 4, "Post-marketing Drug Risk Management in Japan" and Chapter 7, "Post-marketing Pharmacovigilance" were substantially revised. Chapter 8, "Basic Product Information and Information on Proper Use" was newly established in this new version. In addition, Chapter 1 refers to the contents related to "Drug Risk Management in Japan" from the "Draft Summary for Revision of the PMD Act" by the Committee on Pharmaceuticals and Medical Devices which is reviewed every 5 years (to be promulgated in 2019) of the PMD Act enacted in November 2014.

Editing and Planning:

一般財団法人 医薬品医療機器レギュラトリーサイエンス財団
Pharmaceutical and Medical Device Regulatory Science Society of Japan (PMRJ)

古閑　　晃	Kokan, Akira	(Chap.4, 5, 7)
小山　弘子	Koyama, Hiroko	(Chap.1, 2, 3, 8)
津田　重城	Tsuda, Shigeki	(Chap.1, 6)
東宮　秀夫	Tomiya, Hideo	(Chap.1)
平河　　威	Hirakawa, Takeshi	(Chap.4, 7)

(五十音順)

Supervisor of English translation:

Geary, Stewart
エーザイ株式会社 コーポレートメディカルアフェアーズ本部
Corporate Medical Affairs HQ, Eisai Co., Ltd.

Contributors:

大西　昭子　　Onishi , Akiko　　(to Chap.5)
メルクバイオファーマ株式会社 グローバル リサーチ＆ディベロップメント クオリティ部門
Global Research & Development Quality (RDQ), Merck Biopharma Co., Ltd.

慶徳　一浩　　Keitoku, Kazuhiro　　(to Chap.2, 4 and 5)
ファイザー株式会社 医薬品安全性統括部
Japan Drug Safety Unit, Pfizer Japan Inc.

河合　秀晃　　Kawai, Hideaki　　(to Chap.8)
アステラス製薬株式会社 ファーマコヴィジランス部
QA, RA and Pharmacovigilance, Astellas Pharma Inc.

渡部　ゆき子　　Watabe, Yukiko　　(to Chap.2 and 3)
中外製薬株式会社 医薬安全性本部
Drug Safety Division, Chugai Pharmaceutical Co., Ltd.

The above information is sorted alphabetically by last name,
and places of employment as of February, 2019.

目　　次

略語 ……………………………………………………………………… xix

専門用語日英対照表 …………………………………………………… xxiii

専門用語英日対照表 …………………………………………………… xxxix

第1章　わが国の医薬品審査，安全対策をめぐる現状と将来に向けて

1.1　開発や審査の現状と課題 ………………………………………… 4

  1.1.1　治験の現状と課題　*6*

  1.1.2　新薬審査の現状と課題　*6*

  1.1.3　条件付き承認制度　*8*

1.2　市販後安全対策の現状と課題 ………………………………… 12

1.3　新薬の安全性確保と課題 ……………………………………… 18

  1.3.1　薬害再発防止のための医薬品行政等の見直しのその後　*18*

  1.3.2　PMDA の第 3 期 5 か年計画の進捗状況　*26*

  1.3.3　PMDA 第 4 期中期計画への期待　*34*

1.4　医薬品医療機器等法改正への動向 …………………………… 38

  1.4.1　患者アクセスの迅速化に資する承認審査制度の合理化　*38*

  1.4.2　国際的な整合性のある品質管理手法の導入　*42*

  1.4.3　安全対策の充実　*44*

  1.4.4　医薬品，医療機器等の製造・流通・販売に関わる者のガバナンスの強化等　*48*

  1.4.5　その他　*52*

第2章　臨床開発から市販後までの安全体制

2.1　臨床開発時安全体制 …………………………………………… 54

2.2　市販後安全体制 ………………………………………………… 56

  2.2.1　製造販売業三役　*58*

  2.2.2　GVP（改正 GVP）　*62*

  2.2.3　GQP　*64*

CONTENTS

Abbreviation .... **xix**
Terminology Japanese-English .... **xxiii**
Terminology English-Japanese .... **xxxix**

Chapter 1 Current status and future prospects of pharmaceutical approval review and safety policies in Japan

1.1 Current status and issues related to development and approval review
.... **5**
   1.1.1 Current status and issues for clinical trials   7
   1.1.2 Current status and issues related to new drug reviews   7
   1.1.3 Conditional approval system   9
1.2 Current status and issues with post-marketing risk management **13**
1.3 New drug safety assurance and its issues **19**
   1.3.1 Review of drug administration, etc. for prevention of recurrence of incidents of drug-induced suffering   19
   1.3.2 Progress status of the PMDA's third-term five-year plan   27
   1.3.3 Expectations for the PMDA's fourth medium-term plan   35
1.4 Trends towards revision of the Pharmaceutical and Medical Device Act (The PMD Act) **39**
   1.4.1 Rationalization of the review system for speeding up access to patients   39
   1.4.2 Introduction of globally consistent quality control approach   43
   1.4.3 Enrichment of safety measures   45
   1.4.4 Strengthening, etc. of governance over those involved in manufacture, distribution and marketing of pharmaceuticals and medical devices, etc.   49
   1.4.5 Others   53

Chapter 2 Safety system from clinical development to post-marketing

2.1 Safety system during clinical development **55**
2.2 Post-marketing pharmacovigilance system **57**
   2.2.1 Three Officers in Marketing Authorization Holders   59
   2.2.2 GVP (revised GVP)   63
   2.2.3 GQP   65

xii　　目　　次

2.2.4　GPSP（改正 GPSP）　*66*

第3章　臨床開発段階のリスクマネジメント

3.1　臨床開発段階のリスクマネジメント **70**
　3.1.1　規制当局への副作用等緊急報告制度（電子報告）　*70*
　3.1.2　研究報告・外国における措置報告　*72*
　3.1.3　年次報告と DSUR　*72*
　3.1.4　治験実施施設への安全性情報伝達　*76*
　3.1.5　リスク最小化策　*78*
3.2　治験中の安全性情報の活用 **78**

第4章　わが国の市販後リスク管理の概要

4.1　副作用・感染症等報告制度 **82**
　4.1.1　企業報告制度　*84*
　4.1.2　医療機関報告制度　*86*
　4.1.3　患者副作用報告システム　*90*
　4.1.4　WHO モニタリング制度　*90*
　4.1.5　ワクチンの副反応報告制度　*90*
　4.1.5.1　ワクチンの副反応報告制度に関する法的根拠　*92*
　4.1.5.2　報告義務症例の定義と様式　*94*
　4.1.5.3　副反応検討部会による収集データの検討　*94*
4.2　市販直後調査 **94**
　4.2.1　目的　*94*
　4.2.2　調査の対象と実施方法　*100*
4.3　感染症定期報告制度 **102**
4.4　再審査制度 **104**
　4.4.1　再審査期間　*104*
　4.4.2　承認申請から再審査結果通知までの流れ　*106*
　4.4.3　RMP（製造販売後調査等基本計画書）の作成　*106*
　4.4.4　安全性定期報告と PSUR/PBRER　*108*
　4.4.5　再審査結果の判定　*112*
4.5　再評価制度 **116**
　4.5.1　再評価結果の判定　*118*
　4.5.2　品質再評価　*118*
4.6　RMP **120**

2.2.4   GPSP (revised GPSP)   *67*

Chapter 3 Risk management during clinical development

3.1   Risk management during clinical development **71**
   3.1.1   System for expedited reporting of Adverse Drug Reactions (ADRs), etc. to regulatory authorities (electronic reporting)   *71*
   3.1.2   Research reports; Reports on measures taken in foreign countries   *73*
   3.1.3   Annual reporting and the DSUR   *73*
   3.1.4   Transmission of safety information to study sites   *77*
   3.1.5   Risk Minimization Plan   *79*
3.2   Utilization of safety information during clinical trials **79**

Chapter 4 Summary of post-marketing risk management in Japan

4.1   Adverse Drug Reactions and Infections reporting system **83**
   4.1.1   MAH reporting system   *85*
   4.1.2   Medical institution reporting system   *87*
   4.1.3   Patient Adverse Drug Reaction reporting system   *91*
   4.1.4   WHO monitoring system   *91*
   4.1.5   Vaccine Adverse Reactions reporting system   *91*
   4.1.5.1   Legal grounds for vaccine adverse reaction reporting system   *93*
   4.1.5.2   Difinitions of cases for mandatory reporting and forms   *95*
   4.1.5.3   Investigation of collected data by Vaccine Adverse Reaction Review Committee   *95*
4.2   Early post-marketing phase risk minimization and vigilance (EPPV) **95**
   4.2.1   Objective   *95*
   4.2.2   Target and method of EPPV   *101*
4.3   Periodic reporting system for infections **103**
4.4   Reexamination system **105**
   4.4.1   Reexamination period   *105*
   4.4.2   Process from application for approval until notification of Reexamination results   *107*
   4.4.3   Preparation of RMP (Basic Plan for post-marketing studies)   *107*
   4.4.4   Periodic safety reports and the PSUR/PBRER   *109*
   4.4.5   Reexamination results   *113*
4.5   Reevaluation system **117**
   4.5.1   Assessment of Reevaluation results   *119*
   4.5.2   Quality Reevaluation   *119*
4.6   RMP **121**
   4.6.1   Summary of the RMP   *121*
   4.6.2   Preparation and submission of the draft Risk Management Plan at the time of marketing application   *125*

4.6.1 RMP の概要　*120*

4.6.2 申請時における医薬品リスク管理計画書案の作成と提出　*124*

4.6.3 承認条件の付与，解除について　*126*

4.6.4 RMP の見直し　*128*

4.6.5 製造販売後に新たに RMP を作成する場合　*128*

4.6.6 後発医薬品の RMP　*128*

4.6.7 再審査期間終了後の RMP 定期報告　*130*

第5章　ファーマコビジランス査察とファーマコビジランス監査

5.1　GVP および GQP の適合性評価と査察（業査察） **132**

5.2　再審査・再評価申請資料に対する適合性調査（信頼性保証査察） **132**

5.3　自己点検 **134**

5.3.1 手順書およびチェックリストの作成　*136*

5.3.2 GVP の自己点検　*136*

5.3.3 GPSP の自己点検　*136*

5.3.4 自己点検の教育　*136*

5.3.5 その他の自己点検の注意点　*136*

5.4　PV 契約による監査 **138**

5.4.1 EU GVP における PV 監査　*138*

5.4.2 PV 契約の役割　*142*

第6章　医薬品等による健康被害救済制度

6.1　医薬品副作用被害救済制度の概要 **144**

6.1.1 救済の対象　*144*

6.1.2 給付の請求から給付の決定まで　*146*

6.1.3 統計　*148*

6.2　生物由来製品感染等被害救済制度の概要 **152**

6.2.1 救済の対象　*152*

6.2.2 給付の請求から給付の決定まで　*154*

6.2.3 統計　*154*

6.3　予防接種健康被害救済制度 **154**

第7章　市販後安全対策各論

7.1　企業が担う安全管理情報の収集 **158**

4.6.3 Order/removal of conditions for approval   *127*
4.6.4 Readjustment of RMP   *129*
4.6.5 New preparation of RMP after marketing   *129*
4.6.6 RMP for generic medicines   *129*
4.6.7 Periodic reporting on RMP following Reexamination period   *131*

Chapter 5 Pharmacovigilance inspections and pharmacovigilance audits

5.1 GVP and GQP compliance evaluation and inspections (business inspections) **133**
5.2 Compliance Inspection for Reexamination and Reevaluation dossier (reliability assurance inspections/examinations) **133**
5.3 Self inspections **135**
    5.3.1 Preparation of written procedures and checklist   *137*
    5.3.2 GVP self inspections   *137*
    5.3.3 GPSP self inspections   *137*
    5.3.4 Education on self inspections   *137*
    5.3.5 Other points to consider for self inspections   *137*
5.4 Audits under PV contracts **139**
    5.4.1 PV audits under EU GVP   *139*
    5.4.2 Roles of PV contracts   *143*

Chapter 6 Relief Services System for Adverse Health Effects

6.1 Summary of the Relief Service for Adverse Drug Reactions **145**
    6.1.1 Scope of relief   *145*
    6.1.2 Process from application through decision on benefits   *147*
    6.1.3 Statistics   *149*
6.2 Summary of the Relief Service for Infections derived from Biological Products **153**
    6.2.1 Scope of relief   *153*
    6.2.2 Process from application through decision on benefits   *155*
    6.2.3 Statistics   *155*
6.3 Relief Services System for Adverse Health Effects following Vaccination **155**

Chapter 7 General discussion on post-marketing pharmacovigilance

7.1 Collection of safety management information by MAHs **159**

7.1.1 副作用・感染症報告の情報源　*158*

7.1.2 安全管理情報の収集から報告まで　*160*

7.1.3 研究報告の情報源　*162*

7.1.4 措置報告の情報源　*164*

7.2 製造販売後調査・試験 ・・・・・・・・・・・・・・・・・・・・・・・・・・・・・・・・・・・・・・・ **164**

7.2.1 使用成績調査（改正 GPSP 省令では一般使用成績調査に該当）　*166*

7.2.2 製造販売後臨床試験　*168*

7.2.3 製造販売後データベース調査　*170*

7.2.4 製造販売後調査等の実施計画に関する策定の進め方　*172*

7.2.5 製造販売後調査・試験ガイドライン　*174*

7.3 安全管理情報の評価 ・・ **176**

7.3.1 シグナル検出と評価　*176*

7.3.2 個別症例の評価　*178*

7.3.3 集積情報の評価・分析　*180*

7.3.4 医療情報データベース等の利用による評価・分析　*180*

7.4 措置の立案 ・・・ **182**

7.5 行政における安全性情報の評価・分析 ・・・・・・・・・・・・・・・・・・・・・・・・ **184**

7.6 行政が行う安全性情報関連の実施事業・調査 ・・・・・・・・・・・・・・・・・ **184**

第 8 章　製品基本情報と適正使用情報（の内容と伝達）

8.1 製品基本情報 ・・・ **192**

8.1.1 企業中核データシート（CCDS：Company Core Data Sheet）　*192*

8.1.2 添付文書　*194*

8.1.3 患者向医薬品ガイド　*200*

8.2 製品基本情報補完媒体（適正使用情報）・・・・・・・・・・・・・・・・・・・・・・・ **202**

8.2.1 新医薬品の「使用上の注意」の解説　*202*

8.2.2 インタビューフォーム　*204*

8.2.3 医療用医薬品製品情報概要　*204*

8.2.4 くすりのしおり　*204*

8.3 添付文書の改訂等適正使用情報の重要度に応じた情報提供 ・・・・・・・ **204**

8.4 わが国における適正使用情報の提供・伝達の特徴 ・・・・・・・・・・・・・・・ **214**

8.5 PMDA ホームページ ・・・ **216**

和文索引 ・・・ **221**

7.1.1	Information sources of adverse drug reaction and infection reports	*159*
7.1.2	From collection of safety management information to its submission	*161*
7.1.3	Information source of research reports	*163*
7.1.4	Information source of measures-taken reports	*165*

7.2 Post marketing studies **165**

7.2.1	Use-results survey (regarded as General Drug Use Investigations in the revised GPSP ordinance)	*167*
7.2.2	Post-marketing clinical trials	*169*
7.2.3	Post-marketing database studies	*171*
7.2.4	How to create an implementation plan for post-marketing studies	*173*
7.2.5	Guidelines for post-marketing studies	*175*

7.3 Assessment of safety management information **177**

7.3.1	Signal detection and assessment	*177*
7.3.2	Assessment of individual cases	*179*
7.3.3	Assessment and analysis of multiple cases	*181*
7.3.4	Assessment and analysis by use of electronic healthcare database	*181*

7.4 Measures to be taken **183**

7.5 Evaluation and analysis of safety information by MHLW and PMDA ... **185**

7.6 Implementation business/research relating to safety information by MHLW and PMDA **185**

Chapter 8 (The Contents and Communication of) Basic Product Information and Information on Proper Use

8.1 Basic Product Information **193**

8.1.1	Company Core Data Sheet (CCDS)	*193*
8.1.2	Package Inserts	*195*
8.1.3	Drug Guides for Patients	*201*

8.2 Supplementary Materials to Basic Product Information (Information on Proper Use) **203**

8.2.1	Explanation on the "Precautions" of a new drug	*203*
8.2.2	Interview Form	*205*
8.2.3	Ethical Drug Product Information Brochure	*205*
8.2.4	Drug Information Sheet	*205*

8.3 Provision of Information According to the Degree of Importance of Information on Proper Use Such as a Revision of a Package Insert ... **205**

8.4 Characteristics of the Provision and Communication of Information for Proper Use in Japan **215**

8.5 PMDA Website **217**

Alphabetical Index **229**

略語／Abbreviation

略語／Abbr.	正式名称／Long Form	日本語／Japanese
ADR	Adverse Drug Reaction	副作用
AERS	The Adverse Event Reporting System	米国の有害事象報告システム
AESI	Adverse Event of Special Interest	特に注意すべき有害事象
AI	Artificial Intelligence	人工知能
BSE	Bovine Spongiform Encephalopathy	牛海綿状脳症
CAPA	Corrective Action and Preventive Action	是正措置および予防措置
CCDS	Company Core Data Sheet	企業中核データシート
CCSI	Company Core Safety Information	企業中核安全性情報
CDFS	Council on Drugs and Food Sanitation	薬事・食品衛生審議会
CIOMS	The Council for International Organizations of Medical Sciences	国際医学団体協議会
CJD	Creutzfeldt–Jakob disease	クロイツフェルト・ヤコブ病
CRF	Case Report Form	調査票
CTD	Common Technical Document	コモン・テクニカル・ドキュメント／国際共通化資料／承認申請資料
DB	Database	データベース
DCSI	Development Core Safety Information	開発中核安全性情報
DHPLs	Dear Healthcare Professional Letters	医療関係者へのお知らせ
DPC	Diagnosis Procedure Combination	診療群分類包括評価
DSU	Drug Safety Update	DSU
DSU, the Japanese version	Drug Safety Update, the Japanese version	医薬品安全対策情報（日本版 DSU）
DSUR	Development Safety Update Report	治験安全性最新報告
EDC	Electronic Data Capture	電子的データ収集システム

xx　　略　　語

EPPV	Early post-marketing phase risk minimization and vigilance	市販直後調査
EU-RMP	EU-Risk Management Plan	EU のリスク管理計画
FDA	U. S. Food and Drug Administration	米国食品医薬品局
FPMAJ	Federation of Pharmaceutical Manufacturers Association of Japan	日本製薬団体連合会／略称：日薬連
GCP	Good Clinical Practice	臨床試験の実施基準
GHTF	Global Harmonization Task Force on medical devices* * IMDRF is the successor to it from 2013.	医療機器規制国際整合化会合* * 2013 年に IMDRF に移行。
GLP	Good Laboratory Practice	非臨床試験の実施基準
GMP	Good Manufacturing Practice	製造管理及び品質管理基準
GPMSP	Good Post-marketing Surveillance Practice	市販後調査基準
GPSP	Good Post-marketing Study Practice	医薬品の製造販売後の調査及び試験実施基準
GQP	Good Quality Practice	品質管理基準
GVP	Good Vigilance Practice	医薬品，医薬部外品，化粧品及び医療機器の製造販売後安全管理に関する基準
GxP	Good x Practice	適正 x 基準
HCPs	Health Care Professionals	医療関係者
HIV	Human Immunodeficiency Virus	ヒト免疫不全ウイルス
IBD	International Birth Date	国際誕生日
ICH	the International Council on Harmonisation of Technical Requirements for Pharmaceuticals for Human Use	医薬品規制調和国際会議
ICR	Individual Case Report	個別症例報告
ICSR	Individual Case Safety Report	個別症例安全性報告
ICT	Information and Communication Technology	情報通信技術
IF	Interview Form	インタビューフォーム
JADER	Japanese Adverse Drug Event Report database	日本の有害事象報告データベース
JDA	Japan Dental Association	公益社団法人 日本歯科医師会
JMA	Japan Medical Association	公益社団法人 日本医師会

JP	Japanese Pharmacopoeia	日本薬局方
JPA	Japan Pharmaceutical Association	公益社団法人 日本薬剤師会
JPMA	Japan Pharmaceutical Manufacturers Association	日本製薬工業協会 ／略称：製薬協
JPWA	Federation of Japan Pharmaceutical Wholesalers Association	一般社団法人 日本医薬品卸業連合会
JSHP	Japanese Society of Hospital Pharmacists	一般社団法人 日本病院薬剤師会
MAH	Marketing Authorization Holder	製造販売業者 ／医薬品販売承認取得業者
MHLW	Ministry of Health, Labour and Welfare	厚生労働省
MHRA	Medicines and Healthcare products Regulatory Agency	英国医薬品医療製品規制庁
MHW	Ministry of Health and Welfare (which is the precursor of MHLW)	（旧）厚生省
MID-NET	Medical Information Database Network	MID-NET
MIHARI	Medical Information for Risk Assessment Initiative	MIHARI
MR	Medical Representative	医薬情報担当者
MS	Marketing Specialist	医薬品卸販売担当者
OTC drugs	Over The Counter drugs	OTC 医薬品／一般用医薬品
PAL	Pharmaceutical Affairs Law (PAL, which is the precursor of the PMD Act)	（旧）薬事法
PASS	Post-authorisation safety studies	EU における市販後安全性研究
PBRER	Periodic Benefit-Risk Evaluation Report	定期的ベネフィット・リスク評価報告
PIL	Patient Information Leaflet	（英国の）患者向添付文書
PL	Package Leaflet	（EU の）患者向添付文書
(the) PMD Act	Pharmaceutical and Medical device Act/Act on Securing Quality, Efficacy and Safety of Products Including Pharmaceuticals and Medical Devices	医薬品医療機器等法, 医薬品, 医療機器等の品質, 有効性及び安全性の確保等に関する法律
PMDA	Pharmaceuticals and Medical Devices Agency	独立行政法人 医薬品医療機器総合機構
PMS	Post Marketing Surveillance	市販後調査, 市販後監視
PPI	Patient Package Insert	患者用添付文書
PSMF	Pharmacovigilance System Master File	安全性監視（PV） システムマスターファイル

PSUR	Periodic Safety Update Report	定期的安全性最新報告
PV	PharmacoVigilance	医薬品の安全性監視
PVP	PharmacoVigilance Plan	（医薬品）安全性監視計画
QOL	Quality Of Life	クオリティオブライフ
REMS	Risk Evaluation and Mitigation Strategy	リスク評価・リスク緩和戦略（米国）
RMP	Risk Management Plan	医薬品リスク管理計画
SJS	Stevens-Johnson syndrome	スティーブンス・ジョンソン症候群／皮膚粘膜眼症候群
SMON	Subacute Myelo-Optico-Neuropathy	スモン／亜急性脊髄・視神経・末梢神経症
SMT	Safety Management Team	安全性管理チーム
SOP	Standard Operating Procedures	標準業務手順／管理規定
SPC	Summary of Product Characteristics	製品特性概要
TEN	Toxic Epidermal Necrolysis	中毒性表皮壊死症
TERMS	Thalidomide Education and Risk Management System	サリドマイド製剤安全管理手順
vCJD	variant Creutzfeldt-Jakob Disease	変異型クロイツフェルト・ヤコブ病

専門用語日英対照表／ Terminology Japanese-English

* There is also a English - Japanese shown on page xxxix-liv.

日本語	英語
あ	
亜急性脊髄・視神経・末梢神経症	Subacute Myelo-Optico-Neuropathy (SMON)
安全（性）確保	safety assurance
安全確保業務委託者	safety management contractor
安全確保措置	Safety measure
安全管理実施責任者	safety implementation / operational manager
安全管理実施部門	safety implementation division
安全管理情報	safety management information
安全管理責任者	(the) Safety Management Officer
安全管理統括部門	general safety management division
安全性	safety
安全性監視	pharmacovigilance (PV)
（医薬品）安全性監視計画	pharmacovigilance plan
安全性監視（PV）システムマスターファイル	Pharmacovigilance System Master File (PSMF)
安全性管理チーム	Safety Management Team (SMT)
安全性検討事項	safety specification
安全性情報	safety information
安全性情報の評価	evaluation of safety information
安全性情報の分析	analysis of safety information
安全性速報	(the) Blue Letter (the Dear Healthcare Professional Letters of Rapid Safety Communications)
安全性定期報告（制度）	periodic safety report (system)
安全対策	risk minimization measure
安全対策	safety measure
（厚生労働省医薬・生活衛生局）医薬安全対策課	Pharmaceutical Safety Division, Pharmaceutical Safety and Environmental Health Bureau, MHLW (PSEHB/PSD)
（厚生労働省）医薬安全対策課長通知	PSEHB/PSD Notification
い	
EU の医薬品リスク管理計画	EU-Risk Management Plan (EU-RMP)

イエローレター（緊急安全性情報）	(the) Yellow Letter (the Dear Healthcare Professional Letters of Emergent Safety Communications)
医師主導治験	investigator-initiated clinical trial
（厚生労働省）医政局	Health Policy Bureau, MHLW
遺族一時金	Lump-sum benefits for bereaved families
遺族年金	bereaved family pensions
一部変更承認申請／通称：一変申請	partial change approval application
一貫性	consistency
一致性	congruence
一般使用成績調査	general use-results survey
一般患者／一般使用者	general population
一般用医薬品	Over The Counter (OTC) drug
遺伝子解析（手法）	gene analysis (method)
遺伝子組換え製品	genetically-modified product
（人体に対する）異物	foreign substance (to the body)
医薬情報担当者	Medical Representative (MR)
（厚生労働省）医薬・生活衛生局	Pharmaceutical Safety and Environmental Health Bureau, Ministry of Health, Labour and Welfare
（医療法施行規則で要求される）医薬品安全管理責任者	pharmaceutical safety control manager (required by the Ordinance for Enforcement of Medical Care Act)
医薬品安全対策情報	Drug Safety Update, the Japanese version
（医薬品，医薬部外品，化粧品及び医療機器の）製造販売後安全管理に関する基準	Good Vigilance Practice (GVP)
医薬品医療機器情報提供ホームページ	Medical Product Information web page
医薬品医療機器情報配信サービス	Pharmaceuticals and medical devices information e-mail service
独立行政法人 医薬品医療機器総合機構	Pharmaceuticals and Medical Devices Agency (PMDA)
医薬品，医療機器等の品質，有効性及び安全性の確保等に関する法律／医薬品医療機器等法	Act on Securing Quality, Efficacy and Safety of products Including Pharmaceuticals and Medical Devices/(the) PMD Act
医薬品医療機器等法に基づく再評価	reevaluation based on the PMD Act
医薬品卸販売担当者	Marketing Specialist (MS)
医薬品規制調和国際会議	(the) International Council for Harmonisation of Technical Requirements for Pharmaceuticals for Human Use (ICH)
医薬品等安全性情報報告制度	Drugs and Medical Devices Safety Information Reporting System
医薬品等安全対策部会	Committee on Drug Safety
医薬品の安全性監視	pharmacovigilance (PV)

医薬品の市販後調査の基準	Good Post-Marketing Surveillance Practice (GPMSP)
医薬品の製造販売後の調査および試験実施基準	Good Post-Marketing Study Practice (GPSP)
医薬品販売承認取得業者	Marketing Authorisation Holder (MAH)
医薬品副作用被害救済基金（法）	Fund for Adverse Drug Reactions Suffering Relief
医薬品副作用被害救済制度	Relief System for Sufferers from Adverse Drug Reactions
医薬品副作用被害事例	sufffers from ADR
医薬品ライフサイクルマネジメント	drug lifecycle management
医薬品リスク管理計画	Risk Management Plan (RMP)
医薬部外品	quasi-drug
医療安全情報	medical safety information
医療関係者	healthcare professionals (HCPs)
医療関係者へのお知らせ	Dear Healthcare Professional Letter
医療機関	medical institution
医療機関報告制度	medical institution reporting system
医療機関モニター報告制度	(the) medical institution monitoring report system
医療機器	medical device
医療機器安全対策部会	Committee on Medical Device Safety
医療機器規制国際整合化会合* * 2013 年に IMDRF に移行。	Global Harmonization Task Force on medical devices (GHTF) * * IMDRF is the successor to it from 2013.
医療事故	medical accident
医療習慣	medical practice
医療担当者	attending healthcare provider
医療手当	medical allowance
医療費	medical expense
医療法	Medical Care Act
医療用医薬品／処方せん医薬品	ethical drug/prescription drug
医療用医薬品再評価結果	reevaluation result of ethical drug
因果関係	causality
因果関係を支持する実験的なエビデンス	supportive experimental evidence for causality
インタビューフォーム	Interview Form (IF)
インフォームド・コンセント（同意書）	informed consent

う

牛海綿状脳症	Bovine Spongiform Encephalopathy (BSE)
後ろ向きな調査	retrospective investigation

え

英国医薬品医療製品規制庁	Medicines and Healthcare products Regulatory Agency (MHRA)
疫学調査	epidemiological investigation
MR 資格認定制度	qualification certification program for MR

お

OTC 医薬品	over-the-counter (OTC) drug
オーファンドラッグ	orphan drug
追っかけ新薬	separate full application for the same active ingredient as a drug which is still in its reexamination period

か

外国措置情報	information on measures taken overseas
外国措置報告	report of measures taken overseas
外国臨床試験データ	foreign clinical study data
回収	recall
回収処理	recall management
介入研究	interventional study
開発期間	drug development period
開発中核安全性情報	Development Core Safety Information (DCSI)
外部委託	outsourcing
核酸系薬物	nucleic acid agent
学会情報	academic conference report
合併症	complications
観察研究	observational study
患者さんへの服薬説明書	patient medication information
患者向医薬品ガイド	Drug Guides for Patients
患者向製品説明書	Package Leaflet (PL)
（英国の）患者向製品説明書	Patient Information Leaflet (PIL)
患者用添付文書	Patient Package Insert (PPI)
感染症症例報告	infection case reporting
感染症定期報告制度	periodic reporting system for infections
（生物由来製品）感染等被害救済制度	Relief System for Infections Derived from Biological Products
管理規定	administrative rules

き

企業中核安全性情報	Company Core Safety Information (CCSI)
企業中核医薬品リスク管理計画	Core RMP
企業中核データシート	Company Core Data Sheet (CCDS)
希少疾病用医薬品	orphan drug

既承認医薬品	approved drug
規制区分	regulatory classification
規制当局	regulatory authority
既知・重篤症例	expected and serious case
救済給付	relief benefits
給付申請	application for relief benefit
教育訓練	education and training
業査察（医薬品製造業許可に係る調査）	Assessment for manufacturing license of drugs
行政指導	administrative guidance
行政指導に基づく再評価／再審査	reevaluation / reexamination by administrative guidance
行政措置	regulatory measure
業態区分	category of business
強度	strength
業務委託（外部委託）* *日本ではこのように称しているが，内容は外部委託。	outsourcing
許可区分	license category
許可更新	license renewal
許可要件	license condition
局方品	Japanese Pharmacopoeia Drugs (JP Drug)
拠出金（一般，付加）	contribution (general, additional)
拠点医療機関ネットワーク	sentinel medical institution network
記録の保存	retention of records
緊急安全性情報 （通称：イエローレター）	Emergent Safety Communication DHPL / Yellow Letter
緊急措置命令	order for emergency measure
緊急ファックス網	emergency fax network
緊急報告	expedited reporting

く

クオリティオブライフ	Quality Of Life (QOL)
くすりのしおり	patient information leaflet
くすりの適正使用協議会	Risk / Benefit Assessment of Drugs-Analysis and Response (RAD-AR) Council, Japan
国からの補助金	subsidy
クロイツフェルト・ヤコブ病	Creutzfeldt-Jakob disease (CJD)
グローバル RMP	Global RMP
軽微な副作用	mild ADR

け

劇薬	powerful drug

（ワクチンの）研究開発および生産・流通部会	Committee on Vaccine R&D, Manufactureing and Distribution
研究実施計画書	protocol
研究報告	research report
（厚生労働省）健康局	Health Service Bureau, MHLW
健康被害	adverse health effects
原材料	raw material
検証試験	confirmatory trial
兼任	concurrently serve / concurrent service
兼務	concurrent post

こ

抗がん剤併用療法実態把握調査	survey on the actual use of anti-cancer combination therapies
（旧）厚生省	Ministry of Health and Welfare (MHW, which is the precursor of MHLW)
厚生労働省	Ministry of Health, Labour and Welfare (MHLW)
厚生労働白書	annual White Paper on MHLW
抗体医薬品	antibody drug
高度管理医療機器	specially controlled medical device
効能拡大	extend (ed) indication
効能・効果	indications
後発医薬品	generic drugs
国際医学団体協議会	(the) Council for International Organizations of Medical Sciences (CIOMS)
国際医薬品モニタリングセンター	Center for International Drug Monitoring
国際共通化資料	Common Technical Document (CTD)
国際医薬品開発	multi-regional drug development
国際共同治験	multi-regional clinical trial
国際誕生日	International Birth Date (IBD)
国立成育医療研究センター	National Center for Child Health and Development
誇大広告の禁止	prohibition on exaggerated advertisement
個別症例報告	individual case report (ICR)
個別症例安全性報告	Individual Case Safety Report (ICSR)
コモン・テクニカル・ドキュメント	Common Technical Document (CTD)

さ

催奇形性試験	teratogenicity study
再審査	reexamination
再審査期間	reexamination period
再審査結果通知	notification of reexamination result

再審査指定日	date of re-examination designation
再審査申請	re-examination application
再審査申請資料	application dossier for re-examination
再審査制度	reexamination system
再審査対象医薬品	drug to be reexamined
再審査適合性調査	re-examination compliance inspection
再評価申請資料	application dossier for re-evaluation
再評価制度	re-evaluation system
先駆け審査指定制度	SAKIGAKE Designation System
サリドマイド製剤安全管理手順	Thalidomide Education and Risk Management System (TERMs)
参照／参考 RMP	Reference RMP

し

GLP 調査	GLP inspections
GCP 実地調査	GCP on-site inspection
GPSP 実地調査	GPSP on-site inspections
GVP 適合性評価	GVP compliance evaluation
時間の関係	temporality
支給要件	requirement for payment
試験薬（治験薬）	investigational drug / study drug / trial drug
自己点検	self inspection
市場出荷判定	market release decision
実態把握調査	survey on the actual use
実地調査	on-site inspection
情報配信サービス	information E-mail service
自発的情報源	spontaneous information source
自発報告	spontaneous report
（EU における）市販後安全性研究	Post-authorisation safety studies (PASS)
市販後安全対策	post-marketing safety measures
市販後調査／市販後監視	Post Marketing Surveillance (PMS)
（医薬品の）市販後調査の基準	Good Post-marketing Surveillance Practice (GPMSP)
市販後臨床試験審査委員会	Review Committee on Post-Marketing Clinical Trials
市販後臨床試験責任医師	investigator in post-marketing clinical trials
市販直後調査	Early post-marketing phase risk minimization and vigilance / (EPPV)
市販直後の定点観測	fixed-point observation of PV activities in medical institutions at early post-marketing stage
収集症例	collected case

重点監視医薬品	priority monitoring drug
重篤副作用疾患別対応マニュアル	Manuals for Management of Individual Serious Adverse Drug Reactions
重要な基本的注意	important precautions
受託安全管理実施責任者	contracted safety implementation manager
遵守事項	stipulation to be observed
障害児養育年金	Pension for Raising Children with disabilities
障害年金	disability pension
使用期限	expiration date
使用経験	clinical experience
条件付早期承認制度	Conditional Early Approval System
使用限度	limit of use
詳細報告／調査	detailed report / investigation
詳細調査票	detailed CRF
使用上の注意	precautions / precaution for use
使用成績調査	Use-results survey
使用成績比較調査	Use-results survey with comparative group
使用実態調査	Surveys of actual conditions of use
承認基準	approval criteria / standard
承認区分	approval category
承認条件の付与	Order of conditions for approval
承認情報	approval information
承認申請	application for approval
承認申請資料	Application document
使用制限／限定	access restriction / restriction on patient using the drug
情報提供活動	activity to provide information
情報通信技術	Information and Communication Technology (ICT)
症例登録方法	patient enrollment method
症例評価	case assessment
除外医薬品	excluded drug
処方せん医薬品／医療用医薬品	ethical drug/prescription drug
書面調査	Document-based Compliance Assessments / Document-based Assessments
新医療用配合剤	new combination drugs
新効能・効果医薬品	drug with new indication
人工知能	artificial intelligence (AI)
新再評価	new reevaluation

（厚生労働省医薬・生活衛生局）医薬品審査管理課	Pharmaceutical Evaluation Division, Pharmaceutical Safety and Environmental Health Bureau, MHLW
審査期間	review time
人種差	racial difference
申請資料	application dossier
申請前段階	pre-submission stage
診断書	medical certificate
診断情報	diagnostic information
新投与経路医薬品	drug with a new route of administration
真のエンドポイント	true endpoint
新薬使用上の注意解説	explanation of precautions of a new drug
新薬審査体制	(the) new drug review system
新薬審査部（PMDA の一部署）	Office of New Drugs, PMDA
新薬適正使用情報	information on proper use of a new drug
新有効成分医薬品	drug with a new active ingredient / substance
新用法・新用量医薬品	drug with new dosage and administration
信頼性保証査察	reliability assurance inspections / examinations
診療群分類包括評価	Diagnosis Procedure Combination (DPC)

す

スティーブンス・ジョンソン症候群	Stevens-Johnson syndrome (SJS)
スモン	Subacute Myelo-Optico-Neuropathy (SMON)

せ

生活習慣病	lifestyle disease
製造管理及び品質管理基準	Good Manufacturing Practice (GMP)
製造管理者	manufacturing control manager
製造出荷判定	manufacturing release decision
製造承認	manufacturing approval
製造販売業三役	three supervisors in MAH
製造販売業者	Marketing Authorisation Holder (MAH)
製造販売後安全管理業務手順書	SOP on post-marketing safety management
製造販売後調査	post-marketing investigation
製造販売後調査・試験	post-marketing studies
製造販売後調査等管理責任者	Post-marketing Studies Manager
製造販売後調査等基本計画書	basic plan for post-marketing studies
製造販売後調査等業務手順書	SOP on post-marketing studies
製造販売後調査等実施計画書	protocol of post-marketing studies
製造販売後臨床試験	post-marketing clinical trial

製造販売承認	marketing approval
製品回収	product recall
製品情報概要	main product pamphlet
製品情報概要	product information brochure
製品特性概要（EU の製品説明書）	Summary of Product Characteristics (SPC)
生物学的勾配	biologic gradient
生物学的妥当性	biological plausibility
生物由来製品	biological product
生物由来製品感染等被害救済制度	Relief System for Sufferers from Diseases Infected from Biological Products
製薬協	Japan Pharmaceutical Manufacturers Association (JPMA)
是正措置および予防措置	Corrective Action and Preventive Action (CAPA)
専門医	medical specialist
専門医療機関	professional medical institution
専門協議	Expert Discussion
全例調査	all-patient surveillance
全例調査方式	all-patient surveillance system

そ

総括製造販売責任者	(the) Pharmaceutical Officer
総合的適合性評価	overall compliance evaluation
相互作用	drug interaction
葬祭料	funeral expense
措置完了	completion of measures
措置の立案	measures to be taken
ソリブジン事件	Sorivudine incident

た

第一次再評価	first reevaluation
第 1 種製造販売業者	MAH with the first-class marketing license for pharmaceuticals (first-class MAH)
第一報報告	preliminary report
大規模医療情報データベース	large-scale medical information database
大規模長期臨床試験	large scale / long-term clinical trial
第 3 種製造販売業者	3rd-class MAH
耐性菌調査	survey of drug-resistant bacterial strains
代替／代用のエンドポイント	surrogate endpoint
第二次再評価	second reevaluation
第 2 種製造販売業者	2nd-class MAH
対面助言	consultation

Terminology Japanese-English

WHO 国際医薬品モニタリング制度	(the) WHO Programme for International Drug Monitoring
WHO モニタリング制度	WHO monitoring system
担当医療者	medical service provider in attendance

ち

治験	clinical trial for marketing approval
治験安全性最新報告	Development Safety Update Report (DSUR)
治験依頼者	sponsor (of clinical trial)
治験依頼の基準	clinical trial sponsorship criteria
治験基盤整備	establishment of clinical trials infrastructure
治験空洞化	hollowing out of clinical trials
治験契約	clinical trial contract
治験コスト	cost of clinical trial
治験実施医療機関	clinical trial sites
治験成分記号	Investigational New Drug (IND) code
治験相談体制	clinical trial consultation system
治験届出制度	clinical trial notification system
治験薬	investigational drug
致命的な副作用	fatal ADR
中央登録方式	central registration system
中央薬事審議会	Central Pharmaceutical Affairs Council
中毒性表皮壊死症	Toxic Epidermal Necrolysis (TEN)
長期使用に関する調査	long-term use surveillance
調剤薬局	dispensing pharmacy
調査・試験	studies
調査会	subcommittee
調査票	case report form (CRF)

て

DSU	Drug Safety Update (DSU)
TGN1412 事件	the TGN1412 incident
定期接種	routine vaccination
定期的安全性最新報告	Periodic Safety Update Report (PSUR)
定期的再評価	periodic reevaluation
定期的ベネフィット・リスク評価報告	Periodic Benefit-Risk Evaluation Report (PBRER)
定期報告	periodic report
データベース調査	database study/database survey
データ・マイニング手法	data mining method
適応拡大	extend (ed) indication

適合性調査	compliance inspection
適合性評価	compliance evaluation
適正使用情報	information on proper use
適正使用等確保措置	measure to assure proper use
適正 x 基準	Good x Practice (GxP)
電子的データ収集システム	Electronic Data Capture (EDC) system
電子報告	electronic report
添付文書	package insert
添付文書記載要領	guideline instructions for package insert

と

同一成分医薬品	drug with the same ingredient / substance
投薬証明（書）	proof of prescription
特異性	specificity
ドクターレター	Dear Doctor letter
特定使用成績調査	specified use-results survey
特に注意すべき有害事象	Adverse Event of Special Interest (AESI)
特別部会	special committee
毒薬	poisonous drug
ドラッグ・ラグ	drug lag

な

内用固形剤	solid formulation for oral use

に

二次感染者	secondary infection
二重盲検比較試験	double blind comparative study
日薬連	Federation of Pharmaceutical Manufacturers Association of Japan (FPMAJ)
（公益社団法人）日本医師会	Japan Medical Association (JMA)
（一般社団法人）日本医薬品卸業連合会	Federation of Japan Pharmaceutical Wholesalers Association (JPWA)
（公益社団法人）日本歯科医師会	Japan Dental Association (JDA)
日本製薬工業協会（製薬協）	Japan Pharmaceutical Manufacturers Association (JPMA)
日本製薬団体連合会（日薬連）	Federation of Pharmaceutical Manufacturers Association of Japan (FPMAJ)
日本製薬団体連合会 再評価委員会	Reevaluation Committee of the FPMAJ
日本の有害事象報告データベース	Japanese Adverse Drug Event Report database (JADER)
医薬品安全対策情報（日本版 DSU）	Drug Safety Update, the Japanese version
一般社団法人 日本病院薬剤師会	Japanese Society of Hospital Pharmacists (JSHP)
日本標準商品分類番号	Standard Commodity Classification Number of Japan

（公益社団法人）日本薬剤師会	Japan Pharmaceutical Association (JPA)
日本薬局方	Japanese Pharmacopoeia (JP)
任意接種	voluntary vaccination
妊産婦	expectant and nursing mother (s)
妊娠と薬情報センター	Japan Drug Information Institute in Pregnancy
妊婦・産婦・授乳婦への投与	use for pregnant / expectant / nursing women

ね	
年次報告	annual report

は	
配合理由	reason of combination
バリデーション研究	validation study
販売制限	marketing restriction
販売中止	discontinuation of marketing
販売独占期間	(the) period for sales monopoly

ひ	
PMS 制度	PMS system
PMDA メディナビ	PMDA medi-navi
比較臨床試験	controlled clinical trial
被験者	subject
ヒト免疫不全ウイルス	Human Immunodeficiency Virus (HIV Virus)
皮内反応	intracutaneous test
評価指標	endpoint
標準業務手順	Standard Operating Procedure (SOP)
標準製剤	reference preparation
非臨床試験	non-clinical study
非臨床試験の実施基準	Good Laboratory Practice (GLP)
品質管理基準	Good Quality Practice (GQP)
品質管理業務手順書	SOP on quality control
品質再評価	reevaluation for quality
品質保証責任者	(the) Quality Assurance Officer
品質管理責任者	(the) Quality Management Officer
品質保証部門	quality assurance unit

ふ	
ファーマコゲノミクス	pharmacogenomics
ファーマコビジランス査察	PV inspection
不可避的な副作用	unavoidable ADR
副作用	Adverse Drug Reaction (ADR)
副作用感染症等報告制度	Adverse drug reactions and infections reporting system

副作用自発報告	spontaneous ADR report
副作用の警報発信型	reactive issuing mode of warnings for ADRs
副作用の発生頻度	frequency of ADR
副作用の予測・予防型	prediction and prevention style for ADRs
副作用被害者	patient suffering the ADR induced damage
副作用被害判定部会	Committee on Judgement of Suffers from ADRs
副作用報告義務	obligation of ADR reporting
副作用報告義務期間	obligatory ADR reporting term
副作用報告用語	ADR reporting term
副作用モニター制度	ADR monitoring system
副反応	adverse reaction
副反応検討部会	vaccine adverse reaction review committee
プッシュメール	information E-mail service
不適正使用	improper use
ブリッジング試験	bridging study
不良医薬品	adulterated drugs
ブルーレター（安全性速報）	(the) Blue Letter (the Dear Healthcare Professional Letters of Rapid Safety Communications)
プロスペクティブ（前向き）な調査	prospective investigation
プロモーションコード委員会	Promotion Code Committee
文献検索	literature search / retrieval of literature
文献調査	literature searching / searches

へ

米国食品医薬品局	U. S. Food and Drug Administration (FDA)
米国の有害事象報告システム	The Adverse Event Reporting System (AERS)
併用禁止	prohibition of concomitant use
併用薬	concomitant medications
変異型クロイツフェルト・ヤコブ病	variant Creutzfeldt-Jakob disease (vCJD)

ほ

報告期限	reporting time frames
報告期限のタイムクロック	(the) time clock for the reporting timeline
法制化	legalization
（厚生労働省）保険局	Health Insurance Bureau, MHLW
保険薬局	health insurance pharmacy

ま

前向きな調査	prospective investigation

み

未承認薬	unapproved drug
未知・重篤症例	unexpected and serious case
未知の副作用（シグナル）	unexpected ADR (signal)
未知・非重篤定期報告	periodic report for unexpected / non-serious ADR
MID-NET	Medical Information Database Network
MIHARI	Medical Information for Risk Assessment Initiative
民事裁判	civil court (case)
民事責任	civil responsibility
民族差	ethnic difference

も

モニタリングシステム	monitoring system

や

薬害	drug-induced suffering
薬害肝炎事件の検証及び再発防止のための医薬品行政のあり方検討委員会（薬害検証・行政のあり方検討委員会）	Committee for Investigation of Drug-induced Hepatitis Cases and Appropriate Regulatory Administration to Prevent Similar Sufferings
薬害事件	incidents of health damage caused by ADRs
薬剤疫学	pharmacoepidemiology
薬剤疫学的手法	pharmacoepidemiological method
薬事規制	(the) pharmaceutical regulation
薬事・食品衛生審議会	Council on Drugs and Food Sanitation (CDFS) /Pharmaceutical Affairs and Food Sanitation Council
（旧）薬事法	Pharmaceutical Affairs Law (PAL, which is the precursor of PMD Act)
薬物相互作用	drug interaction
薬効群	pharmacological class
薬効問題懇談会	informal conference for discussing drug efficacy

ゆ

有効性	efficacy
有用性	usefulness

よ

要指導医薬品	BTC drugs (behind-the-counter drug) / drug requiring pharmacist's guidance
溶出曲線	dissolution curve
溶出試験	dissolution test
溶出率	dissolution rate

用法・用量	dosage and administration
予防接種	preventive vaccination
予防接種基本方針部会	Commiteee on Immunization Policy
予防接種法	Preventive Vaccinations Act
予防接種・ワクチン分科会	Immunization and Vaccine Section Meeting

ら

ライエル症候群	Lyell syndrome

り

リスク管理	risk management
リスク最小化策（EU）	risk minimization measure
リスク最小化計画（日本）	Risk Minimization Plan
リスク最小化活動	Risk Minimization Activity
リスク評価・リスク緩和戦略（米国）	Risk Evaluation and Mitigation Strategy (REMS) (U. S.)
リスクマネジメント制度	risk management system
臨時の再評価	ad hoc reevaluation
臨床医	physician
臨床研究	clinical research
臨床研究法	(the) Clinical Research Act
臨床検査値	laboratory finding
臨床試験	clinical trial
臨床試験成績	clinical study results
臨床試験データパッケージ	clinical data package
臨床試験の実施基準	Good Clinical Practice (GCP)
臨床評価ガイドライン	(the) new drug clinical evaluation guideline

る

類似性	similarity
類似体	analog

れ

レセプトデータ	claims data
レトロスペクティブ（後ろ向き）な調査	retrospective investigation
連携	liaison
連続調査方式	surveilance system by using consecutive patients

ろ～

（厚生労働省）老健局	Health and Welfare Bureau for the Elderly, MHLW
6か月定期報告	6 month periodic safety report
枠組み警告	boxed warning

Terminology English-Japanese ／専門用語英日対照表

* 日英対照表は，xxiii ～ xxxviii ページにある。

English	Japanese
2nd-class MAH	第 2 種製造販売業者
3rd-class MAH	第 3 種製造販売業者
6 month periodic safety report	6 か月定期報告

A

academic conference report	学会情報
access restriction / restriction on patient using the drug	使用制限／限定
activity to provide information	情報提供活動
(the) Act on Securing Quality, Efficacy and Safety of Pharmaceuticals, Medical Devices, Regenerative and Cellular Therapy Products, Gene Therapy products, and Cosmetics	医薬品医療機器等法，医薬品，医療機器等の品質，有効性及び安全性の確保等に関する法律
ad hoc reevaluation	臨時の再評価
administrative rules	管理規定
ADR monitoring system	副作用モニター制度
ADR reporting term	副作用報告用語
adulterated drugs	不良医薬品
Adverse Drug Reaction (ADR)	副作用
Adverse drug reactions and infections reporting system	副作用・感染症等報告制度
Adverse Event of Special Interest (AESI)	特に注意すべき有害事象
The Adverse Event Reporting System (AERS)	米国の有害事象報告システム
adverse health effects	健康被害
adverse reaction	副反応
all-patient surveillance	全例調査
all-patient surveillance system	全例調査方式
analog	類似体
analysis of safety information	安全性情報の分析
annual report	年次報告
annual White Paper on MHLW	厚生労働白書
antibody drug	抗体医薬品

Application document	承認申請資料
application dossier	申請資料
application dossier for reevaluation	再評価申請資料
application dossier for reexamination	再審査申請資料
application for approval	承認申請
application for relief benefit	給付申請
approval category	承認区分
approval criteria / standard	承認基準
approval information	承認情報
approved drug	既承認医薬品
artificial intelligence (AI)	人工知能
Assessment for manufacturing license of drugs	業査察（医薬品製造業許可に係る調査）
attending healthcare provider	医療担当者

B

basic plan for post-marketing studies	製造販売後調査等基本計画書
bereaved family pensions	遺族年金
biologic gradient	生物学的勾配
biological plausibility	生物学的妥当性
biological product	生物由来製品
(the) Blue Letter (the Dear Healthcare Professional Letters of Rapid Safety Communications)	ブルーレター（安全性速報）
Bovine Spongiform Encephalopathy (BSE)	牛海綿状脳症
boxed warning	枠組み警告
bridging study	ブリッジング試験
BTC drugs (behind-the-counter drug) / drug requiring pharmacist's guidance	要指導医薬品

C

case assessment	症例評価
case report form (CRF)	調査票
category of business	業態区分
causality	因果関係
Center for International Drug Monitoring	国際医薬品モニタリングセンター
Central Pharmaceutical Affairs Council	中央薬事審議会
central registration system	中央登録方式
civil court (case)	民事裁判
civil responsibility	民事責任
claims data	レセプトデータ
(the) Clinical Research Act	臨床研究法

clinical data package	臨床試験データパッケージ
clinical experience	使用経験
clinical research	臨床研究
clinical study results	臨床試験成績
clinical trial	臨床試験
clinical trial consultation system	治験相談体制
clinical trial contract	治験契約
clinical trial for marketing approval	治験
clinical trial notification system	治験届出制度
clinical trial sites	治験実施医療機関
clinical trial sponsorship criteria	治験依頼の基準
collected case	収集症例
Commiteee on Immunization Policy	予防接種基本方針部会
Committee for Investigation of Drug-induced Hepatitis Cases and Appropriate Regulatory Administration to Prevent Similar Sufferings	薬害肝炎事件の検証及び再発防止のための医薬品行政のあり方検討委員会（薬害検証・行政のあり方検討委員会）
Committee on Drug Safety	医薬品等安全対策部会
Committee on Judgement of Suffers from ADRs	副作用被害判定部会
Committee on Medical Device Safety	医療機器安全対策部会
Committee on Vaccine R&D, Manufactureing and Distribution	（ワクチンの）研究開発および生産・流通部会
Common Technical Document (CTD)	国際共通化資料
Common Technical Document (CTD)	コモン・テクニカル・ドキュメント
Company Core Data Sheet (CCDS)	企業中核データシート
Company Core Safety Information (CCSI)	企業中核安全性情報
completion of measures	措置完了
compliance evaluation	適合性評価
compliance inspection	適合性調査
complications	合併症
concomitant medications	併用薬
concurrent post	兼務
concurrently serve / concurrent service	兼任
Conditional Early Approval System	条件付き早期承認制度
confirmatory trial	検証試験
congruence	一致性
consistency	一貫性
consultation	対面助言
contracted safety implementation manager	受託安全管理実施責任者
contribution (general, additional)	拠出金（一般，付加）

controlled clinical trial	比較臨床試験
Core RMP	企業中核医薬品リスク管理計画
Corrective Action and Preventive Action (CAPA)	是正措置および予防措置
cost of clinical trial	治験コスト
(the) Council for International Organizations of Medical Sciences (CIOMS)	国際医学団体協議会
Council on Drugs and Food Sanitation (CDFS) /Pharmaceutical Affairs and Food Sanitation Council	薬事・食品衛生審議会
Creutzfeldt–Jakob disease (CJD)	クロイツフェルト・ヤコブ病

D

database (DB) study/database survey	データベース調査
data mining method	データ・マイニング手法
date of reexamination designation	再審査指定日
Dear Doctor letter	ドクターレター
Dear Healthcare Professional Letter	医療関係者へのお知らせ
detailed CRF	詳細調査票
detailed report / investigation	詳細報告／調査
Development Core Safety Information (DCSI)	開発中核安全性情報
Development Safety Update Report (DSUR)	治験安全性最新報告
Diagnosis Procedure Combination (DPC)	診療群分類包括評価
diagnostic information	診断情報
disability pension	障害年金
discontinuation of marketing	販売中止
dispensing pharmacy	調剤薬局
dissolution curve	溶出曲線
dissolution rate	溶出率
dissolution test	溶出試験
Document-based Compliance Assessments / Document-based Assessments	書面調査
dosage and administration	用法・用量
double blind comparative study	二重盲検比較試験
drug development period	開発期間
Drug Guides for Patients	患者向医薬品ガイド
drug interaction	相互作用／薬物相互作用
drug lag	ドラッグ・ラグ
drug lifecycle management	医薬品ライフサイクルマネジメント
Drug Safety Update (DSU)	DSU
Drug Safety Update, the Japanese version	医薬品安全対策情報（日本版 DSU）

drug to be re-examined	再審査対象医薬品
drug with new dosage and administration	新用法・新用量医薬品
drug with a new route of administration	新投与経路医薬品
drug with a new active ingredient / substance	新有効成分医薬品
drug with new indication	新効能・効果医薬品
drug with the same ingredient / substance	同一成分医薬品
drug-induced suffering	薬害
Drugs and Medical Devices Safety Information Reporting System	医薬品等安全性情報報告制度

E

Early post-marketing phase risk minimization and vigilance (EPPV)	市販直後調査
education and training	教育訓練
efficacy	有効性
ethical drug/prescription drug	処方せん医薬品／医療用医薬品
Electronic Data Capture (EDC) system	電子的データ収集システム
electronic report	電子報告
emergency fax network	緊急ファックス網
Emergent Safety Communication / Yellow Letter	緊急安全性情報 （通称：イエローレター）
endpoint	評価指標
epidemiological investigation	疫学調査
establishment of clinical trials infrastructure	治験基盤整備
ethnic difference	民族差
EU-Risk Management Plan (EU-RMP)	EU の医薬品リスク管理計画
evaluation of safety information	安全性情報の評価
excluded drug	除外医薬品
expectant and nursing mother (s)	妊産婦
expected and serious case	既知・重篤症例
expedited reporting	緊急報告
Expert Discussion	専門協議
expiration date	使用期限
explanation of precautions of a new drug	新薬使用上の注意解説
extend (ed) indication	適応拡大
extend (ed) indication	効能拡大

F

fatal ADR	致命的な副作用
Federation of Japan Pharmaceutical Wholesalers Association (JPWA)	一般社団法人 日本医薬品卸業連合会
Federation of Pharmaceutical Manufacturers Association of Japan (FPMAJ)	日本製薬団体連合会 （略称：日薬連）

first reevaluation	第一次再評価
fixed-point observation of PV activities in medical institutions at early post-marketing stage	市販直後の定点観測
foreign clinical study data	外国臨床試験データ
foreign substance (to the body)	（人体に対する）異物
frequency of ADR	副作用の発生頻度
Fund for Adverse Drug Reactions Suffering Relief	医薬品副作用被害救済基金（法）
funeral expense	葬祭料

G

GCP on-site inspection	GCP 実地調査
gene analysis (method)	遺伝子解析（手法）
general population	一般患者／一般使用者
general safety management division	安全管理統括部門
generic drugs	後発医薬品
genetically-modified product	遺伝子組換え製品
Global Harmonization Task Force on medical devices (GHTF) [*] [*] IMDRF is the successor to it from 2013.	医療機器規制国際整合化会合[*] [*] 2013 年に IMDRF に移行。
Global RMP	グローバル RMP
GLP inspections	GLP 調査
Good Clinical Practice (GCP)	臨床試験の実施基準
Good Laboratory Practice (GLP)	非臨床試験の実施基準
Good Manufacturing Practice (GMP)	製造管理及び品質管理基準
Good Post-Marketing Study Practice (GPSP)	医薬品の製造販売後の調査及び試験実施基準
Good Post-Marketing Surveillance Practice (GPMSP)	（医薬品の）市販後調査の基準
Good Quality Practice (GQP)	品質管理の基準
Good Vigilance Practice (GVP)	（医薬品, 医薬部外品, 化粧品及び医療機器の）製造販売後安全管理に関する基準
Good x Practice	適正 x 基準
GPMSP compliance evaluation [*] [*] Applicable regulations to studies remaining in effect through March 2015.	GPMSP 適合性評価[*] [*] 2015 年 3 月末までに実施される調査に適用される。
GPMSP on-site examination [*]	GPMSP 実地調査
guideline for package insert	添付文書記載要領
GVP compliance evaluation	GVP 適合性評価

H

Health and Welfare Bureau for the Elderly, MHLW	（厚生労働省）老健局
Health Insurance Bureau, MHLW	（厚生労働省）保険局

health insurance pharmacy	保険薬局
Health Policy Bureau, MHLW	（厚生労働省）医政局
Health Service Bureau, MHLW	（厚生労働省）健康局
healthcare professionals (HCPs)	医療関係者
hollowing out of clinical trials	治験空洞化

I

Immunization and Vaccine Section Meeting	予防接種・ワクチン分科会
important precautions	重要な基本的注意
improper use	不適正使用
incidents of health damage caused by ADRs	薬害事件
indications	効能・効果
individual case report (ICR)	個別症例報告
Individual Case Safety Report (ICSR)	個別症例安全性報告
infection case reporting	感染症症例報告
informal conference for discussing drug efficacy	薬効問題懇談会
Information and Communication Technology (ICT)	情報通信技術
information E-mail service	情報配信サービス／プッシュメール
information on proper use	適正使用情報
information on proper use of a new drug	新薬適正使用情報
informed consent	インフォームド・コンセント（同意書）
International Birth Date (IBD)	国際誕生日
(the) International Council for Harmonisation of Technical Requirements for Pharmaceuticals for Human Use (ICH)	医薬品規制調和国際会議
interventional study	介入研究
Interview Form (IF)	インタビューフォーム
intracutaneous test	皮内反応
investigational drug	治験薬
investigational drug / study drug / trial drug	試験薬（治験薬）
Investigational New Drug (IND) code	治験成分記号
investigator in post-marketing clinical trials	市販後臨床試験責任医師
investigator-initiated clinical trial	医師主導治験

J

Japan Dental Association (JDA)	公益社団法人 日本歯科医師会
Japan Drug Information Institute in Pregnancy	妊娠と薬情報センター
Japan Medical Association (JMA)	公益社団法人 日本医師会
Japanese Adverse Drug Event Report database (JADER)	日本の有害事象報告データベース

Japan Pharmaceutical Association (JPA)	公益社団法人 日本薬剤師会
Japan Pharmaceutical Manufacturers Association (JPMA)	日本製薬工業協会（略称：製薬協）
Japanese Pharmacopoeia (JP)	日本薬局方
Japanese Pharmacopoeia Drugs (JP Drug)	局方品
Japanese Society of Hospital Pharmacists (JSHP)	一般社団法人 日本病院薬剤師会

L

laboratory finding	臨床検査値
large scale / long-term clinical trial	大規模長期臨床試験
large-scale medical information database	大規模医療情報データベース
legalization	法制化
liaison	連携
license category	許可区分
license condition	許可要件
license renewal	許可更新
lifestyle disease	生活習慣病
limit of use	使用限度
literature search / retrieval of literature	文献検索
literature searching / searches	文献調査
long-term use surveillance	長期使用に関する調査
Lump-sum benefits for bereaved families	遺族一時金
Lyell syndrome	ライエル症候群

M

MAH with the first-class marketing license for pharmaceuticals (first-class MAH)	第 1 種製造販売業者
main product pamphlet	製品情報概要
Manuals for Management of Individual Serious Adverse Drug Reactions	重篤副作用疾患別対応マニュアル
manufacturing approval	製造承認
manufacturing control manager	製造管理者
manufacturing release decision	製造出荷判定
market release decision	市場出荷判定
marketing approval	製造販売承認
Marketing Authorisation Holder (MAH)	医薬品販売承認取得業者／製造販売業者
marketing restriction	販売制限
Marketing Specialist (MS)	医薬品卸販売担当者
measure to assure proper use	適正使用等確保措置
measures to be taken	措置の立案
medical accident	医療事故

medical allowance	医療手当
Medical Care Act	医療法
medical certificate	診断書
medical device	医療機器
medical expense	医療費
Medical Information Database Network (MID-NET)	MID-NET
Medical Information for Risk Assessment Initiative (MIHARI)	MIHARI
(the) medical institution monitoring report system	医療機関モニター報告制度
(the) medical institution monitoring report system	医療機関モニター報告制度
medical institution reporting system	医療機関報告制度
medical practice	医療習慣
Medical Product Information web page	医薬品医療機器情報提供ホームページ
Medical Representative (MR)	医薬情報担当者
medical safety information	医療安全情報
medical service provider in attendance	担当医療者
medical specialist	専門医
Medicines and Healthcare products Regulatory Agency (MHRA)	英国医薬品医療製品規制庁
mild ADR	軽微な副作用
Ministry of Health and Welfare (MHW, which is the precursor of MHLW)	（旧）厚生省
Ministry of Health, Labour and Welfare (MHLW)	厚生労働省
monitoring system	モニタリングシステム
multi-regional clinical trial	国際共同治験
multi-regional drug development	国際医薬品開発

N

National Center for Child Health and Development	国立成育医療研究センター
new combination drugs	新医療用配合剤
(the) new drug clinical evaluation guideline	臨床評価ガイドライン
(the) new drug review system	新薬審査体制
new reevaluation	新再評価
non-clinical study	非臨床試験
notification of reexamination result	再審査結果通知
nucleic acid agent	核酸系薬物

O

obligation of ADR reporting	副作用報告義務

obligatory ADR reporting term	副作用報告義務期間
observational study	観察研究
Office of New Drugs, PMDA	新薬審査部（PMDA の一部署）
on-site inspection	実地調査
order for emergency measure	緊急措置命令
order of conditions for approval	承認条件の付与
orphan drug	オーファンドラッグ／希少疾病用医薬品
outsourcing	外部委託
Over The Counter (OTC) drug	一般用医薬品／ OTC 医薬品
overall compliance evaluation	総合的適合性評価

P

package insert	添付文書
Package Leaflet (PL)	患者向製品説明書
partial change approval application	一部変更承認申請（通称：一変申請）
patient enrollment method	症例登録方法
patient information leaflet	くすりのしおり
Patient Information Leaflet (PIL)	（英国の）患者向製品説明書
patient medication information	患者さんへの服薬説明書
Patient Package Insert (PPI)	患者用添付文書
patient suffering the ADR induced damage	副作用被害者
Pension for Raising Children with disabilities	障害児養育年金
(the) period for sales monopoly	販売独占期間
Periodic Benefit-Risk Evaluation Report (PBRER)	定期的ベネフィット・リスク評価報告
periodic reevaluation	定期的再評価
periodic report	定期報告
periodic report for unexpected / non-serious ADR	未知・非重篤定期報告
periodic reporting system for infections	感染症定期報告制度
periodic safety report (system)	安全性定期報告（制度）
Periodic Safety Update Report (PSUR)	定期的安全性最新報告
Pharmaceutical Affairs Law (PAL, which is the precursor of PMD Act)	（旧）薬事法
Pharmaceutical Evaluation Division, Pharmaceutical Safety and Environmental Health Bureau, MHLW	（厚生労働省医薬・生活衛生局）医薬品審査管理課
(the) Pharmaceutical Officer	総括製造販売責任者
(the) pharmaceutical regulation	薬事規制
Pharmaceutical Safety and Environmental Health Bureau, Ministry of Health, Labour and Welfare	（厚生労働省）医薬・生活衛生局

Pharmaceutical Safety Division, Pharmaceutical Safety and Environmental Health Bureau, MHLW (PSEHB/PSD)	（厚生労働省医薬・生活衛生局）医薬安全対策課
Pharmaceuticals and Medical Devices Agency (PMDA)	独立行政法人 医薬品医療機器総合機構
Pharmaceuticals and medical devices information e-mail service	医薬品医療機器情報配信サービス
Pharmaceutical Safety control manager (required by the Ordinance for Enforcement of Medical Care Act)	医薬品安全管理責任者（医療法施行規則で要求される）
pharmacoepidemiological method	薬剤疫学的手法
pharmacoepidemiology	薬剤疫学
pharmacogenomics	ファーマコゲノミクス
pharmacological class	薬効群
pharmacovigilance (PV)	医薬品の安全性監視
pharmacovigilance plan (PVP)	（医薬品）安全性監視計画
Pharmacovigilance System Master File (PSMF)	安全性監視（PV）システムマスターファイル
physician	臨床医
PMD Act /Act on Securing Quality, Efficacy and Safety of Products Including Pharmaceuticals and Medical Devices	医薬品，医療機器等の品質，有効性及び安全性の確保等に関する法律／医薬品医療機器等法
PMDA medi-navi	PMDA メディナビ
PMS system	PMS 制度
poisonous drug	毒薬
Post-authorisation safety studies (PASS)	市販後安全性研究（EU における）
Post Marketing Surveillance (PMS)	市販後調査／市販後監視
post-marketing clinical trial	製造販売後臨床試験
post-marketing investigation	製造販売後調査
post-marketing safety measures	市販後安全対策
post-marketing studies	製造販売後調査・試験
Post-marketing studies manager	製造販売後調査等管理責任者
powerful drug	劇薬
precautions / precaution for use	使用上の注意
prediction and prevention style for ADR	副作用の予測・予防型
pre-submission stage	申請前段階
preliminary report	第一報報告
prescription drug/ethical drug	処方せん医薬品／医療用医薬品
preventive vaccination	予防接種
Preventive Vaccinations Act	予防接種法
priority monitoring drug	重点監視医薬品
product information brochure	製品情報概要

product recall	製品回収
professional medical institution	専門医療機関
prohibition of concomitant use	併用禁止
prohibition on exaggerated advertisement	誇大広告の禁止
Promotion Code Committee	プロモーションコード委員会
proof of prescription	投薬証明（書）
prospective investigation	プロスペクティブ（前向き）な調査
protocol	研究実施計画書
protocol of post-marketing studies	製造販売後調査等実施計画書
PSEHB/PSD Notification	（厚生労働省）医薬安全対策課長通知
PV inspection	ファーマコビジランス査察

Q

qualification certification program for MR	MR 資格認定制度
(the) Quality Assurance Officer	品質保証責任者
(the) Quality Management Officer	品質管理責任者
quality assurance unit	品質保証部門
Quality Of Life (QOL)	クオリティオブライフ
quasi-drug	医薬部外品

R

racial difference	人種差
raw material	原材料
reactive issuing mode of warnings for ADRs	副作用の警報発信型
reason of combination	配合理由
recall	回収
recall management	回収処理
reevaluation for quality	品質再評価
reevaluation / reexamination by administrative guidance	行政指導に基づく再評価／再審査
reevaluation based on PMD Act	医薬品医療機器等法に基づく再評価
Reevaluation Committee of the FPMAJ	日本製薬団体連合会 再評価委員会
reevaluation result of ethical drug	医療用医薬品再評価結果
reevaluation system	再評価制度
reexamination	再審査
reexamination application	再審査申請
reexamination by administrative guidance	第一次再評価
reexamination compliance inspection	再審査適合性調査
reexamination period	再審査期間
reexamination system	再審査制度
reference preparation	標準製剤

Reference RMP	参照／参考 RMP
regulatory authority	規制当局
regulatory classification	規制区分
regulatory countermeasure	行政措置
regulatory measure	行政指導
reliability assurance inspections / examinations	信頼性保証査察
relief benefits	救済給付
Relief System for Sufferers from Adverse Drug Reactions	医薬品副作用被害救済制度
Relief System for Sufferers from Diseases Infected from Biological Products	生物由来製品感染等被害救済制度
report of measures taken overseas	外国措置報告
reporting time frames	報告期限
requirement for payment	支給要件
research report	研究報告
retention of records	記録の保存
retrospective investigation	レトロスペクティブ（後ろ向き）な調査
Review Committee on Post-Marketing Clinical Trials	市販後臨床試験審査委員会
review time	審査期間
Risk / Benefit Assessment of Drugs-Analysis and Response (RAD-AR) Council, Japan	くすりの適正使用協議会
Risk Evaluation and Mitigation Strategy (REMS) (U. S.)	リスク評価・リスク緩和戦略（米国）
risk management	リスク管理
Risk Management Plan (RMP)	医薬品リスク管理計画
risk management system	リスクマネジメント制度
Risk Minimization Activity	リスク最小化活動
risk minimization measure	安全対策
risk minimization measure	リスク最小化策（EU）
Risk Minimization Plan	リスク最小化計画（日本）
routine vaccination	定期接種

S

safety	安全性
safety assurance	安全（性）確保
safety implementation / operational manager	安全管理実施責任者
safety implementation division	安全管理実施部門
safety information	安全性情報
safety management contractor	安全確保業務委託者
safety management information	安全管理情報

(the) Safety Management Officer	安全管理責任者
Safety Management Team (SMT)	安全性管理チーム
Safety measure	安全確保措置
safety measure	安全対策
safety specification	安全性検討事項
SAKIGAKE Designation System	先駆け審査指定制度
2nd-class MAH	第2種製造販売業者
second reevaluation	第二次再評価
secondary infection	二次感染者
self inspection	自己点検
sentinel medical institution network	拠点医療機関ネットワーク
separate full application for the same active ingredient as a drug which is still in its reexamination period	追っかけ新薬
similarity	類似性
6 month periodic safety report	6か月定期報告
solid formulation for oral use	内用固形剤
SOP on post-marketing safety management	製造販売後安全管理業務手順書
SOP on post-marketing studies	製造販売後調査等業務手順書
SOP on quality control	品質管理業務手順書
Sorivudine incident	ソリブジン事件
special committee	特別部会
specially controlled medical device	高度管理医療機器
specificity	特異性
specified use-results survey	特定使用成績調査
sponsor (of clinical trial)	治験依頼者
spontaneous ADR report	副作用自発報告
spontaneous information source	自発的情報源
spontaneous report	自発報告
Standard Commodity Classification Number of Japan	日本標準商品分類番号
Standard Operating Procedure (SOP)	標準業務手順
Stevens-Johnson syndrome (SJS)	スティーブンス・ジョンソン症候群（皮膚粘膜眼症候群）
stipulation to be observed	遵守事項
strength	強度
Subacute Myelo-Optico-Neuropathy (SMON)	スモン／亜急性脊髄・視神経・末梢神経症
subcommittee	調査会
subject	被験者

subsidy	国からの補助金
sufffers from ADR	医薬品副作用被害事例
Summary of Product Characteristics (SPC)	製品特性概要（EU の製品説明書）
supportive experimental evidence for causality	因果関係を支持する実験的なエビデンス
surrogate endpoint	代替／代用のエンドポイント
surveilance system by using consecutive patients	連続調査方式
survey of drug-resistant bacterial strains	耐性菌調査
survey on the actual use	実態把握調査
survey on the actual use of anti-cancer combination therapies	抗がん剤併用療法実態把握調査
surveys of actual conditions of use	使用実態調査

T

temporality	時間の関係
teratogenicity study	催奇形性試験
Thalidomide Education and Risk Management System (TERMS)	サリドマイド製剤安全管理手順
the TGN1412 incident	TGN1412 事件
(the) time clock for the reporting timeline	報告期限のタイムクロック
three supervisors in MAH	製造販売業三役
3rd-class MAH	第 3 種製造販売業者
Toxic Epidermal Necrolysis (TEN)	中毒性表皮壊死症
true endpoint	真のエンドポイント

U

U. S. Food and Drug Administration (FDA)	米国食品医薬品局
unapproved drug	未承認薬
unavoidable ADR	不可避的な副作用
unexpected ADR (signal)	未知の副作用（シグナル）
unexpected and serious case	未知・重篤症例
use for pregnant / expectant / nursing women	妊婦・産婦・授乳婦への投与
usefulness	有用性
Use-results survey	使用成績調査
Use-results survey with comparative group	使用成績比較調査

V

vaccine adverse reaction review committee	副反応検討部会
validation study	バリデーション研究
variant Creutzfeldt-Jakob disease (vCJD)	変異型クロイツフェルト・ヤコブ病
voluntary vaccination	任意接種

W - Y

WHO monitoring system	WHO モニタリング制度
(the) WHO Programme for International Drug Monitoring	WHO 国際医薬品モニタリング制度
(the) Yellow Letter (the Dear Healthcare Professional Letters of Emergent Safety Communications)	イエローレター（緊急安全性情報）

日英対訳　日本における医薬品のリスクマネジメント 第3版
－新たな改正GPSP省令への対応と医薬品医療機器等法の改正に向けて－

Drug Risk Management in Japan 3rd ed.

-compatible with Newly revised
GPSP Ordinance and including expectations for the
forthcoming revision of the PMD Act-
（in Japanese and English）

第 1 章

わが国の医薬品審査,
安全対策をめぐる現状と将来に向けて

　わが国は新薬開発国の主要メンバーの 1 つとして, 欧米と協調し, 医薬品規制調和国際会議（ICH：International Council for Harmonisation of Technical Requirements for Pharmaceuticals for Human Use：2015 年, ICH はスイス法に基づく非営利法人となり, さらに参加メンバー（地域）の拡大に伴い, 名称を変更した）における医薬品規制の国際的ハーモナイゼーション推進のために大きく貢献してきた。また, 新薬開発においても, 医療用医薬品世界売上上位 100 品目（2016 年）のうち 13 品目を開発して, 医療分野において国際的な貢献をしてきている（政策研ニュース No.52, 2017 年 11 月 p.51-54）。

　しかしながら, 2000 年代に入り, わが国は国際共同治験等のグローバル開発から取り残され, 欧米で承認された新薬がわが国では遅れて申請され承認されるという, いわゆるドラッグ・ラグが顕在化した。そのため, 欧米に比べて 2 〜 3 年以上遅れて新薬がわが国の医療の場に提供されるという状態が続き, 大きな社会問題となっていた。

　このような課題を解決するため, 厚生労働省（以下, 厚労省）は臨床研究等の推進, 治験推進のための基盤整備, 独立行政法人 医薬品医療機器総合機構（以下, PMDA）における新薬審査体制の強化による審査の迅速化等の施策を強力に進めてきた。その結果, 現在, 欧米の審査当局に比肩する審査の迅速化が図られ, PMDA における審査の遅れ（審査ラグ）はほぼ解消され, 製薬企業からの申請の遅れ（申請ラグまたは開発ラグ）が顕在化している（https://www.pmda.go.jp/files/000222386.pdf）。このような申請ラグの解消とわが国発の新薬開発を推進するため, 厚労省は, 国際共同治験への積極的な参加の推進, 新薬開発環境の整備, 早期承認制度等の施策を講じており, 今後, 新薬開発の面でもわが国は国際的に大きく貢献できるものと期待される。

　一方, 安全対策に関しては, 欧米諸国と同様に, 過去において医薬品副作用による大きな健康被害事件（薬害事件）を経験してきている。サリドマイド事件のように欧米諸国と共通の事例もあるが, わが国独特の背景を有する薬害事件も過去に発生している（詳細については, 「日本の薬害事件：Drug-Induced Suffering in Japan」, 薬事日報社刊　参照）。

　特に, 開発段階における有効性や安全性に関する情報が不足している新薬や, 市

Chapter 1

Current status and future prospects of pharmaceutical approval review and safety policies in Japan

As one of the main countries in new drug development, Japan in collaboration with the United States and European countries has made major contributions to advances in international harmonisation in pharmaceutical regulatory activities via the International Council for Harmonisation of Technical Requirements for Pharmaceuticals for Human Use (ICH; in 2015, ICH became a non-profit corporation under Swiss law, and the name was changed following an increase in the number of participating members [regions]). In new drug development, Japan developed 13 out of the top 100 prescription drugs sold in the world (2016) and is a major international contributor to medical therapy (OPIR: Office of Pharmaceutical Industry Research, Views and Actions, No. 52, November 2017, p. 51–54).

Since entering the 2000s, however, Japan has been left out of global clinical trials and other aspects of global development and a "drug lag" or delay in applications and approvals in Japan for new drugs already approved in the US and European countries has become apparent. Therefore, the situation persisted whereby new drug reached patients in Japan 2–3 or more years after their approvals in the US and Europe, and this became a major social problem.

To solve this issue, the Ministry of Health, Labour and Welfare (MHLW) vigorously pushed forward measures such as promoting clinical research, establishing infrastructure for the promotion of clinical trials, and accelerating reviews by enhancing the new drug review system at the Pharmaceuticals and Medical Devices Agency (PMDA). As a result, rapid reviews comparable to those by regulatory authorities in the US and Europe are now available. The delay in reviews at the PMDA (review lag) has been mostly resolved and a delay in applications from pharmaceutical companies (application lag or development lag) has become apparent (https://www.pmda.go.jp/files/000222386.pdf). In order to resolve this application lag and promote new drug development in Japan, the MHLW has been taking measures such as promoting active participation in global clinical trials, establishing an environment for new drug development, and an organizing early approval system, etc. It is expected that our country can make a major contribution internationally to new drug development.

As for safety measures, Japan has experienced major incidents of health damage caused by adverse drug reactions (ADRs) in the past in the same way as in the US and European countries. Some cases, like that of thalidomide, are similar to those in the US and European countries, but there have also been incidents of damage to health caused by ADRs that had a background peculiar to Japan (For details, see "Drug-Induced Suffering in Japan (published by Yakuji Nippo Ltd.)."

Particularly for new drugs for which information on efficacy or safety in the

販直後に特段の適正使用情報提供の徹底や安全性情報の収集が必要な新薬について
は条件付き承認制度や，市販直後調査制度（EPPV：Early post-marketing phase risk
minimization and vigilance）等を世界に先駆けて導入している（詳細については第4
章参照）。

また，2013年春には，開発から市販後までの一貫したリスクマネジメントの一
環として，医薬品リスク管理計画（RMP：Risk Management Plan）制度の導入が行
われた。さらに，厚労省では，より科学的な安全対策の強化に向けて，電子カルテ
等の医療情報を大規模に収集・解析を行う医療情報データベース「MID-NET」を
PMDA に構築し，2018年春から行政・製薬企業・アカデミアによる利活用が可能
な MID-NET の本格運用が開始された。同時に改正 GPSP 省令が施行され，データ
ベースを活用した製造販売後調査の実施が可能となり，PMDA に「疫学調査相談
窓口」が設置された（詳細については第7章参照）。

1.1 開発や審査の現状と課題

わが国を取り巻く医薬品開発に係る主な問題点としては，

① 世界の医薬品市場に占める日本のシェアの低下，薬価制度改革（特に新薬創
出・適応外薬解消等促進加算適用品目の大幅な絞り込み）による欧米製薬企
業の日本で開発するインセンティブの低下

② 世界的に創薬の中心は低分子化合物からバイオ医薬品へと移行する中で，バ
イオ医薬品に係る基盤整備の遅れ

③ オープンイノベーション推進のための環境整備（産学連携体制，ベンチャー
企業の育成）の遅れ

④ PMDA 独自の要求（グローバル臨床試験における日本人症例の一定割合確
保等）

があげられる。

その結果として，日本企業は海外での開発を先行し，欧米企業もアジアでは日本
以外の国で開発を先行させる傾向が強まり，さらなるわが国での申請の遅れにつな
がっている。このような中にあって，厚労省は，開発の初期段階からの開発支援の
強化，治験環境の整備，わが国の国際共同治験への参加を可能とするための治験相
談体制の強化，審査体制の強化等の施策を講じている。また，2015年4月には国
立研究開発法人 日本医療研究開発機構（AMED）が設立され，基礎研究の支援，
臨床研究等の基盤整備，アカデミア発創薬シーズの実用化に向けた産学連携プロ
ジェクトの推進等に取り組んでいる。

わが国においては，欧米に先駆けて条件付き承認制度を整備し，審査段階におけ
る安全性等に関する情報が限られている新薬についても，一定の条件を付して早期
に承認する路を開いてきた。2013年11月27日に公布された「医薬品，医療機器

development stage are insufficient and new drugs that specially require thorough provision of information on proper use or collection of safety information in the early post-marketing period, Japan was the first in the world to introduce systems such as the conditional approval system and the system for Early post-marketing phase risk minimization and vigilance (EPPV) (For details, see Chapter 4).

In addition, in the spring of 2013, the Risk Management Plan (RMP) was introduced as part of consistent risk management from development through post-marketing. Furthermore, the MHLW has constructed a medical information database, "MID-NET" at the PMDA to make large-scale collection and analysis of medical information such as electronic medical charts, and full-scale operation of the MID-NET began in the spring of 2018 to allow utilization and application of the database by the government, pharmaceutical companies and academia, for strengthened scientific safety measures. At the same time, a revised GPSP Ordinance was enacted to allow implementation of post-marketing studies utilizing databases, and a "Consultation service for epidemiological studies" was established at the PMDA (For details, see Chapter 7).

1.1 Current status and issues related to development and approval review

The main problems related to the development of medical products in Japan are as follows:

[1]   A decrease in the incentive for development of drugs in Japan by US and European pharmaceutical companies due to a decline in the percentage of the global pharmaceutical market occupied by Japan and reformation of the drug pricing system in Japan (considerable narrowing of items for which the premium for new drug development and elimination of off-label drug use is applied in particular)

[2]   A delay in establishment of the infrastructure for biopharmaceuticals against a background of the global shift of the focus of drug development from low-molecular-weight compounds to biopharmaceuticals

[3]   A delay in establishment of an environment for promotion of open innovation (industry-academia collaboration system and development of venture companies)

[4]   The presence of requirements unique to the PMDA (for example, a certain percentage of subjects must be Japanese in global clinical trials)

As a result, there has been a greater tendency for Japanese companies to undertake overseas development first, and the US and European companies to start the development in Asian countries other than Japan, leading to a further delay in applications in Japan. Under such conditions, the MHLW has taken measures such as augmenting support for development from the initial stage of development, establishing an environment for clinical trials, and strengthening the clinical trial consultation system to make possible Japanese participation in global clinical trials. Other improvements being initiated include policies to strengthen the review system. In addition, the Japan Agency for Medical Research and Development (AMED) was established in April 2015 to provide support for basic studies, establish infrastructure for clinical research, etc., and promote industry-academia collaborative projects for practical application of drug seeds developed by the academia.

等の品質，有効性及び安全性の確保等に関する法律」（以下，医薬品医療機器等法）では再生医療等製品の条件及び期限付承認制度が導入され（2014 年 11 月 25 日施行），2015 年 4 月 1 日からは先駆け審査指定制度の試行的実施が開始され，指定された品目に対する優先相談，事前評価，優先審査等により審査期間の短縮を図っている。さらに，2017 年 10 月 10 日には医薬品の条件付き早期承認制度の実施が公表され，即日施行された。

1.1.1　治験の現状と課題

　新薬の創出による治療満足度の向上により，医薬品開発の対象分野ががん，希少疾患，精神疾患等の治療難易度の高い領域に集中しつつある（平成 26 年度＆平成 27 年度国内基盤技術調査報告書「60 疾患の医療ニーズ調査と新たな医療ニーズ」HS 財団）。そのため製薬企業では，薬剤ポテンシャルを早期に見極めることで無駄な臨床開発費用を抑制する必要があり，開発ストラテジーが多様化してきている。ICH でも多様化する臨床試験デザイン，データソースに対応する指針を策定することが合意され（GCP renovation），ICH E8（臨床試験の一般指針）の改定（Modernization），引き続き ICH E6（GCP）の大幅刷新（Renovation）が予定されている。現在の GCP は無作為化比較試験に代表される説明的臨床試験（Explanatory clinical Trials）を想定して作成されているが，GCP renovation では一般化可能性の補強を目的とした実践的臨床試験（Pragmatic clinical Trials），Real World Data を用いた臨床研究，観察研究等の臨床試験／臨床研究全般がスコープに入っている。また，臨床試験／臨床研究の品質管理に関し，Quality by Design（計画に基づいた質の確保）の考え方が反映される予定である。

　GCP renovation では臨床研究全般が対象となるが，わが国では 2017 年 4 月 14 日に臨床研究法が公布され（2018 年 4 月 1 日施行），GCP とは異なる規制の下で臨床研究（「特定臨床研究」に該当する研究）が実施されることになっている。衆参両院の臨床研究法案に対する付帯決議の中に「臨床研究で得られた情報を，医薬品，医療機器等の承認申請に係る資料として利活用できる仕組みについて速やかに検討すること。」との一文が盛り込まれており，承認申請における特定臨床研究結果の活用も今後検討されることになる。

1.1.2　新薬審査の現状と課題

　わが国の審査期間が米国に比べると長すぎるとの指摘がたびたびなされてきたが，PMDA の大幅な体制強化により，承認審査の遅れによるドラッグ・ラグ問題

Japan established a conditional approval system before the US and Europe, and opened the way for early approval with certain conditions for new drugs for which information on safety, etc. are limited at the review stage. Under the PMD Act in Japan (Formal name: the Act on Securing Quality, Efficacy and Safety of Pharmaceuticals, Medical Devices, Regenerative and Cellular Therapy Products, Gene Therapy Products and Cosmetics) promulgated on November 27, 2013, a conditional, fixed-term approval system was introduced for regenerative medicine products (enacted on November 25, 2014). Since April 1, 2015, the SAKIGAKE Designation System has been started experimentally to shorten the review time for designated items by priority consultation, pre-application evaluation and priority review, etc. Furthermore, implementation of conditional early approval system for drugs was promulgated on October 10, 2017 and enacted on the same day.

1.1.1 Current status and issues for clinical trials

In order to focus new drug development on areas of unmet medical need, the target fields for pharmaceutical development have concentrated on areas of high treatment difficulty, such as cancers, rare diseases and psychiatric disorders (Fiscal Year [FY] 2014 & FY 2015 Reports of Surveys on Basic Technologies in Japan, ""Survey on Medical Needs of 60 Disorders and New Medical Needs"", Japan Health Sciences Foundation). To achieve this, pharmaceutical companies must reduce the cost of fruitless clinical development by determining the potential of drugs at an early stage, and developmental strategies are diversifying. The ICH has also agreed to establish guidelines accommodating diverse clinical trial designs and data sources (GCP renovation), and is planning to modernize the ICH E8 Guideline (General Considerations for Clinical Trials), followed by renovation of ICH E6 (GCP). While the current GCP was prepared for explanatory clinical trials represented by randomized controlled trials, the scope of GCP renovation covers pragmatic clinical trials for maximization of generalizability, clinical studies using real world data, and general clinical trials/studies such as observational studies. In addition, the idea of Quality by Design will be reflected in the quality control of clinical trials/studies.

While GCP renovation covers clinical studies in general, the Clinical Research Act was promulgated on April 14, 2017 (enacted on April 1, 2018) and clinical studies (those that are regarded as "Specified clinical studies") are to be conducted under regulations different from GCP in Japan. The supplementary resolution for the proposed Clinical Research Act in both the Houses of Representatives and Councilors included a sentence, "A prompt investigation is required to establish a system which allows application and utilization of the information obtained in clinical studies as the materials for application for approval of drugs and medical devices, etc." Thus, utilization of the results of specified clinical studies in the application for approval will also be considered in the future.

1.1.2 Current status and issues related to new drug reviews

It has often been pointed out that the review period in Japan is longer than that in the US, however, the MHLW is extensively reinforcing the systems in the PMDA, and

はほぼ解決されている。しかし，外資・内資を問わず製薬企業が欧米での開発および申請を先行させ，わが国への申請が遅れること（申請ラグ）により生ずるドラッグ・ラグはいまだに解決されていない。その大きな原因のひとつとして，国際共同治験へのわが国の参加が遅れていることがあげられる。ICH において世界各地域での国際共同治験の受け入れ可能性を高めるためのガイドライン（ICH E17）が合意され，わが国では「国際共同治験の計画及びデザインに関する一般原則」として発出された（2018 年 6 月 12 日）。ドラッグ・ラグ回避のためには国際共同治験への参加が必須であり，当該ガイドラインを踏まえ，製薬企業および PMDA の両者がわが国の国際共同治験への参加を推進していく必要がある。

1.1.3　条件付き承認制度

　医薬品の有効性や安全性を，開発段階の臨床試験により調べ尽くすことは不可能であり，また，開発段階で過剰な調査および検査を課すことは開発の遅延等を招くおそれがある。稀な副作用を検出するためだけの目的で治験の症例数を増やすよりは，むしろ必要に応じて，目的を明確化した全例調査等の実施，製造販売後臨床試験の実施，医療機関を限定した使用等の承認条件を付けたり，販売前に医療機関への新薬の適正使用に関する情報提供の徹底を製造販売業者に義務づけることによる市販後の安全対策を厳重に行うことこそが，新薬開発期間の短縮と，新薬の安全性確保のためには重要である。

　すなわち，開発段階の臨床試験（治験）は，厳重な基準のもとで被験者を選択し，併用薬等についても厳重に管理して行われるという点において，比較可能性を重視した方法である。しかし，市販後の医療の場は，併用薬，合併症，年齢，性別，使用する医療関係者の専門性等さまざまな点で開発段階とは異なっており，治験の結果をそのまま将来の患者集団に適用できない。すなわち，新薬の有効性や安全性を評価するためには，開発段階の評価とともに，市販後段階においてもその有効性や安全性を評価することが重要である。

　わが国における新薬の安全性監視および確保では，多くの場合は豊富な海外安全性データが存在する状況下での対応を考えればよかったが，再生医療等製品の条件及び期限付承認制度（2014 年 11 月 25 日施行，図 1.1 参照），医薬品の条件付き早期承認制度の実施（2017 年 10 月 10 日施行，図 1.2 参照），さらに先駆け審査指定制度の試行的実施（2015 年 4 月 1 日開始，図 1.3 参照）によって，海外安全性データがほとんどない，あるいはわが国で最初に新薬が広く使用されるという状況での安全監視計画を策定し実施していく必要がある。

currently, the drug lag problem due to delays in approval review is almost resolved. Nevertheless, the drug lag due to a delay in submitting applications in Japan (application lag) as both foreign and Japanese domestic pharmaceutical companies first promote development and file applications in the US and Europe, has not yet been resolved. One of the major reasons is a delayed in participation of Japan in global clinical trials. Under ICH, a guidelines (ICH E17) was agreed to increase the acceptability of global clinical trials in each region of the world, and it was issued in Japan as "General Principles for Planning and Design of Multi-Regional Clinical Trials" (June 12, 2018). In order to avoid drug lag, participation in global clinical trials is essential. Based on these guidelines, both pharmaceutical companies and the PMDA must promote participation of Japan in global clinical trials.

1.1.3 Conditional approval system

It is impossible to completely investigate the efficacy and safety of drugs using only clinical trials during development, at the same time, imposing excessive investigations and tests during development may lead to delays and other problems. Rather than increasing the number of trial subjects in order just to detect rare ADRs, implementing the following measures-when necessary—can be important for both shortening the development time and assuring the safety of new drugs: All-patient survey with clear objectives, post-marketing clinical trial, and strict post-marketing safety measures by attaching approval conditions such as allowing use only at limited medical institutions or requiring marketing authorization holders (MAHs) to thoroughly provide information on proper use of new drugs to medical institutions before marketing.

Clinical studies (trials) during development are a method that places importance on comparability, because subjects can be selected based on strict standards and factors such as concomitant medications can be stringently controlled. However, medical practice during marketing differs from the clinical development stage in several respects including concomitant medication use, concomitant diseases, age, gender and the specialization of the healthcare professionals prescribing the drugs. As such, the results of clinical trials cannot be directly applied to the future patient population. Therefore, to assure efficacy and safety of new drugs, it is important to evaluate efficacy and safety not only during clinical development but also in the post-marketing stage. In Japan, in many cases conventional pharmacovigilance and safety assurance for new drugs only had to take account of the situation where abundant overseas safety data were available, however, following the introduction of the conditional and fixed-term approval system for regenerative medicine products (enacted on November 25, 2014, see **Figure 1.1**), implementation of the conditional early approval system for drugs (enacted on October 10, 2017, see **Figure 1.2**), and experimental implementation of the SAKIGAKE Designation System (initiated on April 1, 2015, see **Figure 1.3**), it is now necessary to establish and implement pharmacovigilance plans under circumstances where there are almost no overseas safety data or a new drug is extensively used in Japan before the rest of the world.

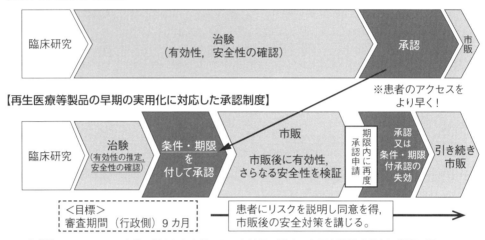

図 1.1 再生医療等製品の条件及び期限付承認制度（PMDA 平成 30 年度第 2 回運営評議会第 4 期中期計画の方向性について（案）[補足資料]）

図 1.2 医薬品の条件付き早期承認制度（PMDA 平成 30 年度第 2 回運営評議会資料 3）

Chapter 1 Current status and future prospects of pharmaceutical approval review and safety policies in Japan

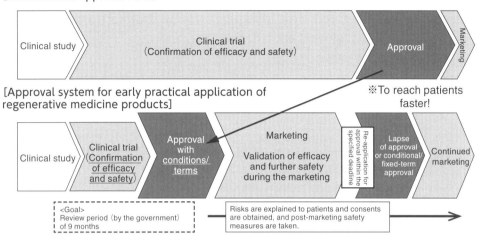

Fig1-1　Conditional and fixed-term approval systems for regenerative medicine products (Directions of the fourth medium-term plan in the PMDA fiscal year 2018 Second Administrative Council (draft) [supplementary document])

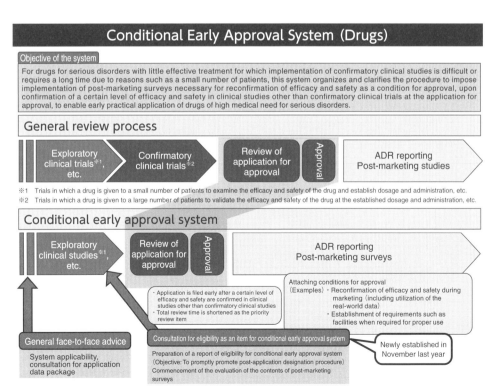

Fig1-2　Conditional early approval system for drugs(Document 3 for the PMDA FY 2018 Second Administrative Council)

先駆け審査指定制度

世界に先駆けて，革新的医薬品・医療機器・再生医療等製品を日本で早期に実用化すべく，世界に先駆けて開発され，早期の治験段階で著明な有効性が見込まれる医薬品等を指定し，各種支援による早期の実用化（例えば，医薬品・医療機器では**通常の半分の6ヶ月間**で承認）を目指す「**先駆け審査指定制度**」を平成27年4月1日に創設。平成29年度も引き続き当該制度を試行的に実施した。

指定基準　※医薬品の例

1. 治療薬の画期性：原則として，既承認薬と異なる作用機序であること（既承認薬と同じ作用機序であっても開発対象とする疾患に適応するのは初めてであるものを含む。）
2. 対象疾患の重篤性：生命に重大な影響がある重篤な疾患又は根治療法がなく社会生活が困難な状態が継続している疾患であること。
3. 対象疾患に係る極めて高い有効性：既承認薬が存在しない又は既承認薬に比べて有効性の大幅な改善が期待できること。
4. 世界に先駆けて日本で早期開発・申請する意思（同時申請も含む。）

指定制度の内容　□：承認取得までの期間の短縮に関するもの　┊┊：その他開発促進に関する取組

①優先相談
〔2か月→1か月〕
○ 資料提出から治験相談までの期間を短縮。

②事前評価の充実
〔実質的な審査の前倒し〕
○事前評価を充実させ，英語資料の提出も認める。

③優先審査
〔12か月→6か月〕
○総審査期間の目標を，6か月に。
※場合によっては第Ⅲ相試験の結果の承認申請後の提出を認め，開発から承認までの期間を短縮

④審査パートナー制度
〔PMDA版コンシェルジュ〕
○審査，安全対策，品質管理，信頼性保証等承認までに必要な工程の総括管理を行う管理職をコンシェルジュとして設置。

⑤製造販売後の安全対策充実
〔再審査期間の延長〕
○通常，新有効成分含有医薬品の再審査期間が8年であるところを，再審査期間を延長し，最長10年までの範囲内で設定する。

図1.3　先駆け審査指定制度（（PMDA平成30年度第2回運営評議会第4期中期計画の方向性について（案）〔補足資料〕）

1.2　市販後安全対策の現状と課題

　わが国では，過去の薬害事件の教訓として，新薬の市販後の安全性を確保するためには，開発・審査段階から市販後段階にいたる一貫したリスク管理が必要であるとの考えから，1980〜90年代において安全対策に係る薬事規制を逐次追加して制度化してきた。製造販売業者に対しては，「副作用・感染症報告制度」，「再審査制度（安全性定期報告制度を含む）」，「再評価制度」を市販後安全対策制度の3本柱として，また，各制度下での安全対策活動の信頼性を確保するために，1997年に「医薬品の市販後調査の基準に関する省令（GPMSP）」を制定，2002年の「製造販売後安全対策の充実と承認・認可制度の見直し」により，GPMSP省令は2005年に製造販売業許可要件のGVP（Good Vigilance Practice：製造販売後安全管理基準）省令と，再審査・再評価申請資料における製造販売後調査・試験の実施の基準であるGPSP（Good Post-marketing Study Practice：製造販売後調査及び試験の実施基準）省令として施行された。一方，2002年の「医薬品・医療機器等安全性情報報告制度」の法制化により「医療機関からの副作用等報告の義務化」と，生物由来製品の安全確保対策の充実を目指した「感染症定期報告制度の導入」が2003年7月に施行された（図1.4参照）。

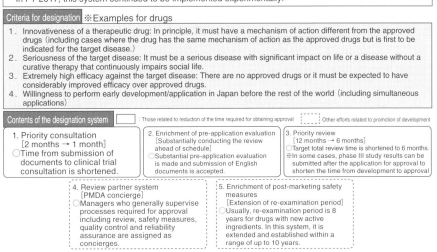

Fig1-3 SAKIGAKE Designation System (Directions of the fourth medium-term plan in the PMDA FY 2018 Second Administrative Council (draft) [supplementary document])

1.2 Current status and issues with post-marketing risk management

In Japan, pharmaceutical regulations related to safety measures were successively added and enacted in the 1980s and 90s based on the policy that consistent risk management was required from the stage of development and review to the post-marketing stage in order to ensure the safety of new drugs during marketing, as lessons learned from drug-induced suffering in the past. For MAHs, the "Adverse drug reaction (ADR) and infection reporting system", "Reexamination system (including the periodic safety update reporting system)" and "Reevaluation system" were established as the 3 core regulations for post-marketing safety measures. In addition, in order to ensure reliability of safety activities under each regulation, the "Good Post-marketing Surveillance Practice (GPMSP) Ordinance" was established in 1997. Following the "Enrichment of Post-marketing Safety Measures and Review of Approval/Authorization System" in 2002, the GPMSP Ordinance was enacted in 2005 as the Good Vigilance Practice (GVP) Ordinance which includes the requirements for manufacturing and marketing authorization and the Good Post-marketing Study Practice (GPSP) Ordinance which sets the standards for implementation of post-marketing studies in the application dossier for reexamination/reevaluation. The "Pharmaceuticals and Medical Devices Safety Information Reporting System" legislation was enacted in 2002, and "Mandatory ADR Reporting by Medical Institutions" and "Introduction of the Periodic Reporting System

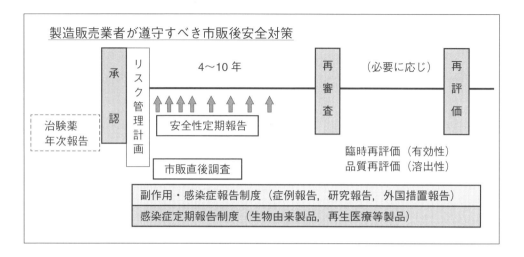

図 1.4 医薬品の市販後安全対策

　その後,「薬害再発防止のための医薬品行政等の見直し」により,「患者からの副作用報告制度」の提言を受けて, 患者からの直接の副作用報告が 2019 年 3 月から正式に開始された。また, 2014 年 10 月改正 GVP 省令, 改正 GPSP 省令が施行, 同年 11 月の医薬品医療機器等法の施行により,「医薬品リスク管理計画（RMP）」の作成は承認条件となり, 2019 年 3 月の時点で 401 製品の RMP が PMDA のホームページに公開されている。RMP は GVP 上必須となったが, 追加の安全性監視計画である製造販売後調査等は GPSP を遵守することになるため, RMP そのもの, および RMP を構成する個別の安全性監視計画／リスク最小化策の再審査における位置づけについて不明確な点もあったが, 2018 年 10 月に開催された医薬品製造販売業等管理者講習会にて, 厚生労働省医薬品審査管理課長より,「安全性監視計画策定の検討の進め方（図 1.5 参照）」における「各対処方法の関連法令下における位置づけの整理」により一部明確化された。しかしながら, 再審査および再評価申請資料の信頼性の確保という GPSP の位置づけについて, 今後厚労省はさらに明確にする必要がある。また, 上記講習会にて医薬品審査管理課長より「製造販売後の有効性の検討」について, 以下が披瀝された。

　○評価すべき具体的な検討事項が存在しない場合は, 製造販売後の有効性評価については, 文献の分析等の製造販売後調査等によらない方法で検討することでよい。

　○具体的な検討事項が生じた場合は, 当該事項を科学的に確認することが可能となる製造販売後調査等を実施する必要がある。

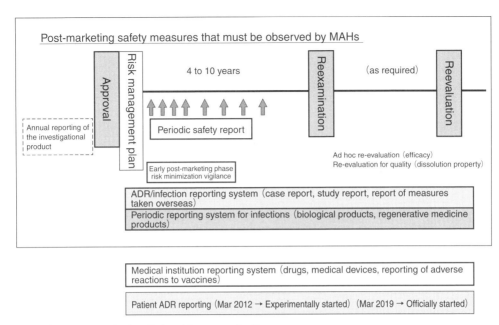

Fig1-4 Post-marketing Safety Measures for Drugs

for Infections" which aimed to enrich the safety assurance measures for biological products was enacted in July 2003 (see **Figure 1.4**). Subsequently, direct reporting of ADRs by patients was officially initiated in March 2019, in response to the proposed "Patient Adverse Drug Reaction Reporting System" by the "Review of Pharmaceutical Administration for Prevention of Recurrence of Incidents of Drug-induced Suffering". In addition, the enforcement of the revised GVP Ordinance and the revised GPSP Ordinance in October 2014, as well as the enforcement of the Pharmaceuticals and Medical Devices Act (the PMD Act) in November the same year made the preparation of a "Risk Management Plan (RMP)" a condition for approval. As of March 2019, RMPs of 401 products are presented on the PMDA's website. While the RMP is requirement under GVP, post-marketing investigations, etc. (additional pharmacovigilance plans) are conducted in compliance with the GPSP and the positioning of the individual pharmacovigilance plan/risk minimization plan comprising the RMP during reexamination was unclear in some respects. However, in the lecture for administrators including MAHs held in October 2018, the Director of the Pharmaceutical Evaluation Division of the MHLW clarified part of the issues in "Organization of the Position of Each Measure under the Relevant Laws and Regulations" in "How to develop pharmacovigilance planning (see **Figure 1.5**)". Nevertheless, the MHLW must further clarify the position of GPSP, which is to ensure the reliability of the reexamination and reevaluation dossiers. The Director of the Drug Evaluation and Licensing Division presented the followings in relation to the "Investigation of Post-marketing Efficacy" at the above lecture:

○ If there are no specific issues that need to be evaluated, the post-marketing efficacy evaluation can be made by methods other than post-marketing studies, such as an analysis of literature.

安全性監視計画策定の検討の進め方

承認時までにステップ3まではPMDAと申請者間で合意される。

ステップ1　各安全性検討事項における製造販売後に明らかにしたい懸念事項の明確化

↓

ステップ2　懸念事項ごとの科学的に適切な対処方法の決定

↓

ステップ3　各対処方法の関連法令下における位置づけの整理

通常の安全性監視	追加の安全性監視			
副作用報告研究・措置報告等	製造販売後臨床試験	使用成績調査（一般，特定，比較）	製造販売後データベース調査	非臨床試験
GVP 省令	GPSP 省令			GLP 省令

↓

ステップ4　詳細な計画（プロトコル）の策定

科学的な観点及び現行の承認審査の過程を考慮し，検討の進め方を4つのステップに分類した。

図 1.5　安全性監視計画策定の検討の進め方（平成 30 年度医薬品製造販売業等管理者講習会資料 17 頁）

　一方，薬剤疫学的手法の導入等による科学的な安全対策等の強化については PMDA が中心となって構築した医療情報データベース（MID-NET）が 2018 年 4 月から行政・製薬企業・アカデミアによる利活用が可能となり，本格運用が開始された（図 1.6 参照）。同時期に施行された改正 GPSP 省令では，これまでの「使用成績調査」および「製造販売後臨床試験」に新たに「製造販売後データベース調査」を加えた計 3 種類の調査・試験が規定され，製造販売後データベース調査に MID-NET の使用が可能となった。しかしながら，公開されている RMP で判断するかぎり，先駆け審査指定制度で承認された医薬品を含めて，追加の安全性監視方法は，従来からの市販直後調査や使用成績調査（特に全例調査）が主流を占めている。条件付き早期承認制度や先駆け審査指定制度の下，製造販売後の安全対策の充実を標榜して承認された画期的な新薬の今後の安全対策の展開を見守りたい（詳細は第 7 章参照）。

Chapter 1 Current status and future prospects of pharmaceutical approval review and safety policies in Japan

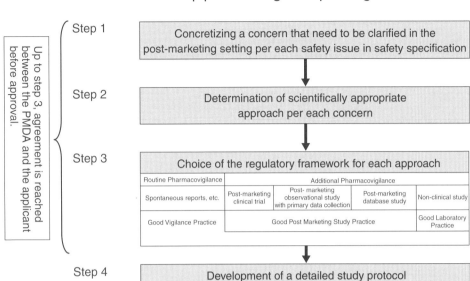

Fig1-5　How to develop pharmacovigilance planning(page 17, document for FY 2018 Lecture for Administrators including MAHs of Drugs)

　○ If specific issues arise, it will be necessary to conduct post-marketing studies, etc. to allow scientific validation of those issues.

　On the other hand, in relation to the strengthening of scientific safety measures by introduction of pharmacoepidemiologic approaches, the medical information database (MID-NET), primarily constructed by the PMDA, has been available for application and utilization by the administration, pharmaceutical companies and academia, and full-scale operation began in April 2018 (see **Figure 1.6**). In the revised GPSP Ordinance enacted around the same time, a total of 3 types of studies were defined, including "Use-results surveys", "Post-marketing clinical trial" and the new "Post-marketing database study", thereby allowing the use of MID-NET in post-marketing database study. However, based on the currently published RMPs, including those of drugs approved by the SAKIGAKE Designation System, conventional early post-marketing phase vigilance and use-results surveys (particularly all-patient survey) account for the majority of additional pharmacovigilance methods. An eye will be kept on the development of future safety measures for newly approved innovative drugs utilizing enrichment of post-marketing safety measures under the conditional early approval and the SAKIGAKE Designation Systems (For details, see Chapter 7).

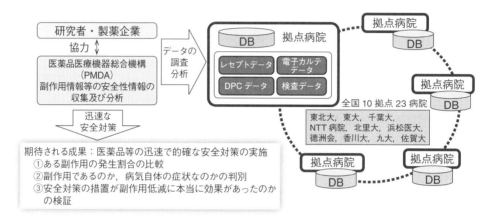

図 1.6　医療情報データベース（MID-NET®）（PMDA 平成 30 年度第 2 回運営評議会第 4 期中期計画の方向性について（案）[補足資料]）

1.3　新薬の安全性確保と課題

1.3.1　薬害再発防止のための医薬品行政等の見直しのその後

本書第 2 版で記したとおり，現在の日本における医薬品のリスクマネジメントに大きな影響を与え続けているのは，2010 年 4 月 28 日に出された薬害肝炎事件の検証及び再発防止のための医薬品行政のあり方検討委員会の最終提言「薬害再発防止のための医薬品行政等の見直しについて」であるが，それから 8 年以上経った現在の「その後」を見てみたい。

なお，本項は，2018 年 6 月 18 日に開催された PMDA 平成 30 年度第 1 回運営評議会資料 1 - 3「平成 29 事業年度業務報告（案）」を参考に最近の状況を加味している。

① 情報収集体制の強化：
　（ア）患者からの副作用情報を活用する仕組みの創設
　　　PMDA では，上記提言に基づき，2012 年 3 月 26 日に患者副作用報告システムを開設し，インターネットを介して，試行的に患者からの医薬品の副作用報告の受付事業を行っていた。本事業では，医薬品により副作用が現れた本人またはその家族から試行的に副作用報告を収集し，医薬品による副作用の発生傾向を把握する等，医薬品の安全対策を進めることを目的としていた。それらの結果を踏まえたうえで，厚労省は 2019

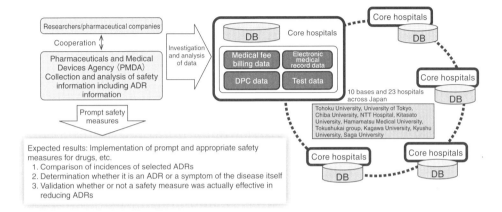

Fig1-6 Medical information database (MID-NET®)(Directions of the fourth medium-term plan in the PMDA FY 2018 Second Administrative Council (draft) [supplementary document])

1.3 New drug safety assurance and its issues

1.3.1 Review of drug administration, etc. for prevention of recurrence of incidents of drug-induced suffering

As stated in the second edition of this document, the current risk management of drugs in Japan has been greatly influenced by the final recommendations of the Review Committee on Drug Administration for Investigation and Prevention of Recurrence of Drug-induced Hepatitis Cases, "Regarding review of drug administration, etc. for prevention of recurrence of incidents of drug-induced suffering" (April 28, 2010). This section discusses the "situation" at present, 8 years or more after the final recommendations.

In addition, this section also takes account of the recent situation with reference to "Annual Business Report for the FY 2017 (draft)", the document 1–3 for the PMDA 2018 First Administrative Council which was held on June 18, 2018.

[1] Strengthening of the information collection system:
    (A) Creation of a mechanism to utilize ADR information from patients
        The PMDA, based on the above recommendations, established the patient ADR reporting system on March 26, 2012. Experimentally, reports of ADRs to drugs were accepted from patients via internet. This operation aimed to promote safety measures for drugs by experimentally collecting ADR reports from patients or their families who have experienced ADRs and ascertaining trends in development of ADRs to drugs. Based on those results, MHLW published "Guidelines for reporting ADRs from patients

年3月26日に「患者からの医薬品副作用報告」実施要領を公表し，正式にPMDAで受け付けることとなった（4.1.3参照）。

2017年度までに収集した患者副作用報告数は下表のとおりであり，順次報告された症例の公表を行っている。

	2013年度	2014年度	2015年度	2016年度	2017年度
患者副作用報告数 （延べ数）＊	122	91	186	50	84

※報告数については各年度末時点の数であり，患者副作用報告の対象外である品目（医薬部外品，化粧品，健康食品等）についての報告は除かれている。

今までの報告数はわずかであり，しかも増加の傾向も見えない。患者からの副作用情報の具体的な活用までの道筋は，まだ見えないのが現状のようである。

（イ）外国規制当局への駐在職員の派遣等の国際連携の強化

海外規制当局との連携については，2016年度（平成28年度）からFDA-EMAファーマコビジランスクラスターへのオブザーバー参加を正式に開始し，より早期からの安全性に係る情報交換に努めているようである。

（ウ）医療機関からの死亡・重篤症例報告についての医療関係者への直接照会等の必要な調査を実施できる体制の整備

医療機関からの副作用等報告については，重篤症例についてPMDAが医療機関に対して直接照会等を行うことにより，情報収集の強化に努めており，具体的には，医薬品による重篤な副作用と疑われる症例のうち，医療機関等から製造販売業者等への情報提供が行われていない症例，またはその有無が不明の症例を原則としてPMDA調査担当症例とし，必要に応じてPMDAにおいて詳細調査を実施している。

これまでのPMDA調査対象症例数は下表のとおりである。

	2013年度	2014年度	2015年度	2016年度	2017年度
PMDA調査対象 症例数	862	1,067	1,100	1,132	1,453

医療機関報告のうち，PMDA調査担当症例については，PMDAが被疑薬と評価した医薬品の製造販売業者にインターネット（情報共有のための専用サーバーを利用）を介して情報共有している。

② 得られた情報の評価

（ア）体制の強化として，「PMDAでは2011年からリスクマネジメント制度を本格導入し，リスクマネージャー（RM）を新薬審査部門に併任することにより，医薬品の開発段階から製造販売後までの安全性を一貫

directly" on March 26, 2019, and patients can report to PMDA by inputting to the web system or by mailed paper (Refer to 4.1.3).

The number of ADRs reported by patients that were collected by FY 2017 are as follows. The reported cases are published as they are received.

	FY 2013	FY 2014	FY 2015	FY 2016	FY 2017
Number of ADRs reported by patients (total number) *	122	91	186	50	84

※ The number of reports indicates the number of ADRs reported by the end of each fiscal year, excluding those on items that are outside the scope of the patient ADR reporting system (quasi-drugs, cosmetics and health foods).

However, the number of reports has been limited and does not appear to increase. The present situation appears to be far from specific utilization of ADR information from patients.

(B) Strengthening international collaborations through dispatching employees to regulatory authorities of foreign countries, etc.

Japan officially started to participate in the FDA-EMA Pharmacovigilance Cluster as an observer since FY 2016 in an effort to exchange safety information at an earlier stage.

(C) Establishment of systems which enable the conduct of necessary investigations such as direct referral from the government to healthcare professionals regarding deaths/serious cases among reports of ADRs, etc. from medical institutions

In relation to ADRs reported directly from medical institutions, efforts are made to reinforce information collection by direct referral from the PMDA to medical institutions for serious cases. Specifically, cases of serious ADRs suspected to be caused by drugs in which information has not been or is not known to have been provided by medical institutions to MAHs are principally regarded as cases subjected to investigation by the PMDA. The PMDA conducts detailed investigations on these cases as needed.

The numbers of cases subjected to investigation by the PMDA thus far are presented in the table below.

	FY 2013	FY 2014	FY 2015	FY 2016	FY 2017
Number of cases subjected to investigation by the PMDA	862	1,067	1,100	1,132	1,453

For cases reported from medical institutions subjected to investigation by the PMDA, the PMDA shares information via the internet (using a dedicated server for information sharing) with the MAH of the drug which is assessed to be a suspect drug by the PMDA.

[2] Evaluation of information obtained

(A) In order to strengthen the system, it is stated in the document for the

して管理できる体制を整備し，2018年3月時点で新薬審査部門の各チームに対応した14名のRMを配置している。」と運営評議会資料に記載されている。

（イ）「予防原則に基づき，因果関係等が確定する前に，安全性にかかわる可能性のある安全性情報を公表し，一層の情報収集を行う」に関しては，PMDAのホームページの「安全対策業務 → 情報提供業務 → 医薬品 → 注意喚起情報 → 評価中のリスク等の情報について」において掲載されている（2018年10月時点）。本情報は，PMDAメディナビとして電子メールで配信されている。「1. 使用上の注意の改訂等につながりうる注目しているリスク情報」については，使用上の注意の改訂を行った場合には「使用上の注意の改訂指示」のページに掲載し，その後，本ページからは一週間程度で削除するとされている。「2. 外国規制当局や学会等が注目し，厚労省およびPMDAが評価を始めたリスク情報」については，2011年に掲載された2つの情報が現時点でも掲載されている。

（ウ）2013年から施行された「医薬品リスク管理計画（RMP）」については，着実に施行されており，2018年10月時点で349製品のRMPがPMDAホームページに公表されている。また「医薬品の製造販売後の調査及び試験の実施の基準に関する省令」（GPSP省令）が新たに改正され，改正省令は2018年4月から施行されている。同改正により，新たに「製造販売後データベース（DB）調査」等が導入された。

　2018年10月時点で，PMDAホームページで公開されているRMPのうち，初回提出年月が2018年4月以降のものは後発品を含めて30件で，そのうちDB調査が含まれているものが安全性に関して2件，有効性に関して1件で，今後調査結果の公表が待たれる。また，その中で30件の市販直後調査で，特定使用成績調査とセットで企画されている一般使用成績調査（全例調査を除く。一部効能に対する調査を含む。）が含まれていたものはわずか9件であった。

（エ）医療情報データベース（MID-NET）の構築は，多くの困難を乗り越えてすでに実用レベルに達し，2018年4月から一般の用にも供されることとなり，9月には初の民間利用が発表された。

　これまでの間，PMDAは多くの若い疫学専門家を採用したといわれ，2009年度からMIHARI（Medical Information for Risk Assessment Initiative）プロジェクトを開始した。MIHARIプロジェクトでは当初，データベースへのアクセス確保・データの検討・データの活用という流れで検討し，薬剤疫学手法の検討を行い，医薬品処方後の有害事象発現リスクの定量的評価や，安全対策措置の影響評価，処方実態調査等が行える体制を構築した（図1.7参照）。2014年度からは，この体制を実際の安全対策

Administrative Council that "The PMDA has officially introduced the risk management system since 2011. Risk managers (RMs) hold the additional post in the Office of New Drugs in order to establish a system for consistent management of safety from the stage of drug development to the post-marketing period. As of March 2018, 14 RMs are assigned to cover each team in the Office of New Drugs".

(B) The statement, "based on precautionary principles information should be further collected with the release of safety information that may be related to safety before determining causal relationships, etc.," is posted on the PMDA's website: "Post-marketing safety measures → Information services → Drugs → PMDA Risk Communications → Drug risk information of ongoing evaluation" as of October 2018. This information is sent via e-mail as PMDA Medi-navi, which is useful. It is stated that "1. Risk information of special interest that may lead to revision of precautions" are posted on the page of "Revisions of PRECAUTIONS" in the case precautions are revised, and deleted from the relevant page after approximately a week. As for "2. Risk information noted by regulatory authorities of foreign countries or scientific academies that is under evaluation by the MHLW and the PMDA", two items posted in 2011 are available.

(C) "Risk Management Plan (RMP)" enacted in 2013 has been steadily operated and the RMPs of 349 products are posted on the PMDA's website as of October 2018. In addition, "Good Post-marketing Study Practice" (GPSP Ordinance) was newly revised and the revised ordinance has been enacted since April 2018. The revised ordinance introduced "Post-marketing database (DB) survey", etc.

As of October 2018, 30 of the RMPs posted on the PMDA's website including generic drugs have initially been submitted since April 2018, of which two RMPs include DB studies in relation to safety and one RMP in relation to efficacy. The publication of study results is awaited. Among 30 RMPs, only 9 RMPs included general drug use-results surveys (excluding all-patient survey, but including surveys on added indications).

(D) The construction of a large-scale medical information database (MID-NET) has already reached a practical level, after overcoming many difficulties. It has been available to the public since April 2018. In September, it was announced that MID-NET was used by a private company for the first time.

Up to now, the PMDA is said to have employed many young epidemiologists, and the Medical Information for Risk Management Initiative (MIHARI) project has been started since FY 2009. In this project, investigation was initially conducted in the following order: securing access to the database; investigating the data; and utilizing the data. In addition, investigation was conducted on pharmacoepidemiologic approaches. Also, a system was constructed to allow quantitative assessment of the risk of onset of adverse events after prescription of drugs, assessment of impacts of safety measures, and investigation of actual prescription practice (see **Figure 1.7**).

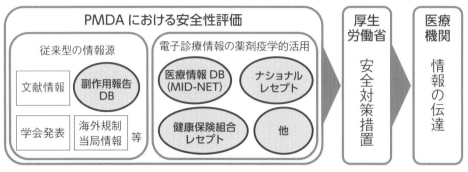

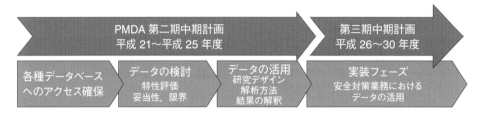

図 1.7　MIHARI プロジェクト（石黒知恵子：第 22 回日本薬剤疫学会学術総会，京都）

措置に活用することを目標とし，個別の医薬品の課題について検討し，専門協議での検討を踏まえて，個別品目の安全対策措置に活用することとしている。また，それと並行し，MIHARI プロジェクトでは新規データソースや，新規手法については引き続き各種試行調査を通じて，その利用可能性について検討を重ねている。

　今までは，医療機関のカスタム設定を含む複雑な電子カルテデータの統合等に多くの労苦を費やしてきたが，今後は MID-NET のさらなる充実とそれを用いた薬剤疫学的評価・解析のレベルを上げていくことが期待される。

③ リスクコミュニケーションの向上のための情報の積極的かつ円滑な提供と患者・消費者の関与

本項目については，1.3.2 項「PMDA の第 3 期 5 か年計画の進捗状況」において触れる。

④ 副作用情報の本人への伝達や情報公開の在り方

本項目については，第 2 版以降の進捗は見られないようである。

⑤ 適正な情報提供および広告による医薬品の適正使用

厚労省から本最終提言が出されたのが 2010 年 4 月，ディオバンに関する臨床研究への疑問が初めて出されたのが 2012 年，ブロプレスの効果に係る臨

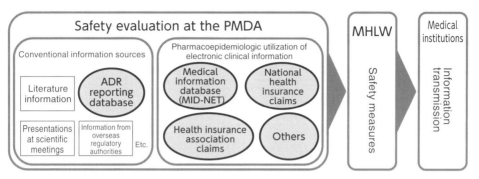

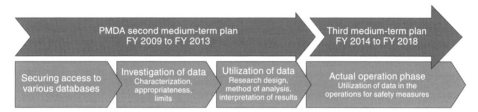

Fig1-7 MIHARI Project (Chieko Ishiguro: The 22nd General Meeting of Japanese Society for Pharmacoepidemiology, Kyoto)

From FY 2014, it was planned to investigate issues of individual drugs in an aim to utilize the system for actual safety measures. Based on advise from consultation with experts, it will be utilized in safety measures for individual items. Simultaneously, it was planned to carry out repeated investigations on the usability of new data sources and new approaches through continuous and various experimental investigations in the MIHARI project.

Thus far, many efforts were made to integrate complex electronic medical record data including custom settings among medical institutions. In the future, it is expected to further enrich MID-NET and to raise the level of pharmacoepidemiologic evaluation and analysis using MID-NET.

[3] Proactive and smooth provision of information for enhancement of risk communication and involvement of patients/consumers

This issue is discussed in Section 1.3.2, "Progress status of the PMDA third-term five-year plan".

[4] Methods of transmission of ADR information to patients and disclosure of information

In relation to this issue, no progress is seen after the second edition of this document.

[5] Proper use of drugs through proper provision of information and advertisements
This final recommendation was issued by the MHLW in April 2010, doubts regarding clinical studies of Diovan first came to notice in 2012, and doubts regarding clinical studies on the effects of Blopress and advertising brochures

床研究およびその結果を紹介した宣伝用パンフレットへの疑問が出されたのが 2014 年である。

最終提言はこれらの問題を予言した形となった。これらの事案を契機として臨床研究法が制定され，2018 年 4 月から施行されたのに加え，2016 年度からは厚労省が「医療用医薬品の広告活動監視モニター事業」を開始した。一方，日本製薬工業協会（製薬協）においても，2015 年 9 月に「医療用医薬品製品情報概要等に関する作成要領」を全面改訂し，2015 年 10 月 1 日に発効されたが，その後も広告活動において医療現場での口頭説明など，証拠が残りにくい事例や明確な虚偽誇大とまでは言えないが，不適正使用を助長すると考えられる事例が発見された。

これらを受け，厚労省は 2018 年 7 月に「医療用医薬品の販売情報提供活動に関するガイドライン（案）」を公表し，意見を求め，9 月 25 日に当該ガイドラインを厚生労働省医薬・生活衛生局長通知として発出した。これにより，今まで業界の自主的な取組みに任されていた販売情報提供（広告）活動にも公的なガイドラインが設けられた。また，製薬協は 2018 年 10 月 18 日の総会で，製薬協企業行動憲章と製薬協コンプライアンス・プログラム・ガイドラインの改定案を承認した。

1.3.2 PMDA の第 3 期 5 か年計画の進捗状況

① 副作用・不具合情報収集の強化

患者からの副作用情報の活用の仕組みについては，1.3.1 ①および 4.1.3 を参照。医薬関係者からの報告の増加を促す対策については，「医療機関からの副作用等報告の増加を促すため，医薬関係者に対する講演による周知を開始するとともに，日本医療研究開発機構（AMED）の当該報告を促すための研究（医薬品等規制調和・評価研究事業）に協力した。」とある。報告件数は，下表に示すとおりであり，2017 年度に大きく増えたが，内容は不明であり，今後の推移に期待したい（4.1.2 参照）。

	2013 年度	2014 年度	2015 年度	2016 年度	2017 年度
医薬関係者からの報告件数	5,420	6,180	6,129	6,047	7,624

副作用情報等の報告システムの強化等については，2013 年に発出された「ICH E2B（R3）実装通知」に基づき，2016 年 4 月から同通知を適用し，2019 年 4 月に完全移行の予定である。なお，2017 年度における PMDA に報告された企業からの医薬品等の副作用・感染症等報告（国内）[*1] の電送化率（オンラインによる報告）は 98.6 ％であった。また，医薬関係者から PMDA へ報告された医薬品副作用等報告[*2] の電送化率（電子メールによる

introducing the relevant results were raised in 2014. It may be said that the final recommendation predicted these problems. Triggered by these cases, the Clinical Research Act was established and enacted in April 2018. In addition, the MHLW started "Surveillance and Monitoring of Advertising Activities for Prescription Drugs" in FY 2016. On the other hand, the Japan Pharmaceutical Manufacturers Association (JPMA) completely revised the "Guidelines for Preparation of Ethical Drug Product Information Brochure" in September 2015 and enacted it on October 1, 2015. Nevertheless, similar cases continued to be found in advertising activities, including those that were less likely to leave evidence, such as oral explanations at the site of medical practice, and those that were thought to promote improper use, although it could not clearly be regarded as false or exaggerated.

In response to these cases, the MHLW published "Guideline for Promotion Information Provision Activities of Prescription Drugs (draft)" in July 2018, invited suggestions, and issued it as a Notification by the Director of the Pharmaceutical Safety and Environmental Health Bureau of MHLW on September 25. Consequently, official guidelines were established for promotion information provision (advertising) activities which had been entrusted to voluntary efforts of the industry. In addition, the JPMA approved the proposed revisions of the JPMA Charter of Corporate Behavior and JPMA Compliance Program Guidelines in a general meeting held on October 18, 2018.

1.3.2　Progress status of the PMDA's third-term five-year plan

[1] Strengthening of collection of ADR/defect information

See [1], Section 1.3.1 and Section 4.1.3 regarding the mechanism to utilize ADR information from patients. In relation to the measures for promotion of an increase in reports from healthcare professions, it is stated that "In order to promote reporting of ADRs, etc. from medical institutions, the operation was begun to disseminate the system through lectures to pharmaceutical personnel, in addition to cooperating in research by the Japan Agency for Medical Research and Development (AMED) for promotion of relevant reporting (Study of Regulatory Coherence and Evaluation of Drugs, etc.)". The actual numbers of reports are as shown in the table below. Although it increased considerably in FY 2017, the contents are unknown and it is expected to increase in the future (See Section 4.1.2).

	FY 2013	FY 2014	FY 2015	FY 2016	FY 2017
Reports from pharmaceutical personnel	5,420	6,180	6,129	6,047	7,624

Regarding strengthening of the ADR information reporting system, "Notification for Implementation of ICH-E2B (R3)" was issued in 2013 and applied from April 2016. The transition will be completed by April 2019. In addition, the electronic transmission rate (online reporting) of reports of ADRs/infections [1] from companies (in Japan) to the PMDA was 98.6% in the FY

報告）は 34.3 % であった。

*1*2 続報など対象外，除外となった報告も含む。

② 副作用等情報の整理および評価分析の体系化

PMDA による調査が必要な医療機関からの報告のすべてについて，フォローアップができる体制を構築できたかは確認できなかったが，1.3.1 ①に示したとおり，調査対象症例は増加している。

③ 医療情報データベース等の構築

1.3.1 ②（エ）参照。医薬品の製造販売業者による MID-NET の活用はこれからであり，成果が期待される。なお，MID-NET の試行的利活用として「ランマーク皮下注 120 mg による重篤な低カルシウム血症のリスクは，安全対策措置後には類薬と同程度であることが確認された」ことを PMDA 関係者は各種講演会で紹介している。

また，医療情報データベース活用の試行結果を踏まえ，医薬品等の製造販売業者が市販後調査等のためにデータベースを利活用する条件についての厚労省の検討結果に基づき，製造販売業者による医療情報データベースの安全対策への活用促進を図るべく，PMDA は 2018 年 2 月に「MID-NET 運用開始記念シンポジウム」を開催し，MID-NET の利活用に際しては以下の研修を受けることを要求している。

・利活用申出前研修
・利活用開始前研修
・オンサイトセンター研修

さらに有用な医療機器・再生医療等製品を迅速かつ安全に国民に提供するため，関係学会，関係企業等との連携により，長期に安全性を確認する患者登録システム（レジストリ）を構築することによる市販後情報収集体制を整えることとなっている。

④ 情報のフィードバック等による市販後安全体制の確立

医療機関に提供される情報の緊急性・重大性を判別しやすくする方策は，具体化されたようには思われなかった。しかし，企業からの副作用報告のラインリストの公表は，報告からおおむね 4 か月の期間で行い，調査した医療機関からの当局への直接報告等の公表も行っている。2012 年 4 月から公開している調査・研究に利用可能な CSV 形式の副作用症例データセット（Japanese Adverse Drug Event Report database（JADER））についても，報告からおおむね 4 か月後に公開を行っている。

添付文書改訂指示情報は，発出から 2 日以内に PMDA ホームページに掲載し，即日，PMDA メディナビ配信を行っている。また，当該添付文書とリンクさせている。

医薬品医療機器情報配信サービス（PMDA メディナビ，図 1.8 参照）に

Chapter 1 Current status and future prospects of pharmaceutical approval review and safety policies in Japan

2017. Also, the electronic transmission rate (reporting via e-mail) of reports of ADRs [*2] from pharmaceutical personnel to the PMDA was 34.3%.

[*1*2] Including reports that were outside the scope or excluded, such as follow-up reports.

[2] Organization of information on ADRs, etc. and systematization of evaluations/analyses

Although it could not be confirmed whether or not a system has been constructed to enable the implementation of PMDA's follow-up investigations on all reports from medical institutions that need to be investigated, the number of cases subjected to investigation is increasing as shown in [1], Section 1.3.1.

[3] Creation of medical information database, etc.

See (D), [2], Section 1.3.1. The utilization of MID-NET by MAHs has just begun and fruitful results are expected. As a trial application and utilization of MID-NET, PMDA personnel presented that "the risk of serious hypocalcemia associated with Ranmark Subcutaneous Injection 120 mg was confirmed to be comparable to those of similar drugs after safety measures were taken." at various lecture meetings.

In addition, taking account of the results of experimental utilization of the medical information database, the PMDA held a "Commemorative Symposium for Initiation of MID-NET" in February 2018 in order to promote the utilization of the medical information database by MAHs in safety measures based on the results of the investigation by the MHLW on conditions for application and utilization of the database by MAHs in post-marketing studies, etc. The following trainings must be completed before utilizing MID-NET:

Training before applying for utilization of MID-NET

Training before utilizing MID-NET

On-site center training

Furthermore, in order to provide useful medical devices and regenerative medicine products to people promptly and safely, it is planned to organize a structure to collect post-marketing information in cooperation with the relevant scientific societies and companies, through construction of a patient registration system (registry) for confirmation of long-term safety.

[4] Establishment of post-marketing pharmacovigilance system with information feedback, etc.

It did not appear that measures for easier determination of the urgency and significance of information provided to medical institutions were realized. However, the line lists of ADR case reports from companies is released within approximately 4 months after reporting, and direct reports of ADRs, to the authority etc. from medical institutions which conducted investigations are also released. In addition, the Japanese Adverse Drug Event Report database (JADER) in CSV format has been released and available for investigations and researches since April 2012 and is also released approximately 4 months after reporting.

Information on instructions to revise package inserts is posted on the PMDA website within 2 days of issuance and delivered through PMDA Medi-navi on the same day. In addition, it is linked to the relevant package insert.

The pharmaceuticals and medical devices information e-mail service (PMDA

おいては，2017年7月からはOTC医薬品使用上の注意改訂情報を配信している。「RMP掲載のお知らせ」についても，メール本文から各品目のRMPにリンクを貼るなど，利用者の利便性向上が図られている。その登録件数は，2013年度末の102,790件から，2017年度末には164,821件（約1.6倍）に増加した。これは計画より若干遅いペースではあるものの，今後もさらに登録件数を伸ばすための努力に期待したい。

⑤ 医薬品・医療機器等の安全性に関する国民への情報提供の充実
PMDAのホームページは，患者や一般の消費者がより見やすい・使いやすいものへと継続的に改善が図られていると思われる。平成29年度業務報告（案）にも，「日々発出される安全性情報のうち，使用上の注意の改訂等の重要な安全性情報については迅速にPMDAホームページに掲載し，添付文書情報等の各種の安全性情報についても，同様にPMDAホームページに掲載し，情報提供の充実強化に努めている。」と記載されている。また，2017年度末現在の患者向医薬品ガイドの掲載件数は3,873件であり，患者向医薬品ガイドの作成・改訂時に使用する「一般の方が理解しやすい副作用用語集」の改訂に向けた案を作成した。

国民・医療関係者に対するより効果的な情報伝達の方策に関する調査研究の実施と具体的な方策の検討については，AMEDの「患者及び医療関係者

図1.8 PMDAメディナビ（PMDA 平成30年度第1回運営評議会資料1-3）

Medi-navi, see **Figure 1.8**) delivers information on revision of precautions for OTC drugs from July 2017. For "Notice of posting of RMP", efforts have been made to increase convenience for users, such as posting a link in the e-mail text to the RMP of each item. The number of subscriptions for the service increased from 102,790 at the end of FY 2013 to 164,821 at the end of FY 2017 (approximately 1.6-fold). Although the increase is slightly slower than planned, it is expected that efforts will be made to further increase the number of subscriptions.

[5] Improvement of information provision to the public regarding safety of pharmaceuticals and medical devices, etc.

It appears that the PMDA website has continuously been improved to make it more easy-to-understand and -use for patients and general consumers. It is also stated in the Annual Report for FY 2017 (draft) that "Out of safety information that are released daily, important safety information including the revision of precautions are promptly posted on the PMDA website. Similarly, various safety information including the information on package inserts are also posted on the PMDA website in an effort to enrich and strengthen information provision". In addition, 3,873 Drug Guides for Patients were posted as of the end of FY 2017. Also, a draft revision was prepared for the "Glossary of Adverse Drug Reactions that are Easier to Understand by General Population" for use at the preparation/revision of Drug Guides for Patients.

In addition, for implementation of surveys and studies on more efficient

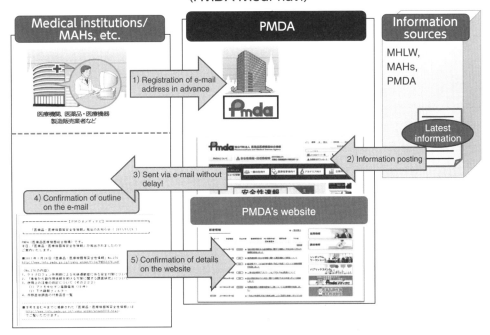

Fig1-8 PMDA Medi-navi (Document 1-3 for the PMDA FY 2018 First Administrative Council)

に向けた医薬品等のリスク最小化情報の伝達方法に関する研究」班との共催により，患者を含めた関係者間でのリスクコミュニケーションの向上をめざし，2017 年 11 月に公開フォーラムを開催したと報告されている。

⑥ RMP に基づく適切な安全対策の実施

1.3.1 ②（ウ）を参照。

⑦ 新たな審査制度の導入に対応した安全対策の強化および審査から一貫した安全性管理の体制

救済部門と安全対策部門間で情報を共有し，救済給付請求事例等を通じ，すでに添付文書などで注意喚起してきているにもかかわらず繰り返されている同様の事例などについて，「PMDA からの医薬品適正使用のお願い」として PMDA ホームページに掲載し，医療従事者等が活用しやすいように，安全に使用するための注意点などをわかりやすく解説して適正使用のさらなる徹底を呼びかけている。新再生医療等製品については，審査過程（治験相談，製造販売後調査計画の検討，添付文書案の検討，専門協議等）への安全第一部，第二部職員の参加等の取組みを実施している。承認条件として全例調査が付された医薬品については，市販後に得られた安全性情報等を迅速に評価し，適宜当該企業と協議しつつ，必要に応じて情報提供資材の利用関係者への配布等を指導した。

他は，1.3.1 ②（ア）を参照。

⑧ 講じた安全対策措置のフォローアップの強化・充実

2017 年度は，2014 年度および 2015 年度にそれぞれ実施した病院，薬局における医薬品安全性情報の入手・伝達・活用状況等に関する調査のフォローアップ等を目的に，病院（全国の病院のうち 10％を対象）および薬局（全国の保険薬局のうち 5％を対象）における医薬品安全性情報の入手・伝達・活用状況等に関する調査を 2018 年 1 ～ 2 月に実施した。

調査結果からは，病院・薬局とも，情報伝達対象・手段等の手順化，PMDA メディナビを活用した重要な情報の網羅的な入手，リスクコミュニケーションツール，特に RMP（医薬品リスク管理計画）に述べられている追加のリスク最小化活動の資材の積極的な活用があげられており，PMDA のホームページで公表されている（8.6 参照）。

information transmission methods to the public and healthcare professionals and for examination of specific measures, it has been reported that a public forum was held in November 2017 together with the "AMED Research group for method of transmission of drug risk minimization information to patients and healthcare professionals" with the aim to improve risk communication among relevant parties including patients.

[6] Implementation of appropriate safety measures based on RMP

See (C), [2], Section 1.3.1.

[7] Strengthening of safety measures compatible with introduction of new review system and consistent safety management system from review stage

Some cases are repeatedly observed despite information sharing between the Relief and Safety Measure Sections through claims for financial relief and cautions provided in package inserts, etc. These cases are posted on the PMDA website as "PMDA Alert for Proper Use of Drugs". For easier utilization by healthcare professionals, precautions for safe use are explained in an easy-to-understand manner to appeal for further proper use. For new regenerative medicine products, employees of the Office of Safety I and II participate in the review process (clinical trial consultation, examination of post-marketing studies plan, examination of draft package insert, and expert discussion, etc.) along with other approaches. For products that require an All-patient investigation as an approval condition, safety information, etc. obtained from post-marketing studies are promptly evaluated, and through appropriate discussions with the company, instructions are provided to distribute information provision materials to the relevant parties as needed.

See (A), [2], Section 1.3.1 for others.

[8] Strengthening and enrichment of follow-up of safety measures

In FY 2017, an investigation was conducted between January and February 2018 on the status of acquisition, transmission and utilization of pharmaceutical safety information in hospitals (10% of all hospitals in Japan) and pharmacies (5% of all health insurance pharmacies in Japan) with the aim to follow-up the same investigations conducted in hospitals and pharmacies in FY 2014 and FY 2015, respectively.

As a result, both hospitals and pharmacies reported establishing procedures on the scope and method of information transmission, comprehensive acquisition of important information utilizing PMDA Medi-navi, risk communication tool particularly proactive utilization of additional risk minimization activity materials mentioned in the RMP. The results are posted on the PMDA website (See Section 8.6).

1.3.3　PMDA 第 4 期中期計画への期待

　2018 年 10 月 17 日に開催された 2018 年度第 2 回運営評議会に，「第 4 期中期計画（2019 年度〜2023 年度）の方向性について（案）」が提出された。その基本的考え方において，「世界最先端の医薬品等が海外での使用経験なくわが国の医療現場で使用される状況を想定し，保健衛生上の危害発生の防止，発生時の的確かつ迅速な対応を行い，医薬品等がその役割をより長期にわたって果たせるようにするための安全対策業務」が謳われている。

　「基本的な副作用等情報の収集・整理・評価分析の実施」においては，端緒についたばかりとは言えるが，MID-NET® 等の医療情報データベースを活用した薬剤疫学的調査に基づく安全性評価の推進，「医療関係者，患者・一般消費者への安全性情報の提供と講じた安全対策措置のフォローアップ」においては，新たに，リスクコミュニケーションの強化（一般国民向けシンポジウムの開催など，一般国民向けの適切な情報提供の実施）があげられている。

　なお，同【補足資料】においては，RMP に基づき作成した資材については，順次「RMP マーク」を表示し，2019 年度より PMDA ホームページに掲載予定としたほか，日本薬剤師会，日本病院薬剤師会等と協力して，RMP の位置づけを含め内容についての理解向上および資材の活用について周知を図るとされている。

　本項の最初で示した，今までに日本があまり経験したことのない「安全対策業務」を本格的に実施していくためには，これらの内容には若干の不満が残ると言わざるを得ない。例えば，以下にあげる課題は従来から指摘されてきたものが多く，短期間で解決できるものではないであろうが，一刻も速い本格的な取組みが，切に望まれる。

　1）安全対策の科学レベルの向上および欧米諸国の動向の注視

　　　2018 年 8 月にようやく措置が取られたオセルタミビルの 10 代への使用に関する禁忌および枠付きの警告の解除は，当初から他の抗インフルエンザ薬と違いはあるのか，原疾患でも重篤な「異常行動」は発現することが知られているが，医薬品服用時と比較して頻度に差はあるのかといった疑問があり，当局においても調査が長期間行われていた。しかし，解除の措置が相当時間遅れたのは否めない。本措置は欧米諸国では取られておらず，もちろん常に欧米諸国と同じ措置が正しい訳ではないが，安全対策の科学レベルのさらなる向上と，やはり安全対策の科学面においては進んでいると認めざるを得ない欧米諸国の動向の注視・研究が必要と考えられる。

　2）医療情報データベースの開発・活用に関する国際的実態との乖離の回避

　　　1.3.1 ②（エ）でも若干触れたが，MID-NET を構築し，それをさらに充実させることの意義には非常に大きなものがある。しかし，MID-NET や日本における民間等の医療情報 DB の構築について考慮すると，はるかに先行している欧米諸国の DB の実態と医療情報 DB の活用についてかけ離れた規制等

1.3.3 Expectations for the PMDA's fourth medium-term plan

In the 2018 Second Administrative Council held on October 17, 2018, the "Directions of the fourth medium-term plan (FY 2019 to FY 2023) (draft)" was submitted. The basic strategy proposes "Safety measures for prevention of health and hygiene hazards, for appropriate and prompt handling of such hazards, and for enabling drugs, etc. to carry out their roles for a longer period of time, assuming the situation where the world's most advanced drugs, etc. are used in clinical practice in Japan before being used in the rest of the world".

"Implementation of collection, organization, evaluation and analysis of basic ADR information" includes promotion of safety assessments based on pharmacoepidemiologic investigations utilizing medical information database such as MID-NET®, which may be said to be just beginning. For "Provision of safety information to healthcare professionals, patients and general consumers and follow-up of safety measures taken", reinforcement of risk communication (implementation of appropriate information provision to the general population, such as holding a symposium for the general population) is proposed.

In addition, in the same [supplementary document], it is stated that materials prepared based on the RMPs will sequentially be labeled with an "RMP mark" and posted on the PMDA website from FY 2019. In addition, efforts will be made to promote understanding of the contents of the RMP including the position of the RMP and utilization of the materials in cooperation with Japan Pharmaceutical Association and Japanese Society of Hospital Pharmacists, etc.

For full-scale implementation of "safety measures" described in the first paragraph of this section which have rarely been conducted in Japan, it must be said that the above contents are not completely satisfactory. For example, many of the following tasks have long been pointed out and must be addressed in earnest, although they would not be solved in a short period of time.

1) Improvement of the scientific level of safety measures and close monitoring of trends in the US and Europe

Finally, in August 2018, the contraindication of oseltamivir for use in children aged 10 to 19 years and a boxed warning were removed. From the beginning, there were some uncertainties, whether there were differences between oseltamivir and other anti-influenza drugs and whether there was a difference in the incidence of serious "abnormal behavior" with and without the use of oseltamivir, although it was known that such behavior also occurred in association with the primary disease. The regulatory authority also conducted long-term investigations. Nevertheless, it cannot be denied that measures to remove the contraindication and warning were considerably delayed. Such a contraindication and warning were not issued in the US or European countries. Of course, that does not mean that measures taken in the US and European countries are always correct; however, it is considered necessary to further improve the scientific level of safety measures and perform close monitoring and research on trends in the US and European countries that are undeniably more advanced in terms of scientific aspects

は避けるべきである。例えば，薬剤疫学的リサーチクエスチョンへの取組みについて，少なくとも教科書的には，医療情報DBの活用は「仮説検出」のために用いられ，「仮説検証」のためにはDB研究のみに頼るのではなく，いくつかの適切な薬剤疫学的な調査を総合して判断する，あるいは最近増加している大規模単純化試験などが必要とされている。官民の医療情報DBの構築や活用については，この点を踏まえ，信頼性確保などが過剰にならないようにする必要がある。また，RMPや再審査において，国内DBのことしか話題になっていないようであるが，特に日本において医療情報DBの数が極めて限られる現在，国民の公衆衛生の保護を第一課題とする医薬品等の行政においては，豊富に存在する欧米諸国等の医療情報DBの適切な活用が必要であると考えられる。この点について，日本の情報と海外の情報をことさら分けて考えるのは，本分野の科学的常識と相容れないように考えられる。さらには第1次データを用いるフィールド研究の重要性も忘れてはならない。

3）医薬品安全対策の本質的な変化（国際的な潮流）の把握と対応への準備

ICHにおいては，E19（（ある（some）後期承認前臨床試験や製造販売後臨床試験における)安全性データ収集の最適化)ガイドラインが議論されている。これは，薬剤の一般的な副作用が十分に理解され，示されている場合には，患者の安全性が損なわれないかぎり，安全性データの収集に関して，目標を定めた（targeted）アプローチをいつ，どのように適用すればよいのかに関するものである。被験者や医療従事者，製薬企業や規制当局の無駄な負荷を，軽減できないかというものである。

このように，ICT技術の発達，データ量の増加や各国の薬事規制の強化等に伴い，副作用等のイベント報告が急速に増加している中で，従来の「投網的な」情報収集・処理・評価の方法が限界に来ていることは，多くの規制当局・製薬企業の認識となっている。一部の外資系企業では，緒についたばかりではあるが，拡大する安全性管理規制と安全性監視業務の中で，AI・機械学習をコンプライアンス支援の一翼を担える手段と認識し，検討を開始している。一部の検討結果は国際学会でも発表されるようである。想像できるように，これは簡単なプロセスではないが，また，PMDAにおいても，新たに第4期中期計画で「ホライゾン・スキャニング」*の方法論の分析の推進を掲げているので，このような国際的な動きに遅れることなく，新たな方向を確実に追い，将来実行していくことが，本項の最初に掲げた野心的な課題への挑戦に不可欠と考えている。今後のがんばりに，大いに期待したい。

---

* レギュラトリーサイエンスに基づき，どのような革新的技術が登場しつつあるのかの網羅的調査と，それが規制に及ぼす影響の評価を行い，革新的技術に対する適切な規制構築に役立てる取組み。

of safety measures.

2) Prevention of divergence from global standards for development and utilization of medical information database

As touched on in (D), [2], Section 1.3.1, construction and further enrichment of MID-NET are extremely significant. However, taking into consideration of the construction of MID-NET and private information database in Japan, regulations etc. that differ from the actual situation of foreign databases in the US and European contrives where such practice is much more advanced should be avoided. For example, in order to address a pharmacoepidemiologic research question, it is considered necessary, at least according to textbooks, to utilize a medical information database for "hypothesis generation", instead of solely depending on the database survey, comprehensive judgment must be made based on several appropriate pharmacoepidemiologic surveys or recently increasing large-scale simple trials must be conducted. For construction and utilization of official and private medical information databases, precautions should be taken to avoid excessive reliance with consideration to the above. In addition, although it appears that only Japanese databases are discussed in relation to RMPs and reexamination, the number of medical information databases is extremely limited at present, particularly in Japan. Thus, it is considered necessary to appropriately utilize the abundant medical information databases in the US and European countries in pharmaceutical governance in which the protection of the public health is the most important issue. It is thought that thinking about Japan information and foreign information is isolation is incompatible with scientific common sense in this field. Moreover, the importance of field studies using primary data must not be forgotten.

3) Ascertainment of essential changes (global trends) in pharmaceutical safety measures and preparation of corresponding measures

The ICH is discussing the E19 guidelines (optimization of safety data collection in some late-stage pre-approval or post-marketing clinical studies). It concerns when and how a targeted approach should be applied for collection of safety data, as long as patient safety is not compromised, in the case where the common ADRs of a drug are already fully understood and demonstrated. It aims to reduce unnecessary burdens on subjects, healthcare professionals, pharmaceutical companies and regulatory authorities.

The reporting of events including ADRs is rapidly increasing following the development of ICT technology, increased data, and strengthened pharmaceutical regulations in various countries. Under such circumstances, many regulatory authorities and pharmaceutical companies recognize that conventional "rounding up" information collection, processing and assessment are limited. Some foreign companies are beginning to regard AI and machine learning as means that can bear a part of the compliance support and have started investigation their use, in response to expanding safety management regulations and pharmacovigilance operations. Some of the results of the investigation will be presented at global scientific meetings. As expected, it is not an easy process. In addition, the PMDA has also proposed promotion of analysis by "horizon

1.4 医薬品医療機器等法改正への動向

2019年11月に施行から5年目を迎える医薬品医療機器等法は，付則に「施行後5年をめどに改正後の実施状況を勘案し，必要があると認めるときは検討を加え，その結果に基づいて必要な措置を講ずる」と記載されていることから，2018年度の厚生科学審議会・医薬品医療機器制度部会では，医薬品医療機器等法改正に関連する議論が本格化してきている。

そこで，本項では2018年12月14日開催の第10回医薬品医療機器制度部会に提出された「薬機法等制度改正に関するとりまとめ」から，「日本における医薬品のリスクマネジメント」に関連すると思われる個所を以下に記載する。

1.4.1 患者アクセスの迅速化に資する承認審査制度の合理化

① 先駆け審査指定制度，条件付き早期承認制度の法制化

　○ 革新的な医薬品・医療機器等や小児用法用量設定など医療上充足されていないニーズを満たす医薬品・医療機器等について速やかな患者アクセスを確保するためには，企業が当該分野において開発を円滑に進められるよう，「先駆け審査指定制度」，「条件付き早期承認制度」について，医薬品医療機器等法に基づく制度として規定し，審査の迅速化等により，関連する製造販売業者の承認申請を促すとともに，併せて製造販売後の有効性・安全性を適切に確認する制度を整備する必要がある（図1.9参照）。また，法制化する制度の運用に当たっては，適用の条件や判断プロセスを明確にして透明性を高めることが重要である（図1.10参照）。

　○ 上記制度を導入する際には，製造販売後の安全対策の重要性が増すことから，製造販売後調査を含めた市販後の情報収集活動とその評価を充実させる必要がある（図1.11参照）。

　▼ 対象となる医薬品医療機器等法関係条文は第77条の2（指定等）ほか。

② 治験手続の明確化と被験者の安全性の確保

　○ 治験において，対照薬等や併用薬等として未承認薬等が用いられる場合の

Chapter 1 Current status and future prospects of pharmaceutical approval review and safety policies in Japan 39

scanning"* methodology as a new task in its fourth medium-term plan. In order to challenge ambitious tasks presented in the first paragraph of this section, it is essential to follow new developments intently and realize them in the future, without lagging behind global trends. There are great expectations for future efforts.

* An approach to conduct comprehensive investigation on emerging innovative technologies based on regulatory science and to assess their impacts on regulations in an aim to establish appropriate regulations for innovative technologies.

1.4 Trends towards revision of the Pharmaceutical and Medical Device Act (The PMD Act)

In November 2019, the PMD Act marks the fifth year since its enactment. Since it is stated in the supplementary provision that "Approximately 5 years after enactment, additional investigation should be carried out as necessary, taking account of the implementation status after the revision, and necessary measures should be taken based on the results of the investigation". Thus, discussion on the revision of the PMD Act has started in earnest in the FY 2018 Committee on Pharmaceuticals and Medical Devices, Health Science Council, MHLW.

Therefore, this section refers to issues that are considered relevant to "Drug risk management in Japan" from the "Summary for Revision of the PMD Act" submitted to the 10th Committee on Pharmaceuticals and Medical Devices held on December 14, 2018.

1.4.1 Rationalization of the review system for speeding up access to patients

[1] SAKIGAKE Designation System legistlation and Conditional Early Approval System

○In order to ensure that innovative drugs and medical devices, etc. and those that meet unmet medical needs such as establishment of the dosage and administration for children are promptly delivered to patients, the "SAKIGAKE Designation System" and "Conditional Early Approval System" should be legislated as regulations based on the PMD Act to enable companies to promote smooth development in these fields. It is necessary to promote applications by relevant MAHs by speeding up the review process, in addition to establishing a system for appropriate confirmation of post-marketing efficacy and safety (See **Fig. 1.9**). Also, for operation of legislated systems, it is important to increase the transparency of the systems by clearly specifying the conditions for application and the assessment process (See **Fig. 1.10**).

○When the above systems are introduced, post-marketing safety measures will be more important. Therefore, it is necessary to enrich post-marketing information collection activities and assessment of such information, including post-marketing studies (See **Fig. 1.11**).

▼The relevant articles of the PMD Act include Article 77-2 (Designation, etc.).

[2] Clarification of clinical trial procedures and assurance of subject safety

現状と課題
○医療上必要性が高い医薬品・医療機器に対して，優先的に審査する制度や，税制上の優遇措置・助成金の交付を行う制度といった，様々なインセンティブが設定され，対象となる医薬品・医療機器の特性等に応じて適応されている。
○革新的な医薬品医療機器等の速やかな患者アクセスを確保するためには，どのような承認審査制度が必要か。
（第2回制度部会より）

（参考）現行の医薬品等の承認審査における実用化促進制度と根拠規定

優先審査	審査期間短縮（12→9ヶ月）	薬機法第14条第7項 第23条の2の5第9項
希少疾病用医薬品等	審査期間短縮，助成金交付，税制措置，再審査期間延長（医療機器を除く）	薬機法第77条の2
条件付き早期承認制度	探索的臨床試験成績による申請，審査期間短縮，承認条件による製造販売後調査実施	なし（通知）
先駆け審査指定制度	優先相談，事前評価，コンシェルジュによる支援，審査期間短縮（12→6ヶ月）	なし（通知）

[主な意見]
○希少疾病用医薬品・医療機器等が，臨床現場に対して大きな成果を上げる一方で，現在でも妊婦の安全性，小児等への医薬品の用量設定等，医薬品・医療機器等の承認には，医療上充足されていないニーズがあるのではないか。
○「条件付き早期承認制度」及び「先駆け審査指定制度」の2つの制度については，この機会に法律に基づく制度ということを希望。
○医薬品開発や製造販売後安全対策に関する制度上の財政的な支援を検討してほしい。
○「条件付き早期承認制度」「先駆け審査指定制度」「希少疾病用医薬品」「優先審査」等，類似している制度の関係を明確にしてほしい。
○「条件付き早期承認制度」を制度化する場合，どういうものが対象になるかが重要。際限なく広がるおそれを懸念しており，適応の条件やその判断プロセスを明確にして透明性を高めるべき。
○条件付き早期承認制度のように審査を早める場合には安全対策の観点で市販後調査の重要性が増すことから，市販後調査の対応を充実させなければならない。
等

図1.9　医薬品医療機器等法改正への動向（平成30年10月18日第7回医薬品医療機器制度部会資料1）

医療上の必要性の高い医薬品等の分類の考え方とイメージ（案）

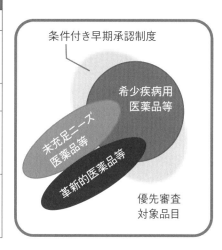

分類	考え方	要件		
		患者数 少ない	医療上 必要性	画期性 革新性
優先審査対象品目	医療上特にその必要性が高いと認められるもの	ー	○	ー
条件付き早期承認制度	医療上必要性が高く，検証的臨床試験の実施が困難，長期間を要するもの			
希少疾病用医薬品等	本邦における対象患者が5万人未満又は指定難病	○	○	ー
革新的医薬品等	①画期性あり ②対象疾患が重篤 ③対象疾患に対して極めて高い有効性 ④（世界同時を含め）世界に先駆けて日本で早期開発・申請するもの	ー	◎	◎
未充足ニーズを満たす医薬品等	医療上特に優れた使用価値を有し，既承認のものとは異なる効能・効果／用法・用量が医療上に必要とされているもの （例）小児用法・用量，AMR対策の用法変更等		◎	×

○：必要要件　ー：考慮を要しない要件　×：多くの場合存在しない

図1.10　医薬品医療機器等法改正への動向（平成30年10月18日第7回医薬品医療機器制度部会資料1）

Chapter 1 Current status and future prospects of pharmaceutical approval review and safety policies in Japan

Present situation and issues

○For drugs/medical devices of high medical need, various incentives including the priority review system, tax-relief system and subsidy system are established and applied according to the properties of the relevant drug/medical device

○What kind of review system is required to ensure that innovative drugs/medical devices are promptly delivered to patients? (from the Second Committee on the System)

(Reference) Systems and provisions for promotion of practical application in the present review process for drugs, etc.

Priority review	Reduction of review time（12 months → 9 months）	Article 14, Paragraph 7 of PMD Act Article 23-2-5, Paragraph 9 of PMD Act
Orphan drugs, etc.	Reduction of review time, subsidy, tax-relief measure, extension of reexamination period（excluding medical devices）	Article 77-2 of PMD Act
Conditional early approval system	Application based on the results of exploratory clinical trials, reduction of review time, implementation of post-marketing studies as the condition for approval	None（Notification）
SAKIGAKE Designation System	Priority consultation, pre-application evaluation, support by concierges, reduction of review time（12 months → 6 months）	None（Notification）

[Major opinions]

○While orphan drugs/medical devices have brought significant achievements to clinical practice, there may still be some unmet medical needs in relation to approval of drugs/medical devices, such as safety in pregnant women and establishment of dosage for children, etc.

○Two systems, "Conditional early approval system" and "SAKIGAKE Designation System" should take this oppotunity to be established as regulations with a legal basis.

○Regulatory financial support should be provided for pharmaceutical development and post-marketing safety measures.

○Relationships with similar systems, such as "Conditional early approval system", "SAKIGAKE Designation System", "Orphan drugs", and "Priority review" should be clarified.

○If "Conditional early approval system" is going to be systematized, the scope of the system will be important. There is a concern that the scope may be expanded without limit. The conditions for application and the process for judgment of eligibility should be clarified to increase transparency.

○If the review is going to be accelerated as in the conditional early approval system, the importance of post-marketing studies will increase with respect to the safety measures. Therefore, measures for post-marketing studies must be enriched.

Etc.

Fig1-9 Trends for revision of Pharmaceutical and Medical Device Act(October 18, 2018, document 1 for the 7th Committee on Pharmaceuticals and Medical Devices)

How to Categorized of Drugs of High Unmet Medical Need and its Image（Draft）

Category		Description	Requirements		
			Small number of patients	Medical need	Innovative-ness
Items eligible for priority review		Those that are found to be of particularly high medical need	—	○	—
	Conditional early approval system	Those of high medical need for which implementation of confirmatory clinical trials is difficult or requires a long time			
Orphan drugs, etc.		Diseases that affect <50,000 patients in Japan or designated orphan diseases	○	○	—
Innovative drugs, etc.		1. Innovative 2. Target disease is serious 3. Extremely high efficacy against the target disease 4. Early development and application in Japan before the rest of the world（including globally simultaneous application）	—	◎	◎
Drugs, etc. that satisfy unmet need		Those of medically excellent use value with indication/dosage and administration different from approved drugs that are considered to be of high medical need（Examples）Dosage and administration for children, change in usage against AMR, etc.	—	◎	×

○: Necessary requirements, —: Requirements that do not require consideration, ×: Not present in many cases

Fig1-10 Trends for revision of the Pharmaceutical and Medical Device Act (October 18, 2018, document 1 for the 7th Committee on Pharmaceuticals and Medical Devices)

- 重篤で有効な治療方法が乏しい疾患の医薬品等で，患者数が少ない等の理由で検証的臨床試験の実施が困難なものや，長期間を要するものについて，承認申請時に検証的臨床試験以外の臨床試験等で一定程度の有効性及び安全性を確認した上で，製販後に有効性・安全性の再確認等のために必要な調査等を実施すること等を承認条件により付与することにより，重篤な疾患に対して医療上の有用性が高い医薬品の速やかな患者アクセスの確保を図る。
- あわせて，承認後に実施される調査等の結果を再審査を待たずにタイムリーに評価し，安全対策等に反映させる仕組みを導入。

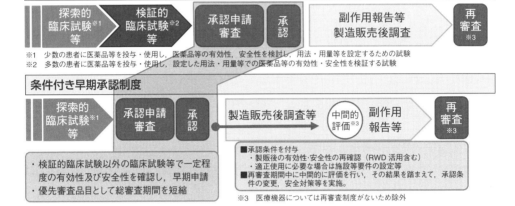

図 1.11　医薬品等の条件付き早期承認制度の考え方について（案）（平成 30 年 10 月 18 日第 7 回医薬品医療機器制度部会資料 1）

副作用・不具合報告や医療機関への情報提供等の義務を明確化することや，複数の治験薬を同時にそれぞれ異なる患者集団に投与するような複雑な治験を効率的かつ適切に管理するための運用の改善などを通じて，被験者の安全の確保を図るべきである。

▼　対象となる医薬品医療機器等法関係条文は第 80 条の 2（治験の取扱い）ほか。

1.4.2　国際的な整合性のある品質管理手法の導入

① 製造所ごとの GMP・GCTP（Good Gene, Cellular and Tissue-based Products Manufacturing Practice）適合性調査の導入

○ 医薬品，医薬部外品および再生医療等製品の承認後，製造販売業者は，品目ごとに GMP・GCTP 適合性調査を定期的（5 年ごと）に申請し，調査を受ける必要がある。この調査については，品目に共通な項目の重複調査回避，国際整合性を踏まえた品質管理の効率化・重点化等の観点から，調査項目は維持しつつ，製造業者の申請に基づき，製造所単位の調査を受けることも可能とすべきである。なお，製造所単位の調査では，剤形（固形剤，

Chapter 1 Current status and future prospects of pharmaceutical approval review and safety policies in Japan

- For drugs for serious disorders with little effective treatment for which implementation of confirmatory clinical studies is difficult or requires a long time due to reasons such as a small number of patients, implementation of post-marketing surveys necessary for reconfirmation of efficacy and safety is imposed as a condition for approval, upon confirmation of a certain level of efficacy and safety in clinical studies other than confirmatory clinical studies in the marketing application, to ensure that drugs of high medical need for serious disorders are promptly delivered to patients.
- At the same time, a system is introduced to evaluate the results of surveys conducted after approval in a timely manner without waiting for re-examination and to reflect them in safety measures, etc.

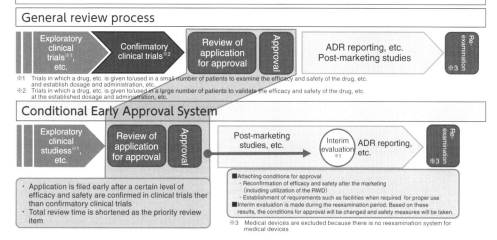

Fig1-11 Description of Conditional Early Approval System for drugs, etc. (draft) (October 18, 2018, document 1 for the 7th Committee on Pharmaceuticals and Medical Devices)

○In global clinical trials, it is necessary to ensure the safety of subjects by clearly specifying obligations, such as reporting of ADRs/defects and provision of information to medical institutions when unapproved drugs, etc. are used as control drugs or concomitant medications. In addition, the management of clinical trials should be improved for efficient and appropriate conduct of complex trials in which multiple investigational products are simultaneously administered to different patient populations.

▼The relevant articles of the PMD Act include Article 80-2 (Handling of clinical trials).

1.4.2 Introduction of globally consistent quality control approach

[1] Introduction of GMP/GCTP (Good Gene, Cellular and Tissue-based Products Manufacturing Practice) compliance inspection on each manufacturing site

○After the approval of drugs, quasi drugs and regenerative medicine products, the MAHs must regularly (every 5 years) apply for GMP/GCTP compliance inspections for each item and undergo the inspection. For this inspection, while maintaining the items of inspection, the MAHs should be allowed to undergo the inspection at manufacturing site level based on their applications in order to avoid overlapping inspection of items common among products, from the perspective of optimization and prioritization of quality control based on global consistency. In addition, in the inspection at manufacturing site level, compliance

液剤等）や製造工程の技術特性に合わせた区分を設けて適合性を確認すべきである。

▼　対象となる医薬品医療機器等法関係条文は第 14 条（医薬品等の製造販売の承認）ほか。

② QMS 適合性調査の見直し

○　医療機器および体外診断用医薬品の製造販売業者が，安定供給や組織改編によるバックアップ等を目的とし，同一の製造工程を複数の製造所で行うことがあるが，その後，製造の安定等により，基準適合証に記載された一部の製造所を利用しなくなる場合がある。このように，QMS 適合性調査を受けた製造所のうち同一工程を複数の製造所で行っていたものの一部を利用しなくなる場合には，改めて当該調査を受けることまでは要しないこととすべきである。

▼　対象となる医薬品医療機器等法関係条文は第 23 条の 2 の 5（医療機器及び体外診断用医薬品の製造販売の承認）ほか。

③ リスクに応じた品質に係る承認事項の変更管理手法

○　製造技術のイノベーションの活用やグローバル化したサプライチェーンの効率的な管理を促進するため，製造方法等に関する承認事項の変更手続を円滑に行えるようにする必要がある。このため，PACMP（承認後変更管理計画書）を活用した品質に係る承認事項の変更管理手法を導入し，当該計画に沿った変更を行う場合は，より柔軟な手続を可能とするとともに，リスクに応じた予見可能性の高い変更管理手法を検討すべきである。

○　医薬品等の製造過程における保管のみを行う製造所については，製造販売業者による適切な管理が行われ，当局による調査の実施が可能であることを前提として，サプライチェーンにおける変更内容を迅速かつ合理的に承認書等へ反映する方法を検討すべきである。

▼　対象となる医薬品医療機器等法関係条文は第 14 条（医薬品，医薬部外品及び化粧品の製造販売の承認）ほか。

1.4.3　安全対策の充実

① 添付文書情報の提供

○　医薬品・医療機器等の適正使用に資する最新の情報を速やかに医療現場へ提供するとともに，納品されるたびに同じ添付文書が一施設に多数存在するといった課題を解決するため，添付文書の製品への同梱を廃止し，電子的な方法による提供を基本とすることが適当である。

○　同梱に代わる確実な情報提供の方法として，製造販売業者の責任において，必要に応じて卸売販売業者の協力の下，医薬品・医療機器等の初回納品時に紙媒体による提供を行うものとする。また，最新の添付文書情報へのア

Chapter 1 Current status and future prospects of pharmaceutical approval review and safety policies in Japan

should be confirmed by each category based on dosage forms (solid preparations, liquid preparations, etc.) and technical properties of the manufacturing processes.

▼The relevant articles of the PMD Act include Article 14 (Approval of manufacturing and marketing of drugs, etc.).

[2] Review of QMS compliance inspection

◯In some cases, MAHs of medical devices and in vitro diagnostics go through the same manufacturing process at multiple manufacturing sites to ensure stable supply and backup for organizational changes. However, the MAHs may discontinue using a part of the manufacturing sites stated on the compliance certificate due to stable manufacture, etc. In such cases where the same process takes place at multiple manufacturing sites in which QMS compliance inspection already took place and the MAHs stop using some of these sites, it should be specified that these sites do not need to be subjected to a new inspection.

▼The relevant articles of the PMD Act include Article 23-2-5 (Approval of manufacturing and marketing of medical devices and *in vitro* diagnostics).

[3] Risk-based change management approach for quality-related approved matters

◯In order to promote utilization of technological innovation in manufacturing and efficient management of a globalized supply chain, it is necessary to ensure that approved matters related to manufacturing methods, etc. can be changed smoothly. For this purpose, a change management approach utilizing a PACMP (post-approval change management plan) should be introduced for quality-related approved matters. When changes are made according to a PACMP, procedures should be more flexible. In addition, consideration is required to establish a risk-based, highly predictable change management approach.

◯For manufacturing sites that are only used for storage in a manufacturing process of drugs, etc., a measure should be established to reflect contents of changes in the supply chain in the approval certificate, etc. promptly and reasonably, provided that such manufacturing sites are appropriately managed by the MAHs and can be inspected by the authority.

▼The relevant articles of the PMD Act include Article 14 (Approval of manufacturing and marketing of drugs, quasi-drug and Cosmetics).

1.4.3 Enrichment of safety measures

[1] Provision of package insert information

◯In order to provide the latest information for proper use of drugs and medical devices, etc. promptly to clinical practices and to address issues such as the presence of multiple copies of the same package insert in an institution, accumulating each time products are delivered, in principle it would be appropriate to provide package inserts by electronic means, instead of attaching them to products.

◯As a reliable mean of information provision replacing attachments, paper package inserts should be provided at the first delivery of drugs and medical devices, etc. under the responsibility of MAHs, in cooperation with the wholesale distributors

■添付文書情報の提供方法の在り方（医薬品の例）

○製造販売業者又は卸売販売業者は，医療機関・薬局が医薬品を納入する場合，医療機関・薬局に赴く際に，原則紙媒体を提供する。あわせて，添付文書情報の電子的入手方法を伝達する。
○添付文書情報が改訂された場合は，電子的方法及び紙媒体の提供等を通じて，改訂後の情報を医療機関・薬局に速やかに提供する。
○また，製造販売業者は製品の外箱等に QR コード等を表記し，医療機関・薬局がアクセスした場合に，最新の添付文書情報を確実に入手できる状態を確保する。

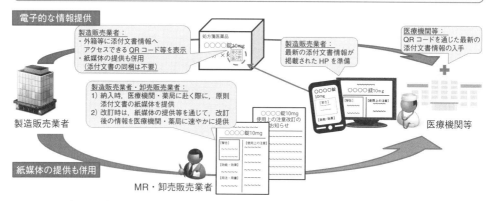

図 1.12　添付文書情報の提供方法（平成 30 年 11 月 8 日医薬品医療機器制度部会資料 1）

　　　　　クセスを可能とする情報を製品の外箱に表示し，情報が改訂された場合には紙媒体などにより医療機関・薬局等に確実に届ける仕組みを構築する必要がある（図 1.12 参照）。
　　○　また，一般用医薬品等の消費者が直接購入する製品は，使用時に添付文書情報の内容を直ちに確認できる状態を確保する必要があるため，現行のままの対応とすることが適当である。
　　▼　対象となる医薬品医療機器等法関係条文は第 52 条（添付文書等の記載事項）ほか。
　②　トレーサビリティ等の向上
　　○　医療安全の確保の観点から，製造，流通から，医療現場に至るまでの一連において，医薬品・医療機器等の情報の管理，使用記録の追跡，取り違えの防止などバーコードの活用によるトレーサビリティ等の向上が重要である。このような取組みによる安全対策を推進するため，医薬品・医療機器等の直接の容器・被包や小売用包装に，国際的な標準化規格に基づくバーコードの表示を義務化することが適当である。
　　○　バーコード表示を求めるに当たっては，医薬品・医療機器等の種類や特性に応じた効率的・段階的な対応や一般用医薬品などを含めた現状のコード規格の普及状況などを考慮する必要がある。
　　○　また，バーコード表示の義務化と合わせて製品情報のデータベース登録などを製造販売業者に求めるとともに，医療現場などにおけるバーコードを

■Desirable method of provision of package insert information (for drugs)

○In principle, MAHs or wholesalers provide a paper medium to medical institutions and pharmacies when delivering drugs. In addition, medical institutions and pharmacies are informed how to obtain the package insert information electronically.
○When the package insert information is revised, revised information is promptly provided to medical institutions and pharmacies electronically and via provision of the paper medium.
○Also, MAHs indicate QR code, etc. on the outer box of the product, etc. to ensure that medical institutions and pharmacies can obtain the latest package insert information by accessing the relevant site.

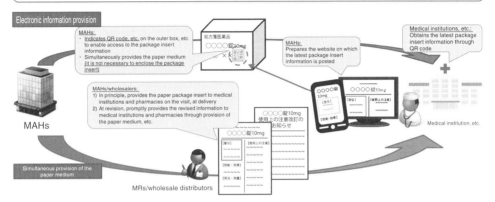

Fig1-12 Method of provision of package insert information (document 1 for the Subcommittee on Pharmaceuticals and Medical Devices on November 8, 2018)

as required. Also, a system should be constructed to indicate relevant information on the outer box of the product to enable access to the latest package insert information and to ensure that any revision in the information is reported to medical institutions and pharmacies, etc. using the paper medium, etc. (See **Fig. 1.12**).

○The current measures are appropriate for products including over-the-counter (OTC) drugs that are directly purchased by consumers, because it is necessary to ensure that the contents of the package insert information can readily be confirmed at the time of use.

▼The relevant articles of the PMD Act include Article 52 (Matters to be included in package inserts, etc.).

[2] Improvement of traceability, etc.
○For assurance of medical safety, it is important to improve traceability, etc. utilizing barcodes throughout the process of manufacture, distribution and delivery to clinical practices to control drug/medical device information, to trace use records, and to prevent misidentification of drugs and medical devices, etc. In order to promote safety measures by these efforts, it would be appropriate to mandate barcode labeling on the direct container/package and retail package of drugs and medical devices, etc. based on international standard specifications.
○Before mandating barcode labeling, it is necessary to take account of efficient and stepwise measures based on types and properties of drugs and medical devices, etc. and the usage of present code specifications including the OTC drugs.
○Also, it is necessary to require MAHs to register product information in a

活用した安全対策の取組みを推進していく必要がある。

▼　対象となる医薬品医療機器等法関係条文は「直接の容器等の記載事項」に関する医薬品（第50条），医療機器（第63条）ほか。

③　疾患登録レジストリ等の情報の安全対策への活用

○　疾患ごとに患者情報が集積されている疾患登録レジストリ等の情報について，医薬品・医療機器等の安全対策に十分活用できるよう，製造販売業者がそれらの情報を収集しやすくすることが必要である。

▼　対象となる医薬品医療機器等法関係条文は第68条の2（情報の提供等）ほか。

1.4.4　医薬品，医療機器等の製造・流通・販売に関わる者のガバナンスの強化等

①　許可等業者・役員の責務の明確化

○　医薬品，医薬部外品，化粧品，医療機器および再生医療等製品の製造・流通・販売に関わる医薬品医療機器等法上の許可等業者が，法令を遵守して業務を行うことを確保する必要がある。このため，許可等業者について，法令遵守のための体制整備等の必要な措置，必要な能力および経験を有する責任者，管理者等の選任等の義務を明確化すべきである。

○　許可等業者が法人である場合には，その役員が許可等業者の法令遵守に責任を有することを明確にするため，以下の点を規定すべきである。

・許可等業者の薬事に関する業務に責任を有する役員（責任役員）を薬機法上位置づけること。

・責任役員による許可等業者の法令遵守を担保するため，必要な場合に，当該責任役員の変更を命じることができるものとする措置を定めること（その後，法案から本項目は削除された）。

▼　対象となる医薬品医療機器等法関係条文は第73条（総括製造販売責任者等の変更命令）ほか。

○　許可等業者が，必要な能力および経験を有する技術責任者の選任義務を果たすことができるようにするため，医薬品の製造販売業者が選任する総括製造販売責任者に求められる要件を，以下のように整理すべきである。

・現行制度を基本に，薬剤師であり，かつ一定の従事経験を有し，品質管理業務または安全確保業務に関する総合的な理解力および適正な判断力を有する者が任命されるよう，要件を明確化すること。

・総括製造販売責任者としての責務を果たすことが可能な職位を有する薬剤師が確保できない場合などに限り，薬剤師以外の者を選任できるような例外規定を設けること。

・その場合であっても，例外規定が長く続かないように，専門的見地から総括製造販売責任者を補佐する社員たる薬剤師の配置，薬剤師たる医薬

Chapter 1 Current status and future prospects of pharmaceutical approval review and safety policies in Japan   49

database together with mandatory barcode labeling, in addition to promoting safety measures utilizing barcodes in clinical practices.

▼The relevant articles of the PMD Act include Article 50 for drugs and Article 63 for medical devices (Matters to be stated on the direct container, etc.).

[3] Utilization of information including disease registry for safety measures

○In relation to information including disease registry which accumulates patient information for each disease, it is necessary to make it easier for MAHs to collect such information so that it can be fully utilized for safety measures for drugs and medical devices, etc.

▼The relevant articles of the PMD Act include Article 68-2 (Information provision, etc.).

1.4.4 Strengthening, etc. of governance over those involved in manufacture, distribution and marketing of pharmaceuticals and medical devices, etc.

[1] Clarification of responsibilities of authorized vendors and executives

○It is necessary to ensure that authorized vendors involved in manufacture, distribution and marketing of drugs, quasi drugs, cosmetics, medical devices and regenerative medicine products as specified by the PMD Act fulfil their duties in compliance with laws and regulations. For this purpose, responsibilities of the authorized vendors must be clarified, including measures such as establishment of systems necessary for conforming to the laws and regulations, and assignment of officers/management and administrators with required capabilities and experiences.

○When authorized vendors are corporations, the followings must be specified to clarify that respective executives have responsibilities to ensure that the authorized vendors conform to the laws and regulations.

· Define executives responsible for pharmaceutical affairs of the authorized vendors (responsible executives) in the PMD Act.

· Specify measures to allow ordering changes in responsible executives as required in order to ensure that the authorized vendors conform to laws and regulations under the responsibility of the responsible executives. [This item was deleted in the proposal version]

▼The relevant articles of the PMD Act include Article 73 (Ordering changes in the Pharmaceutical Officer, etc.).

○In order to enable the authorized vendors to complete the obligation to assign technical managers with necessary capacity and experience, requirements of the pharmaceutical officer assigned by an MAHs should be organized as follows:

· Based on the present system, requirements should be specified such that a person who is a pharmacist with a certain level of experience and comprehensive understanding and appropriate judgment in relation to quality management and/or safety assurance operations is assigned.

· An exception should be provided to allow assignment of those who are not pharmacists only when it is not possible to assign a pharmacist with a position which enable accomplishment of responsibilities as the Pharmaceutical Officer.

· Even in such a case, a system should be established to allocate pharmacists as

品等総括製造販売責任者の社内での継続的な育成などの体制を整備すること。

▼　対象となる医薬品医療機器等法関係条文は第17条（総括製造販売責任者等の設置）ほか。

② 経済的利得の是正を通じた違法行為の抑止

○　経済的利得を主たる目的とするものと考えられる広告違反等の違反行為が，医薬品医療機器等法上の業許可を持たない事業者によっても行われるなど，現行の行政処分によっては抑止効果が機能しにくい実態があることを踏まえ，違法行為の抑止を図るため課徴金制度を検討すべきである。

○　課徴金制度については，行政処分が機能しにくい業許可を持たない事業者等に対する取締りを実効的に行うことができるようにするとともに，その執行が適正に行われることを確保するため，以下のような明確な要件を検討すべきである。なお，納付された課徴金を医療費等に還元する可能性についても検討すべきであるとの指摘があった。

・他の行政処分が機能している場合等には課徴金納付命令を行わないことができるものとする除外規定を設けること。

・不当な経済的利得が一定規模以上の事案を課徴金納付命令の対象とすること。

・課徴金の額の算定については，違法行為の対象となった製品の売上額に一定の算定率を乗じる簡明な算定方式を採用すること。

・納付命令の実施主体については，国と都道府県等の双方に権限を付与すること。

○　加えて，広告違反行為に対しては，訂正広告等を命じる措置命令を検討すべきである。

○　また，違反広告と併せて行われることが多い未承認の医薬品・医療機器等の販売，授与等の禁止への違反行為に対する十分な抑止措置も検討すべきである。

▼　対象となる医薬品医療機器等法関係条文は，薬機法第66条（虚偽・誇大広告），第68条（未承認医薬品等の広告），第72条（改善命令等）ほか。

③ 卸売販売業者に対する規制の見直し

○　医薬品を中心とした流通における品質管理の観点から，医薬品営業所管理者が適切な機能を発揮することが重要である。このため「物の出入り」のみならず，全体業務の把握と管理を医薬品営業所管理者の業務として業務手順書に位置づけるとともに，業務を遂行するための勤務体制，不在時の連絡体制の確保等を卸売販売業者の義務として明確化すべきである。

○　また，返品等を含めた流通全体における品質管理については，トレーサビリティの確保も活用しつつ，卸売販売業者のみならず関係者との連携を含

Chapter 1 Current status and future prospects of pharmaceutical approval review and safety policies in Japan

employee who assist the Pharmaceutical Officer from a specialists' viewpoint and to continue development of the future the Pharmaceutical Officer who is a pharmacist within the company such that the exception will not be used for a long period of time.

▼The relevant articles of the PMD Act include Article 17 (Establishment of the the pharmaceutical officer).

[2] Prevention of illegal acts through correction of economic profit

○Under the present administrative disposition it is difficult to prevent illegal acts in some cases. For example, an illegal act such as illegal advertising primarily aiming to obtain economic profit is taken by vendors not approved by the PMD Act. Given these situations, investigations should be conducted to establish an administrative monetary penalty system for prevention of illegal acts.

○For the administrative monetary penalty system, the following requirements should be considered to enable effective control of unauthorized vendors for which administrative disposition is less likely to function, as well as to ensure to appropriate control.

○Furthermore, it was pointed out that consideration should be given on a possibility to use paid administrative monetary penalty so as to contribute to medical expenses, etc.

・To establish an exception that an order for payment of monetary penalty may not be made in cases where other administrative penalties are functioning.

・To include cases with a certain level of unjust economic profit in the scope of the order for payment of a monetary penalty.

・To employ a plain calculation system for calculation of monetary penalty, in which the revenue of the product involved in the illegal act is multiplied by a fixed estimated value.

・To grant authority to both the country and prefectures as responsible organizations for the order for payment.

○In addition, for illegal advertising, an order for corrective advertising, etc. should be considered. Also, investigations should be carried out to establish adequate preventive measures against illegal acts including marketing or delivery of unapproved drugs and medical devices, etc. which is often performed together with illegal advertising.

▼The relevant articles of the PMD Act include Article 66 (False or misleading advertising), Article 68 (Advertisement of unapproved drugs, etc.) and Article 72 (Order for improvement, etc.).

[3] Review of regulations on wholesalers

○From the perspective of quality management in distribution of drugs in particular, business office managers for pharmaceuticals must exert appropriate actions. For this purpose, not only "ascertainment of incoming and outgoing resources" but also supervision and management of the overall operation should be specified as the duties of business office managers for pharmaceuticals with in the operating procedures. In addition, establishment of work shift for completion of the operation and a contact system in case the person in charge is absent should be specified as the duties of wholesalers.

めた対応について検討すべきである。

▼　対象となる薬機法関係条文は，薬機法第 34 条（卸売販売業の許可）ほか。

1.4.5　その他

○　「薬害肝炎事件の検証及び再発防止のための医薬品行政のあり方検討委員会」の指摘した「第三者組織」については，医薬品・医療機器等にかかわる行政の透明性の向上等の観点から，医薬品・医療機器等の安全対策の実施状況を評価・監視し，必要に応じて厚生労働大臣に意見を述べることができる組織として，実効性のある組織を検討したうえで厚生労働省に設置すべきである。

○　「医療用医薬品の販売情報提供活動に関するガイドライン」については，その施行後の運用および遵守状況の調査・分析を実施し，その結果に応じて適切な方策を講じることとすべきである。

Chapter 1 Current status and future prospects of pharmaceutical approval review and safety policies in Japan

○Furthermore, for quality management of the entire distribution including returned products, etc., investigations should be conducted to establish measures involving not only the wholesalers but also cooperating relevant parties, utilizing the assurance of traceability.

▼The relevant articles of the PMD Act include Article 34 (Approval of wholesalers).

1.4.5 Others

○The "third-party organization" pointed out by the "Review Committee on Drug Administration for Investigation and Prevention of Recurrence of Drug-induced Hepatitis Cases" should be established at the MHLW upon consideration of effective organization, as an organization which evaluates and supervised the status of implementation of safety measures for drugs and medical devices, etc. and provides opinions to the Minister of Health, Labour and Welfare as required, from the perspective of improved transparency of the government with respect to drugs and medical devices, etc.

○For the "Guideline for Promotion Information Provision Activities of Prescription Drugs", the status of operation and compliance after the enactment should be examined and analyzed, and appropriate measures should be taken based on the results.

第 2 章

臨床開発から市販後までの安全体制

　日本では 1990 年以降, GCP（Good Clinical Practice：医薬品の臨床試験の実施基準）が導入され, 臨床開発時の被験者の安全確保に寄与している。また, 市販後安全体制としては, 1988 年 GPMSP（Good Post Marketing Surveillance Practice：新医薬品等の再審査の申請のための市販後調査の実施に関する基準）案の公表以降, GPMSP の省令施行（1997 年）, その後, 製造販売業許可要件の GVP（Good Vigilance Practice：製造販売後安全管理基準）省令と再審査・再評価申請資料における製造販売後調査・試験の実施の基準である GPSP（Good Post-marketing Study Practice：製造販売後調査及び試験の実施基準）省令として, 2005 年に施行されている。

2.1　臨床開発時安全体制

　GCP は被験者の保護, 安全の保持および福祉の向上を図り, 治験（医薬品の製造販売承認申請の際に提出すべき資料のうち, 臨床試験の試験成績に関する資料の収集を目的とする試験）の科学的な質および成績の信頼性を確保することを目的として, 治験および製造販売後臨床試験に関する計画, 実施, モニタリング, 監査, 記録, 解析および報告等に関する遵守事項を定めている。なお, 欧米では GCP は介入研究として実施される臨床試験全般に適用されているが, 日本では GCP の法的拘束力は, 企業および医師主導の治験および製造販売後臨床試験のみに適用される。

　日本において GCP は 1990 年 10 月に最初に導入されたが, 当時の GCP には法的な基盤がなく, また, その運用も当時の日本の治験を取り巻く環境に配慮したものであった。その後, 1996 年に ICH E6 ガイドラインとして日米欧で合意した GCP ガイドラインが発表されたのを受け, 日本でも 1997 年 3 月に法的効力のある GCP 省令が発表され, これにより, ICH 水準の GCP 環境下で治験が実施されることとなった。その後, 日本における国際共同治験の実施数も年々増加し, GCP 等の治験の基準をより国際基準に近づけていくこと, および治験の手続き等の一層の効率化が課題とされた。

　これに対し, 治験における GCP の具体的な運用を定めた通知が 2012 年 12 月に改訂（「医薬品の臨床試験の実施の基準に関する省令」のガイダンスについて（2012

Chapter 2

Safety system from clinical development to post-marketing

In Japan, GCP (Good Clinical Practice) was introduced in 1990 and has contributed to ensuring safety for subjects during clinical development. Regarding post-marketing safety, after the draft of GPMSP (Good Post Marketing Surveillance Practice) was released in 1988, the GPMSP ministerial ordinance came into force (1997), and subsequently the GVP (Good Vigilance Practice) ministerial ordinance on marketing license conditions and GPSP (Good Post-marketing Study Practice) which provides implementation standards for post-marketing surveys and studies in reexamination and reevaluation application materials came into force in 2005.

2.1 Safety system during clinical development

GCP contains stipulations to be observed related to the planning, conduct, monitoring, auditing, recording, analysis and reporting of clinical trials and post-marketing clinical trials with the aim of protecting, ensuring the safety of and improving the welfare of subjects and assuring the scientific quality and reliability of the results of clinical trials for marketing approval (i.e. clinical trials performed prior to marketing approval to collect data which will be submitted in the application for marketing approval for drugs). In Japan, the legal binding power of GCP applies only to company-initiated and investigator-initiated clinical trials and post-marketing clinical trials, while in the US and EU, GCP applies to all interventional clinical studies.

In Japan, GCP was first introduced in October 1990, but there was no legal infrastructure for GCP at that time, and GCP was applied with consideration to the environment for clinical trials in Japan at that time. After that, the GCP Guideline agreed upon as the ICH E6 Guideline in 1996 among Japan, the US, and Europe was released, and in reaction to this, the legally-effective GCP ministerial ordinance was released in Japan in March 1997. This led to the implementation of clinical trials under GCP according to ICH standards. Since then, the number of global clinical trials performed has been increasing every year. Bringing the standards for clinical trials such as GCP closer to international standards and further increasing the efficiency of clinical trial procedures, etc. have been regarded as issues.

In response, a notification which concretely specifies the use of GCP in clinical trials was revised in December 2012 (Guidance on "Ministerial Ordinance on Good Clinical Practice for Drugs [PFSB/ELD Notification No. 1228-7 dated December 28, 2012],

年〔平成 24 年〕12 月 28 日付 薬食審査発 1228 第 7 号，一部改正：2013 年〔平成 25 年〕4 月 4 日付 薬食審査発 0404 第 4 号））され，新通知は GCP 運用の "ガイダンス" の位置付けとなった。これにより，GCP 省令の規定に合致し，被験者の人権の保護，安全の保持および福祉の向上が図られ，治験の科学的な質および試験の成績の信頼性が確保されるのであれば，本ガイダンス以外の適切な運用により治験を実施することが可能となり，新しいシステムでの臨床試験に，よりフレキシブルに対応することが可能となっている。

ICH E6 ガイドラインは 2016 年 11 月に補遺が追加される形で改定された。この背景には，1996 年に最初の ICH GCP が合意され 20 年間を経る間に，臨床試験の国際化，複雑な臨床試験デザインの増加，そして電子化システム等の発展に伴い，臨床試験の実施方法が大幅に変化し，GCP の刷新が期待された。ガイドラインに新たに追加された項として「Quality Management」があり，治験依頼者は臨床試験の実施にあたり，その品質を維持管理するシステム（Quality Management System：QMS）を構築する責務が明記された。治験依頼者は QMS の構築にあたり，被験者の安全確保において重要な臨床試験のプロセスやデータを Critical Process，Critical Data として特定し，ここで発生し得るリスクについて，これを低減するための方策を講じることを求められている。

2.2　市販後安全体制

日本における市販後安全対策は，薬害防止の観点から薬事法（医薬品医療機器等法）改正のたびに強化されてきたが，1988 年 11 月に GPMSP 案が公表されたことが転機となり GxP 化が始まった。しばらくの間は，行政指導レベルでの GPMSP 運用が続き，1997 年 4 月に GPMSP 省令が施行されたことにより法令に位置付けられることとなった。その後，GPMSP 省令は，製造販売業の許可要件の GVP 省令と，再審査・再評価申請資料における製造販売後調査・試験の基準である GPSP 省令に分けられ，2005 年 4 月に施行された。

また，薬害肝炎訴訟における原告と国との和解などを契機に，さらなる市販後安全対策の強化に取り組むこととなり，厚生労働大臣が設置した薬害肝炎事件の検証および再発防止のための医薬品行政のあり方検討委員会の最終提言が 2010 年 4 月に公表された。この最終提言を受けて，法改正について検討するために設置された厚生科学審議会医薬品等制度改正検討部会により 2012 年 1 月に公表された報告を踏まえて薬事法の改正が検討され，2013 年 11 月に医薬品医療機器等法（正式名称：医薬品，医療機器等の品質，有効性及び安全性の確保等に関する法律）が公布され，2014 年 11 月 25 日に施行された。

この改正法律の目的は，以下の 3 点である。

①　医薬品，医療機器等に係る安全対策の強化

partly revised: PFSB/ELD Notification No. 0404-4 dated April 4, 2013). The new notification is positioned as a "guidance" on the use of GCP. As a consequence, it has become possible to conduct a clinical trial with appropriate use of regulations other than this guidance as long as the provisions of the GCP ministerial ordinance are met, the protection of human rights, maintenance of safety, and enhancement of welfare in subjects can be performed, and the scientific nature of the clinical trial and the reliability of the study results can be ensured. It has become possible to flexibly deal with clinical studies under this new system.

The ICH E6 guideline was revised in November 2016 with the addition of an addendum. Over the 20 years since the agreement on the first ICH GCP in 1996, clinical studies have globalized, complex clinical study designs have increased, and electronic data capture systems have been developed, resulting in substantial changes to the methods of implementation of clinical studies. As such, renewal of GCP was desired. New sections that have been added to the guideline include "Quality Management". It has been stated that sponsors have a responsibility to construct a Quality Management System (QMS) and to identify the processes and data which constitute a "Critical Process" or "Critical Data" and take measures to reduce potential risks associated with them when performing clinical studies. In the construction of the QMS, the sponsors are required to identify clinical study processes and data that are important for assurance of subject safety as critical processes and data, and take measures to reduce potential risks associated with these processes and data.

2.2 Post-marketing pharmacovigilance system

From the viewpoint of prevention of drug-induced suffering, post-marketing safety measures in Japan have been strengthened each time the Pharmaceutical Affairs Law (PMD Act) was revised, but with the release of the proposal for GPMSP in November 1988 as a turning point, the application of GxP was started. For a while, the use of GPMSP was continued on the level of administrative guidance, and with the enforcement of the GPMSP ministerial ordinance in April 1997, these ordinances became positioned as laws and regulations. After that, the GPMSP ministerial ordinance was divided into the GVP ministerial ordinance on marketing license conditions and the GPSP ministerial ordinance which provides standards for post-marketing surveys and studies performed for Reexamination and Reevaluation applications, which came into force in April 2005.

With changes such as the amicable settlement between the plaintiffs and the government in the lawsuit over drug-induced hepatitis as a turning point, efforts have been made to further strengthen post-marketing safety measures, and the final recommendation by the Review Committee on Drug Administration for Investigation and Prevention of Recurrence of Drug-induced Hepatitis Cases established by the Minister of Health, Labour and Welfare was released in April 2010. In response to this final recommendation, revising the Pharmaceutical Affairs Law was considered taking into account a report released in January 2012 by the Review Committee on Revision of Systems for Drugs, etc., The Health Science Council, which was established to consider revision of the law, and the PMD Act (formal name: The Act on Securing Quality,

58　第 2 章　臨床開発から市販後までの安全体制

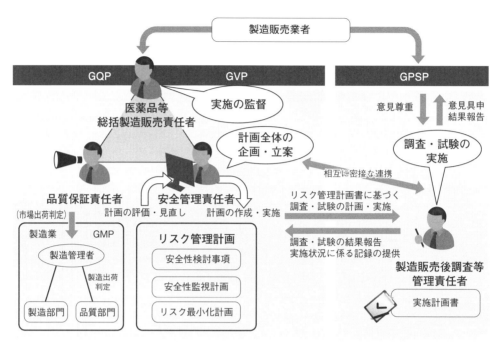

図 2.1　製造販売業三役と製造販売後調査等管理責任者（文献 1）より一部改変）

② 医療機器の特性を踏まえた規制の構築
③ 再生医療等製品の特性を踏まえた規制の構築

2.2.1　製造販売業三役

　2005 年 4 月に施行された旧薬事法では，欧米の状況を踏まえて製造承認から製造販売承認へと制度が変更された．これにより，製造業と製造販売業が分離され，製造所をもたなくても医薬品の販売が可能となった．製造販売業の許可は 5 年ごとに更新される．また，同じくこの際に総括製造販売責任者，安全管理責任者および品質保証責任者のいわゆる製造販売業三役の設置，GVP，GQP（Good Quality Practice：製品の市場への出荷時の品質管理基準）遵守の体制整備が業許可の要件となった．それ以前からある GMP（Good Manufacturing Practice：製造管理及び品質管理基準）は，製品の製造所からの出荷時の品質管理（製造出荷判定）に関するものである．製造販売業三役の位置付けと役割分担は図 2.1 に示すとおりである．

　改正 GVP・GPSP の施行（2014 年 10 月 1 日）後は，医薬品リスク管理計画書に基づく調査・試験の計画，実施のため，安全管理責任者と製造販売後調査等管理責任者との連携が求められている．なお，製造販売業三役は，製造販売業者における

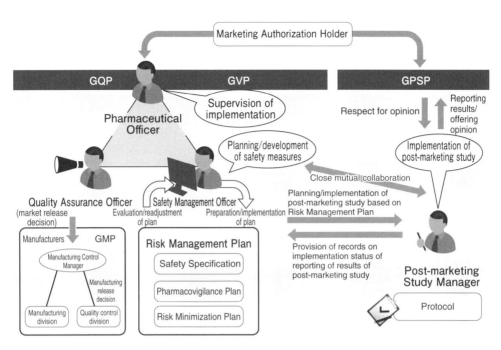

Fig.2.1 Three Officers in Marketing Authorization Holders and Post-marketing Study Manager (partially modified from Reference [1])

Efficacy and Safety of Pharmaceuticals, Medical Devices, Regenerative and Cellular Therapy Products, Gene Therapy Products and Cosmetics) was promulgated in November 2013 and came into force on November 25, 2014.

The objectives of the revised law are the following 3 issues:

[1] Strengthening of safety measures for pharmaceuticals, medical devices, etc.
[2] Creation of regulations taking into account the characteristics of medical devices
[3] Creation of regulations taking into account the characteristics of regenerative medicine products.

2.2.1 Three Officers in Marketing Authorization Holders

Under the old Pharmaceutical Affairs Law that came into force in April 2005, the system underwent a change from manufacturing approval to marketing approval, taking into account the situations in the US and Europe. With this change, the manufacturing business and marketing business were separated, thereby making it possible to sell drugs without having a manufacturing site. The manufacturing business license is to be renewed every five years. At the same time, appointment of three Officers - the Pharmaceutical Officer, the Safety Management Officer and the Quality Assurance Officer - and establishment of a system to comply with GVP and GQP (Good Quality Practice: standards for quality control at the time of release of products to the market) became license conditions. Good Manufacturing Practice (GMP), which had been in existence from before then, is related to quality control at the time of release of the product from the plant (manufacturing release decision). The division of responsibilities for the three Officers in an MAH is shown in **Fig. 2.1**.

After the enforcement of revised GVP/GPSP (October 1, 2014), collaboration between

60   第 2 章　臨床開発から市販後までの安全体制

表 2.1　GVP 省令と製造販売業の許可区分ごとの規制の状況[2)]（○は規制あり，×は規制なし）

許可区分	安全管理統括部門	安全管理責任者	安全管理実施責任者	安全管理業務手順書	三役の兼務
第 1 種製造販売業 ・処方せん医薬品 ・高度管理医療機器 ・再生医療等製品	○	○ （3 年以上の業務経験）	○	○	兼務不可
第 2 種製造販売業 ・処方せん医薬品以外の医療用医薬品 ・一般用医薬品 ・体外診断用医薬品 ・管理医療機器	×	○	×	○	二役兼務可。ただし，安全管理責任者と品質保証責任者の兼務は不可
第 3 種製造販売業 ・医薬部外品 ・化粧品 ・一般医療機器	×	○	×	×	三役兼務可

注）許可区分をまたがる医薬品等総括製造販売責任者，安全管理責任者と品質保証責任者の兼務は認められるが，その場合には最も上位の許可区分の要件に従う。

製造販売後安全管理および品質管理業務の統括管理と健康被害発生等の防止のための措置決定に必要な体制である。したがって，製造販売業三役の緊密な連携は製造販売業者にとって不可欠であり，製造販売業三役の管理規定および製造販売後安全管理業務手順書や品質管理業務手順書にそのことを明記しておく必要がある。

Chapter 2 Safety system from clinical development to post-marketing   61

Table2.1   GVP ministerial ordinance and regulations for each license category of MAH[2]
(○ = Regulation applies, × = Regulation does not apply)

License category	General safety management division	Safety Management Officer	Safety Management Implementation Manager	Safety Management SOP	Concurrent posts
Type 1 marketing business · Prescription drugs · Highly controlled medical devices ·Regenerative medicine products	○	○ (Experience of at least 3 years)	○	○	Concurrent positions not allowed
Type 2 marketing business · Ethical drugs other than prescription drugs · OTC drugs · In vitro diagnostics · Controlled medical devices	×	○	×	○	Two concurrent positions possible. Concurrent safety Management Officer and Quality Assurance Officer not allowed.
Type 3 marketing business · Quasi-drugs · Cosmetics · General medical devices	×	○	×	×	Three concurrent positions allowed

Note) Holding the posts of the Pharmaceutical Officer, the Safety Management Officer and the Quality Assurance Officer concurrently across the licensing categories is permitted, but in such cases, the regulation should be based on the highest licensing category.

the Safety Management officer and the Post-marketing Study Manager became required for planning and implementation of surveys or studies based on the Risk Management Plan. The three Officers in Marketing Authorization Holders are necessary for overall control of post-marketing safety management and quality control activities and for deciding measures to prevent incidents such as those that could lead to damage of health. Therefore, close liaison among these three Officers is indispensable for MAHs and it is essential to clearly outline these points within corporate management codes and standard operating procedures (SOP) covering post-marketing safety management and quality management.

2.2.2 GVP（改正 GVP）

GVP 省令は，**表 2.1** に示すように，医薬品，医薬部外品，化粧品，医療機器および再生医療等製品に分かれて，製造販売業の許可区分ごとに規定されている。

本項では，処方せん医薬品を取り扱う第 1 種製造販売業者に関する要件を中心に述べるが，処方せん医薬品以外の医療用医薬品と一般用医薬品を取り扱う第 2 種製造販売業者，および医薬部外品や化粧品を取り扱う第 3 種製造販売業者にあっても，GVP 省令における要件が定められている。なお，第 1 種および第 2 種製造販売業の総括製造販売責任者は，医薬品医療機器等法第 17 条により薬剤師でなければならないとされている。ただし，厚労省令で定める医薬品についてのみ，その製造販売をする場合においては，厚労省令で定めるところにより薬剤師以外の技術者をもってこれに代えることができる。

製造販売業者は GVP 省令に基づいて販売部門から独立した安全管理統括部門を設置し，安全管理責任者の指導のもと，安全管理情報を入手してから，安全管理情報の評価・分析・検討を行い，その結果に基づく安全確保措置を立案，決定し，安全対策措置を講じる。処方せん医薬品の安全管理責任者には，安全管理業務あるいはこれに類する業務等に 3 年以上の経験が求められる。なお，それぞれの業務については，遅滞なく実施できるように標準的事務処理期間を設けて，製造販売後安全管理業務手順書に明記しておく必要がある。また，MR が所属する販売部門（安全管理実施部門）等には安全管理実施責任者を設置し，安全管理統括部門と連携して，医療機関から安全性情報を収集し，必要な安全性情報を伝達・提供する。

GVP 省令では，製造販売後安全管理業務を適正かつ円滑に実施するために，下記の手順書を定めるように規定されている。

① 安全管理情報の収集に関する手順

② 安全管理情報の検討およびその結果に基づく安全確保措置の立案に関する手順

③ 安全確保措置の実施に関する手順

④ 安全管理責任者から総括製造販売責任者への報告に関する手順

⑤ 安全管理実施責任者から安全管理責任者への報告に関する手順

⑥ 市販直後調査に関する手順（2014 年 10 月施行改正 GVP 省令においては医薬品リスク管理に関する手順〔市販直後調査に関する手順を含む〕に変更された）

⑦ 自己点検に関する手順

⑧ 製造販売後安全管理に関する業務に従事する者に対する教育訓練に関する手順

⑨ 製造販売後安全管理に関する業務に係る記録の保存に関する手順

⑩ 品質保証責任者その他の処方せん医薬品，高度管理医療機器または再生医療等製品の製造販売に係る業務の責任者との相互の連携に関する手順

2.2.2 GVP (revised GVP)

As shown in **Table 2.1**, the GVP ordinance is specified for each license category of MAHs classified by drugs, quasi-drugs, cosmetics, medical devices, and regenerative medicine products.

This section concentrates on requirements for a type 1 marketing business which concerns prescription drugs, but requirements are also specified within the GVP ordinance for type 2 marketing businesses which handle ethical drugs other than prescription drugs and OTC drugs and type 3 marketing businesses which handle quasi-drugs and cosmetics. The Pharmaceutical Officer of type 1 and type 2 marketing businesses must be a pharmacist as specified in Article 17 of the PMD Act. However, if such marketing is done only for a drug specified in the MHLW ordinance, technicians other than pharmacists may replace them pursuant to the provisions of the MHLW ordinance.

Under the GVP ordinance, MAHs must establish a general safety management division independent of the marketing division and, under the guidance of the Safety Management Officer, must evaluate, analyze and examine all safety management information after its collection. Based on the results of that analysis safety assurance measures must be drafted, decided and implemented. Safety Management Officer of prescription drugs must have at least 3 years of experience in safety management or related work. Standard processing times for all activities must be specified so that the work is completed without delay and these must be details in the SOPs covering post-marketing safety management. Also, Safety Management Implementation Managers are appointed in divisions such as the marketing division (safety implementation division) which employ Medical Representatives (MRs) and MRs to collect safety information from medical institutions and communicate and provide necessary safety information in cooperation with the general safety management division.

The GVP ordinance specifies that the following SOPs must be prepared to assure appropriate and smooth post-marketing safety management.

[1] SOP on collection of safety management information
[2] SOP on examination of safety management information and drafting of safety assurance measures accordingly
[3] SOP on implementation of safety assurance measures
[4] SOP on reporting by the Safety Management Officer to the Pharmaceutical Officer
[5] SOP on reporting by the Safety Management Implementation Managers to the Safety Management Officer
[6] SOPs on Early Post-marketing Phase Risk Minimization and Vigilance (EPPV) (In the revised GVP ministerial ordinance that will come into force in October 2014, the SOPs were modified to SOPs on Drug Risk Management [including SOPs for EPPV])
[7] SOP on self inspections
[8] SOP on education and training of personnel related to post-marketing safety management
[9] SOP on retention of records on work related to post-marketing safety management

⑪ 製造販売後調査等管理責任者との相互の連携に関する手順（2014年10月施行改正GVP省令で追加された）

⑫ その他製造販売後安全管理に関する業務を適正かつ円滑に行うために必要な手順

このほか，再生医療等製品および生物由来製品の製造販売業者においては，感染症定期報告を行うことが求められるので，「感染症定期報告に関する手順」を定める必要がある。なお，GVP関連業務の委託については，GVP省令とは別に医薬品医療機器等法施行規則で規定されている。

2.2.3　GQP

GQP省令も，医薬品，医薬部外品，化粧品または再生医療等製品（医薬品等）に分けて制定されているが，本項では医薬品に関するGQPについて述べる。

製造販売業者は，GQP省令に基づいて総括製造販売責任者の監督の下，販売部門から独立した品質管理統括部門として品質保証部門を設置し，品質保証責任者の監督のもとに市場への出荷のための品質管理を行う。具体的には，品質情報の収集に努め，品質不良の場合には適切な処理を行い，製品回収にあっても適切に処理しなければならない。品質保証責任者は安全管理責任者と同様に，品質管理業務等に3年以上の経験が求められる。製造業者と製造販売業者が同一の場合であって，品質保証責任者がその業務を行う事業所と同一施設内に製造所を有する場合には，品質保証責任者と，GMPで製造所ごとに設置する製造管理者を兼任することが可能である。製造業者と製造販売業者が異なる場合にあっては，両者の役割分担について取り決め，品質管理業務手順書等に定めなければならない。なお，医薬品の製造管理者は医薬品医療機器等法第17条により薬剤師でなければならない（例外規定あり）とされている。

GQP省令では，品質管理業務を適正かつ円滑に実施するために，下記の手順書を定めるように規定されている。

① 市場への出荷の管理に関する手順

② 適正な製造管理及び品質管理の確保に関する手順

③ 品質等に関する情報及び品質不良等の処理に関する手順

④ 回収処理に関する手順

⑤ 自己点検に関する手順

⑥ 教育訓練に関する手順

⑦ 医薬品の貯蔵等の管理に関する手順

⑧ 文書及び記録の管理に関する手順

⑨ 安全管理統括部門その他の品質管理業務に関係する部門又は責任者との相互の連携に関する手順

[10] SOP on liaison with Quality Assurance Officer and other managers related to manufacturing and marketing of prescription drugs, highly controlled medical devices or regenerative medicine products

[11] SOPs on Mutual Collaboration with Post-marketing Study Manager (added to the revised GVP ministerial ordinance that will come into force in October 2014)

[12] Other SOPs necessary for appropriate and smooth conduct of work related to post-marketing safety management

Since periodic infection reports are also required for MAHs of regenerative medicine products and biological products, it is necessary to specify an "SOP for periodic infection reports." Out-contracting of GVP related work is also specified in the Enforcement Regulation of the PMD Act separate from the GVP ministerial ordinance.

2.2.3 GQP

The GQP ordinance is also divided into drugs, quasi-drugs, cosmetics, regenerative medicine products (drugs), but in this section, only GQP related to drugs is discussed.

Under the GQP ordinance, MAHs must establish a quality assurance unit independent of the marketing division as the general quality management division under the supervision of the Pharmaceutical Officer, and quality management must be performed for release on the market under the Supervision of the Quality Assurance Officer. They must make an effort to collect quality information, and must handle any cases of poor quality appropriately and also handle product recalls appropriately. The Quality Assurance Officer, similar to the Safety Management Officer, must have at least 3 years of experience in quality management work. When the manufacturer and the MAH are the same and the manufacturing plant is located at the same facility as the office where the Quality Assurance Officer performs its duties (PFSB Notification No.070900 isseud on July 9, 2004), the Quality Assurance Officer can concurrently serve as the Manufacturing Control Manager in each facility applying GMP. When the manufacturer and the MAH are the same, the Quality Assurance Officer can concurrently serve as Manufacturing Control Manager in each facility applying GMP. When the manufacturer and the MAH are the Quality Assurance Officer and Manufacturing Control Managers must be decided and this must be specified in the SOP for quality management. A Manufacturing Control Manager of drugs must be a pharmacist as specified in Article 17 of the PMD Act (with exemptions).

The GQP ordinance specifies that the following SOPs must be prepared to assure appropriate and smooth post-marketing quality management work.

[1] SOP on control of product release to the market

[2] SOP on assurance of appropriate manufacturing control and quality management

[3] SOP on processing of quality-related information and quality defects

[4] SOP on management of recalls

[5] SOP on self inspections

[6] SOP on education and training

[7] SOP on control of storage of drugs

[8] SOP on control of documents and records

[9] SOP on liaison with the general safety management division and other divisions or managers related to quality management

⑩　その他品質管理業務を適正かつ円滑に実施するために必要な手順

2.2.4　GPSP（改正 GPSP）

　製造販売業者等は，GPSP 省令に基づいて製造販売後の調査・試験の実施にかかわる業務を統括する製造販売後調査等管理責任者を，販売にかかわる部門から独立して設置しなければならない。RMP の導入に伴い改正された（2014 年 10 月 1 日施行）GPSP は，医療情報データベースを利用した製造販売後の調査を再審査および再評価申請に利用可能にするためさらに改正され，2017 年 10 月 26 日に公布，2018 年 4 月 1 日に施行された[3,4]。改正 GPSP では，これまでの「使用成績調査」および「製造販売後臨床試験」に新たに「製造販売後データベース調査」を加えた計 3 種類の調査・試験が規定された。さらに，「使用成績調査」の細分類として，これまでの「特定使用成績調査」の他「一般使用成績調査」および「使用成績比較調査」が加わった。「製造販売後データベース調査」は「医療情報データベース」の情報を二次利用する調査であることに対して，「使用成績調査」は医療機関から直接収集する情報を用いる調査であることが明示的に規定された。「使用成績比較調査」は，これまでも「使用成績調査」のひとつとして実施されてきたものだが，特定の医薬品を使用する患者の情報だけでなく，当該医薬品等を使用していない患者の情報についても医療機関から収集し，比較を行う使用成績調査の実施が可能であることを明確にするため，新たに規定された。「一般使用成績調査」は，特定使用成績調査および使用成績比較調査以外の使用成績調査（いわゆる従来型の使用成績調査）が該当する。これらの調査・試験は承認された効能・効果，用法・用量の範囲内で製造販売後調査等管理責任者が企画・立案した製造販売後調査等実施計画書等に従って実施される。医療情報データベースや調査票により情報を収集し，集計・評価の上，結果を取りまとめて，医薬品の有効性，安全性に関する根拠資料として再審査・再評価申請資料等に活用するとともに，必要に応じて医療関係者に提供する。なお，安全確保措置のために実施する調査等の企画・立案の決定は，安全管理責任者または総括製造販売責任者の責務であり，委託できないことが GVP 省令で規定されているので，そこで決定された調査等について製造販売後調査等管理責任者が製造販売後調査等実施計画書に盛り込むことになる。

　GPSP 省令では，製造販売後調査等業務を適正かつ円滑に実施するために，下記の手順を記載した製造販売後調査等業務手順書を定めるように規定されている。

①　使用成績調査に関する手順
②　製造販売後データベース調査に関する手順
③　製造販売後臨床試験に関する手順
④　自己点検に関する手順
⑤　製造販売後調査等業務に従事する者に対する教育訓練に関する手順

Chapter 2 Safety system from clinical development to post-marketing   67

[10] Other SOPs necessary for appropriate and smooth implementation of other quality management operations

2.2.4 GPSP (revised GPSP)

Under the GPSP ordinance, the Marketing Authorization Holder must appoint a Post-marketing Study Manager independent of the division related to marketing who oversees work related to the conduct of post-marketing studies. GPSP, which was revised (coming into force on October 1, 2014) following the introduction of RMP, was further revised to make post-marketing studies using medical information databases possible for applications for Reexamination and Reevaluation, promulgated on October 26, 2017, and effective on April 1, 2018.[3, 4]. In the revised GPSP, a total of 3 types of studies were specified: "Use-results survey," "post-marketing clinical trials" and the newly added "post-marketing database studies." Furthermore, as sub-classifications of "Use-results survey" in addition to the existing "Specified use-results survey". "Use-results survey" and "Use-results survey with comparative group" were newly added. It was clearly specified that "post-marketing database studies" are studies that make secondary use of the information within a "medical information database," while "Use-results survey" are studies that use information directly collected from medical institutions. Although "Use-results survey with comparative group" has been conducted as a type of the "Use-results survey," it was newly specified to clarify that it is possible to conduct a Use-results survey by collecting information from medical institutions not only on patients who are using a specific drug but also on those who are not using the relevant drug and comparing this information. "General use-results survey" refer to Use-results survey other than Specified use-results survey and Use-results survey with comparative group (i.e., conventional drug use-results survey). These studies are performed in accordance with the Post-marketing Studies Implementation Plan which is planned and drafted by the Post-marketing Studies Manager within the approved indications, dosage and administration. The information is collected from the medical information database and case record forms, aggregated and evaluated. The results are compiled and used as evidence of efficacy and safety in applications for Reexamination and Reevaluation. The data is also supplied to healthcare professionals (HCPs) when required. Decisions on drafting of plans for studies performed as safety assurance measures must be made by the Safety Management Officer or Pharmaceutical Officer. Because such decisions cannot be outsourced to others according to the GVP ordinance, the Post-marketing Study Manager will include the study decided in the Post-marketing Studies Implementation Plan.

The GPSP ordinance specifies the following SOPs for post-marketing studies to conduct appropriate and smooth post-marketing studies.

[1] SOP on Use-results survey
[2] SOP on post-marketing database studies
[3] SOP on post-marketing clinical trials
[4] SOP on self inspections
[5] SOP on education and training of personnel involved in post-marketing studies
[6] SOP on outsourcing of post-marketing studies
[7] SOP on retention of records related to post-marketing studies
[8] Other SOPs necessary for appropriate and smooth conduct of work related to

⑥　製造販売後調査等業務の委託に関する手順

⑦　製造販売後調査等業務に係る記録の保存に関する手順

⑧　その他製造販売後調査等を適正かつ円滑に実施するために必要な手順

なお，製造販売後臨床試験の実施にあたっては，GCP 省令に基づき行う。

文　　献

1)　磯崎正季子：医薬品医療機器レギュラトリーサイエンス財団 2014 年製造販売後安全管理・調査，基礎研修講座資料，2014

2)　高橋春男：安全管理，製造販売後調査の実施のための医薬品の適正使用と安全対策－ PMS の歴史，じほう，2011，p.86

3)　医薬品医療機器等安全性情報, No.351：医療情報データベース「MID-NET」について，2017

4)　医薬品医療機器等安全性情報, No.355：参考資料・GPSP 省令の改正と製造販売後調査等について，2018

5)　厚生労働省医薬・生活衛生局長通知，2017 年（平成 29 年）6 月 26 日付，薬生発 0626 第 3 号

post-marketing studies

Post-marketing clinical trials are to be implemented based on the GCP ministerial ordinance.

References

1) Makiko Isozaki: Materials for the basic training course on post-marketing safety management/surveillance in 2014, Pharmaceutical and Medical Device Regulatory Science Society of Japan, 2014

2) Haruo Takahashi: Proper use of drugs and safety measures for implementation of safety management/post-marketing surveys - History of PMS; Jiho, Inc. 2011, p.86

3) Pharmaceuticals and Medical Devices Safety Information, No. 351: Medical Information Database MID-NET (Medical Information Database NETwork), 2017

4) Pharmaceuticals and Medical Devices Safety Information, No. 355: (Reference) Revision of the Ministerial Ordinance on Good Post-marketing Study Practice (GPSP Ordinance), 2018

5) PSEHB Notification No. 0626-3, June 26, 2017

第3章

臨床開発段階のリスクマネジメント

　日本では治験中の安全性情報に関する規制として，規制当局への治験薬副作用等緊急報告制度，治験薬の年次報告制度があり，また，GCP に従い，治験責任医師および治験実施施設の長への情報伝達の義務がある。

　本章ではこれらの規制を紹介するとともに，治験中のリスク最小化策について考えるべきポイントを述べる。

3.1　臨床開発段階のリスクマネジメント

3.1.1　規制当局への副作用等緊急報告制度（電子報告）

　治験中に得られる安全性情報の取り扱いについては，ICH E2A ガイドラインが 1994 年 10 月に合意されている。これを受け，日本において，治験薬の副作用・感染症症例報告が旧 薬事法で定められ（医薬品医療機器等法第 80 条の 2，医薬品医療機器等法施行規則第 273 条），1997 年 4 月以降，治験依頼者に義務付けられている（表 3.1）。

　ICH E2A ガイドラインでは規制当局への副作用報告の対象を「治験薬概要書から予測不可能な重篤副作用」としているが，日本の規制ではこれに加え，「治験薬概要書から予測可能な死亡，死亡のおそれのある副作用」についても報告対象としている点が大きな相違点の 1 つである。また，規制当局への個別症例報告の対象として，当該治験薬の使用によるものと疑われる感染症の発生もこれに含まれる。

　治験薬副作用報告の対象は，国内症例は国内で治験依頼者が実施する治験が対象

表 3.1　治験に係る副作用・感染症等症例の規制当局への報告

予測性	重篤性	国内症例	外国症例 [注]
予測できない	死亡・死亡につながるおそれ	7 日以内	7 日以内
	その他重篤	15 日以内	15 日以内
予測できる	死亡・死亡につながるおそれ	15 日以内	15 日以内
	その他重篤	不要	不要

注）国内で承認取得している医薬品の一変治験を実施する際の外国症例の報告は，市販後の外国副作用症例報告に代えることができる。

Chapter 3

Risk management during clinical development

I n Japan, regulations related to safety information during clinical trials include the system for expedited reporting of Adverse Drug Reactions (ADRs), etc. to regulatory authorities and the system for annual reporting for investigational drugs. Also, there is an obligation to transmit information to investigators and heads of study sites in accordance with GCP.

In this chapter, these regulations are introduced, and points to consider for risk minimization measures during clinical trials are described.

3.1 Risk management during clinical development

3.1.1 System for expedited reporting of Adverse Drug Reactions (ADRs), etc. to regulatory authorities (electronic reporting)

The ICH E2A Guideline on the handling of safety information obtained during clinical trials was agreed upon in October 1994. In response to this, in Japan, investigational drug ADR/infection case reporting is stipulated in the old Pharmaceutical Affairs Law (Article 80-2 of PMD Act; Article 273 of the Enforcement Regulations of PMD Act), and since April 1997, sponsors have been obliged to make those reports (**Table 3.1**).

In the ICH E2A Guideline, ADRs subject to reporting to the regulatory authorities are "serious ADRs unexpected from investigator's brochure," but one of the major differences in the Japanese regulations, "deaths and life-threatening ADRs expected from investigator's brochure" are also subject to reporting in addition to the above. Occurrences of infections suspected to be due to the use of a relevant investigational drug are also to be reported as individual case reports to the regulatory authorities.

Table3.1　Reporting of ADRs, Infections, etc. from Clinical Trials to Regulatory Authorities

Expectedness	Seriousness	Japanese case	Foreign case [Note]
Unexpected	Fatal/life-threatening	Within 7 days	Within 7 days
	Other serious	Within 15 days	Within 15 days
Expected	Fatal/life-threatening	Within 15 days	Within 15 days
	Other serious	Not necessary	Not necessary

Note) Reporting of foreign cases, if a clinical trial for partial change of a drug approved in Japan, can be replaced with reporting of post-marketing foreign ADRs.

であるが，外国症例については，治験薬と成分が同一性を有すると認められるものであれば，投与経路，用法・用量，効能・効果等が異なる場合も対象となる。治験依頼者となる企業が既に国内で承認取得している医薬品の一変治験（用法・用量または効能・効果の追加，変更または削除に係る承認事項一部変更を目的とする治験）を実施する際には，当該製品に関する市販後の外国副作用等症例報告を活用し，治験薬副作用報告に代えることができる。

3.1.2　研究報告・外国における措置報告

前述の個別症例の副作用報告に加え，その他の安全性情報の緊急報告として研究報告，外国における措置報告が義務付けられている。研究報告は，当該被験薬等の副作用もしくはそれらの使用による感染症により，がんその他の重大な疾病，障害もしくは死亡が発生するおそれがあること，当該被験薬等の副作用によるものと疑われる疾病等，もしくはそれらの使用によるものと疑われる感染症の発生数，発生頻度，発生条件等の発生傾向が著しく変化したこと，または当該被験薬等が治験の対象となる疾患に対して効能もしくは効果を有しないことを示すものが該当する。

外国における措置報告の対象は，通知においては「外国で使用されている物であって被験薬と成分が同一性を有すると認められるものに係る製造，輸入または販売の中止，回収，廃棄その他保健衛生上の危害の発生または拡大を防止するための措置の実施」とされているが，具体的な例として，外国における有効性または安全性の観点からの製造等の中止のほか，効能もしくは効果，用法もしくは用量または製造方法の変更，医薬関係者へのお知らせの配布を伴う重要な使用上の注意の改訂等が含まれると説明されている。治験薬についてはいずれの報告も治験依頼者が情報を知りえた日から 15 日以内に報告することとされている。

治験薬副作用等症例報告，研究報告・措置報告の規制当局への報告義務期間は，初回治験計画届出日から承認取得日または開発中止届出の提出日までとなっている。なお，治験計画届の提出を要しない場合，治験実施計画書の治験開始日から承認日または開発中止届出の提出日までとなる。

また，日本においては副作用・感染症症例報告に加え，研究報告や外国措置報告についても ICH E2B/M2 に基づいて電子報告を行うこととされており，これは2019 年 4 月 1 日より ICH E2B（R3）での報告が必須となる。

3.1.3　年次報告と DSUR

日本における治験薬の定期報告は 2009 年 4 月に施行された 6 か月ごとの定期報

Chapter 3 Risk management during clinical development   73

Investigational drug ADR reports for domestic (Japanese) cases are to be made in clinical trials conducted by sponsors in Japan, but reports for foreign cases are also to be made for any drugs that are considered to have the same ingredient as an investigational drug even if the administration route, dosage and administration, and indications are different. If a company as a sponsor conducts a clinical trial for a partial change (a clinical trial intended to make a partial change in approved items for dosage/administration or addition, change, or deletion of indication) for a drug which was already approved in Japan, this may be replaced with investigational drug ADR reports by utilizing post-marketing foreign ADR case reports related to the product.

3.1.2 Research reports; Reports on measures taken in foreign countries

In addition to the above-mentioned ADR reports in individual cases, there is an obligation to make research reports as expedited reports of safety information as well as reports of measures taken overseas. Research reports correspond to those of a cancer or other significant disease/disorder or death that may occur due to an ADR to a relevant test drug, etc. or infection associated with the use of such drug, those of a substantial change in tendency of occurrence such as the number/frequency of cases, occurrence conditions, etc. of a disease suspected to be associated with an ADR to a relevant test drug or infection suspected to be associated with the use of such drug, or those showing that a relevant test drug, etc. has no effect for a disease that is the target for the clinical trial.

According to notifications, reports of measures taken overseas are to be made for "discontinuation of manufacturing, import, or selling, recall, disposal due to a product used in a foreign country with the same ingredient as a test drug or implementation of other measure to prevent the occurrence or spread of a hazard in health and hygiene" As concrete examples, it is explained that items for those reports include a change in indication, dosage/administration, or manufacturing method and modification of important precautions for use associated with distribution of a "Dear Healthcare Professional Letters" in addition to discontinuation of manufacturing, etc. from the viewpoint of efficacy or safety in a foreign country. For an investigational drug, all of those reports are to be made within 15 days after the day when the sponsor initially receives the information.

The period during which there is an obligation to make investigational drug ADR case reports and research reports or reports on foreign measures to the regulatory authorities is from the date of initial clinical trial plan notification to the date of obtainment of approval or the date of submission of the development discontinuation notification. If submission of a clinical trial plan notification is not needed, the period is from the start date of the clinical trial in the protocol to the date of approval or date of submission of the development discontinuation notification.

Also in Japan, research reports and reports of measures taken overseas, in addition to ADR/infection case reports, are to be made electronically according to ICH E2B/M2 and from April 1, 2019 reporting according ICH E2B (R3) will be mandatory.

3.1.3 Annual reporting and the DSUR

In Japan, periodic reports for investigational drugs were required for the first time

告制度（以下，6か月定期報告）が最初である。この6か月定期報告は，これに先立ち厚生労働省（以下，厚労省）に設置された「治験のあり方に関する検討会」が2007年9月に提出した報告書の提言の1つ，「治験中の副作用等報告の整理と定期報告制度の導入」を受け，導入された。本検討報告書の作成当時，同時にICHではICH E2F（DSUR：Development Safety Update Report）ガイドラインの検討が進められていたことから，報告書には「ICH E2F ガイドラインの導入時には，DSUR と半年ごとの定期報告との位置付けを見直す」とされていた。

ICH E2F ガイドラインは2010年9月にICHで合意され，日本では2012年12月にこれに基づく治験薬の年次報告（以下，年次報告）を導入する通知が発出された。日本における年次報告の構成は，

① 治験安全性最新報告概要（以下，年次報告概要）
② 国内重篤副作用等症例の発現状況一覧（以下，国内重篤副作用一覧）
③ 治験安全性最新報告（以下，DSUR）

の3部からなり，この③が ICH E2F ガイドラインに基づいて作成された DSUR に該当する（図3.1）。

DSUR が英語で作成されている場合は，英語で提出することが可能であるが，年次報告概要と国内重篤副作用一覧は和文で作成することとされている。年次報告概要の「重篤副作用及びその他の安全性情報の集積評価を踏まえた見解及び安全対策」欄の記載は DSUR の内容（特に，エグゼクティブサマリー）を基本とし，国内における状況，治験依頼者の見解等を追加して記載することとされている。年次報告

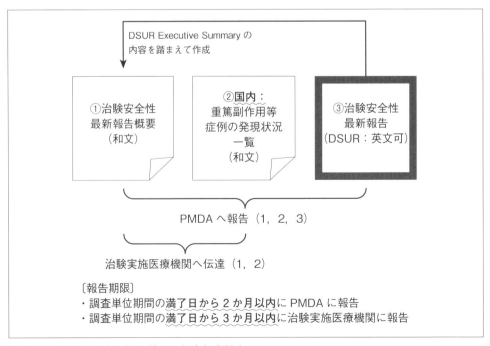

図3.1　DSUR：国内通知に基づく年次報告提出

under the system for periodic reporting at six month-intervals that came into force in April 2009 (hereinafter, six-month periodic reporting). Six-month periodic reporting was introduced with the "organizing of ADR reports during clinical trials and introduction of periodic reporting system," which was one of the recommendations on reporting submitted in September 2007 by the "Review Committee on Ways of Clinical Trials" which was established at the Ministry of Health, Labour and Welfare (hereinafter, MHLW). At the time when this review report was prepared, the ICH E2F Development Safety Update Report (DSUR) Guideline was also being considered within ICH, and with that background, the report included the statement, "At the time of introduction of the ICH E2F Guideline, the positioning of the DSUR and period reports at six month-intervals will be readjusted."

The ICH E2F Guideline was agreed upon at the September 2010 ICH meeting, and in Japan, a notification of the introduction of annual reporting for investigational drugs based on the guideline (hereinafter, annual reporting) was issued in December 2012. In Japan, annual reporting is composed of:

[1] A summary of the clinical trial safety updated report (hereinafter, summary of the annual report)
[2] A list of the current status of domestic serious ADRs (hereinafter, list of domestic serious ADRs)
[3] The clinical trial safety updated report (hereinafter, DSUR)

Part [3] corresponds to DSURs prepared based on the ICH E2F Guideline (**Fig. 3.1**).

If a DSUR is prepared in English, it is possible to submit it in English, but the summary of the annual report and list of domestic serious ADRs should be prepared in

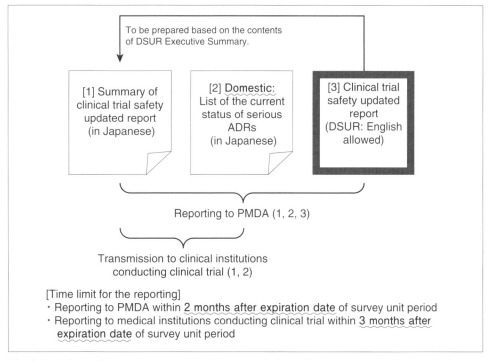

Fig.3.1 DSUR: Submission of Annual Report based on Domestic Notifications

の報告期限は開発国際誕生日をもとに設定した調査単位期間ごとに，その期間の満了した日から2か月以内に規制当局へ前述の①〜③の資料を提出する。

年次報告の規制当局への報告義務期間は，初回治験計画届出日から承認取得日，または開発中止届出の提出日までである。承認取得または開発中止届提出の際には，その日を起算に2か月以内に最後の年次報告として年次報告概要および国内重篤副作用一覧を提出する必要がある。

3.1.4　治験実施施設への安全性情報伝達

治験実施施設への安全性情報伝達の範囲はGCP省令第20条に定められており，治験依頼者は治験薬概要書から予測できない重篤副作用症例報告，研究報告，措置報告について，直ちに治験責任医師および治験実施医療機関の長に通知する必要がある。また，年次報告については，調査単位期間の満了後3か月以内に，治験責任医師および実施医療機関の長へ，年次報告概要および国内重篤副作用一覧（3.1.3項で説明した①，②の資料）を提出することとされている。

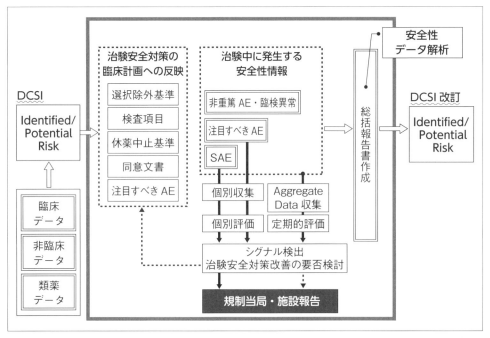

図3.2　臨床試験におけるリスクマネジメント

Japanese. The description in the column, "View and safety measures based on cumulative evaluation of serious ADRs and other safety information" in the summary of the annual report is to be based on the contents of the DSUR (particularly, the Executive Summary). The status of the program in Japan, the sponsor's view, etc., are to be added to the description. The above-mentioned materials [1] to [3] are to be submitted to the regulatory authorities within two months from the date of completion of each reporting period which is based on the development International Birth Date (IBD).

The obligation to make annual reports to the regulatory authorities extends from the date of the initial clinical trial plan notification to the date of approval of or the date of submission of the notification of discontinuation of development. The summary of the annual report and a list of domestic serious ADRs must be submitted as the final annual report within two months from the time of approval or submission of the notification of discontinuation of development.

3.1.4 Transmission of safety information to study sites

The scope of transmission of safety information to study sites is defined in Article 20 of the GCP ministerial ordinance. Sponsors need to immediately notify investigators and heads of medical institutions conducting clinical trials about reports of serious ADRs which are unexpected based on the investigator's brochure, and also research reports and reports of measures taken in foreign countries. In addition, the summary of the annual report and list of domestic serious ADRs (materials [1] and [2] explained in section 3.1.3) are to be submitted to investigators and the heads of medical institutions within three months from the completion of the reporting period.

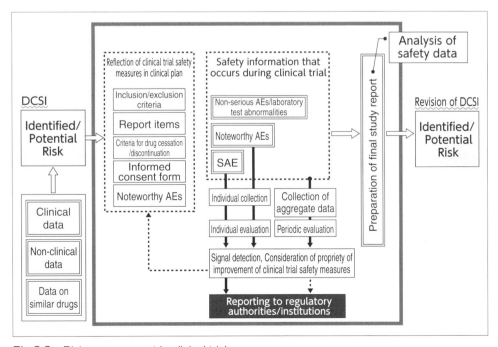

Fig.3.2　Risk management in clinical trials

3.1.5 リスク最小化策

治験中のリスクマネジメントについて，独立したリスク管理計画（RMP：Risk Management Plan）等の作成を求める国内規制は存在しない。しかしながら，GCP を遵守し，適切に計画された治験実施計画書をもとに治験を実施することが最大の治験中のリスクマネジメントになることは明らかである。治験実施計画書の選択・除外基準，治験薬の中止基準，適切な間隔での問診・臨床検査の実施は副作用発現の予知・予防策となりうるし，同意説明文書に予想される副作用やリスクを適切に反映させることで，被験者およびその家族とリスクコミュニケーションをとることができる。

なお，2005 年に発表された国際医学団体協議会（CIOMS：Council for International Organizations of Medical Science）Working Group VI 報告「臨床試験からの安全性情報の取り扱い」では，医薬品の研究開発期間を通じて得られるデータを具体的な安全対策につなげるために治験依頼者が留意すべき事項が具体的に述べられている。例えば，

- 非臨床データ，類薬情報，臨床試験のデータをもとに治験薬の安全性プロファイルをまとめた治験中核安全性情報（DCSI：Development Core Safety Information）を作成し，臨床開発期間を通じて管理すること
- 治験中に収集すべき安全性情報として，有害事象，重篤有害事象，臨床検査値等の一般的なデータに加え，特に注目すべき有害事象（AESI：Adverse Event of Special Interest）を設定し，当該治験薬で特に懸念される有害事象について評価に有用なデータを速やかに収集する仕組みをつくること
- 治験薬の安全性について包括的かつ科学・医学的な評価を可能にするために，機能横断的な安全性管理チーム（SMT：Safety Management Team）を構成し，定期的な安全性データの評価を行うこと

があげられている。

また，世界共通に使用可能な新たな治験中の年次報告として DSUR が検討されたのも本報告書の提案をもとにしている。わが国でも国際共同治験への参画などをきっかけに，CIOMS-VI を参考にしたリスクマネジメント（図 3.2）を行う試験が増加してきている。

3.2 治験中の安全性情報の活用

治験中に安全性情報を収集することの第一の目的は，治験中の被験者の保護である。治験の実施が医薬品の承認申請の際に使用する臨床試験成績の資料の収集を目的としていることから，有効性データとともに安全性データについても申請用の資料収集が意識されるが，臨床開発期間中であっても，収集された安全性データを速やかに治験中のリスクマネジメントに反映させていくことが重要である。

3.1.5 Risk Minimization Plan

There are no regulations in Japan that require the preparation of an independent risk management plan (RMP：Risk Management Plan), etc., during clinical trials. However, it is obvious that implementing clinical trials in compliance with GCP based on an appropriately-planned protocol can be the optimal risk management plan during clinical development. Inclusion/exclusion criteria, the criteria specified in the protocol for interruption of the investigational drug, and conduct of study visits and laboratory tests at appropriate intervals can be preventive measures for ADRs. Appropriately reflecting expected ADRs and risks in the informed consent document enables communication with subjects and their families.

The CIOMS (Council for International Organizations of Medical Science) Working Group VI Report "Handling of Safety Information from Clinical Studies" released in 2005 concretely describes what sponsors should do in order to apply data obtained throughout the drug research & development period to concrete safety measures. For example,

- Development Core Safety Information (DCSI) which summarizes the safety profile of investigational drugs based on non-clinical data, information on other drugs in the same class, and data from clinical studies should be prepared and updated throughout the clinical development period;
- Adverse Events of Special Interest (AESI) should be specified in addition to general data such as adverse events, serious adverse events, and laboratory test values, and a mechanism to promptly collect data useful for evaluation should be created for adverse events of particular concern for the relevant investigational drug;
- A cross-functional Safety Management Team (SMT) should be organized to enable comprehensive and scientific/medical evaluation for the safety of investigational drugs and periodic safety data should be evaluated.

Consideration of DSURs as a new annual report during clinical trials which could be available for common use throughout the world was begun based on the proposals in this report. In Japan as well, in the wake of such things as participation in global clinical trials, risk management in clinical studies with reference to CIOMS-VI (**Fig. 3.2**) has been increasing.

3.2 Utilization of safety information during clinical trials

The primary purpose for collection of safety information during clinical trials is to protect subjects during clinical trials. Clinical trials are intended to collect data to be used when making applications for marketing approval for drugs, and therefore there is an awareness of collection of safety data in addition to efficacy data for those applications, but even during the clinical development period, it is important to promptly reflect newly collected safety data in risk management during clinical trials.

また，医薬品開発のスピードアップは全世界的な潮流であり，国際共同治験の実施による世界同時開発，同時申請は開発期間の短縮を可能にするが，従来の承認申請準備のように，十分な日本人データを中心に市販後安全対策を検討するということは困難になる。したがって，臨床試験終了時に入手された副作用データのみを注視することなく，臨床開発計画全体や各治験がどのようにデザインされ実施されているか，また，収集されたデータが臨床開発期間を通じてどのように評価されているかを理解した上で，申請用の安全性データパッケージの強み，弱みを把握し，市販後安全対策につなげていくことが重要であろう。

Acceleration of drug development is a worldwide trend. Worldwide simultaneous development and applications through performing global clinical trials enables a shortening of the development period, but under these circumstances, it can be more difficult to obtain sufficient Japanese data for planning post-marketing safety measures compared to the previous way of making preparations for marketing applications. For this reason, it is important to grasp the strengths and weaknesses of the safety data package used for the marketing application and plan post-marketing safety measures with an understanding of how the entire clinical development plan and each clinical trial have been designed and implemented and how the data collected were evaluated throughout the clinical development period, instead of only paying close attention to the final ADR data itself.

第4章

わが国の市販後リスク管理の概要

　厚生労働大臣が設置した「薬害肝炎事件の検証及び再発防止のための医薬品行政のあり方検討委員会」から，最終提言が2010年4月に公表された。最終提言では，医薬品の市販後安全対策をさらに強化するために何をすべきかの提言が盛り込まれている。そこには，「開発段階から市販後に懸念される課題を抽出し，市販後において個々の懸念される課題に対応した安全性確保の措置や安全性監視活動が必要かを検討する仕組みが必要であり，欧米における制度を参考に，リスクマネジメントを適切に実施すべきである」とされている。これを受けて2013年4月1日以降に製造販売承認申請される新医薬品とバイオ後続品から医薬品リスク管理計画（RMP）の策定が求められることになった。

　このように，市販後安全対策の強化策として，わが国に医薬品リスク管理計画（RMP：Risk Management Plan）が導入された背景は，薬害再発防止のための取り組みに起因している。

　ただし，RMPは導入されたものの，その構成を成すのは，従来のわが国のPMS制度の3本柱である「副作用・感染症報告制度」，「再審査制度」，「再評価制度」である。

　本章ではこれら軸となる制度の概要を述べたのちに，RMPについて言及する。

4.1　副作用・感染症等報告制度

　1960年代初頭のサリドマイド薬害の広がりを契機として，世界的に自発報告制度が開始された。日本の副作用・感染症等報告制度は，厚生労働省（以下，厚労省），医師，歯科医師，薬剤師等の医薬関係者と製造販売業者等が協力して安全性情報を収集し，報告することが医薬品医療機器等法（旧称：薬事法）で定められている。この5年間の製造販売業者からの報告，医薬関係者からの副作用報告数について**表4.1**に示す。加えて，2010年4月28日に公表された「薬害再発防止のための医薬品行政等の見直しについて（最終提言）」を受けて，試行的に患者からの副作用報告制度を開始した。その後，2019年3月26日からウェブシステムへの入力または紙媒体の郵送による患者からの医薬品の副作用報告をPMDAにて受け付けることとなった（4.1.3 参照）。

Chapter 4

Summary of post-marketing risk management in Japan

The "Review Committee on Drug Administration for Investigation and Prevention of Recurrence of Drug-induced Hepatitis Cases" established by the Minister of Health, Labor and Welfare released its final recommendations in April, 2010. These final recommendations include proposals for what to do to further strengthen post-marketing safety measures for drugs. The recommendations include the statement, "It is necessary to have mechanisms to extract issues from the development stage which will be of concern in the post-marketing setting and to consider whether safety assurance measures and pharmacovigilance activities are necessary during marketing in response to individual issues of concern. Risk management should be appropriately implemented with reference to systems in the US and Europe." In response to these recommendations, it has been decided to require establishment of a pharmaceutical Risk Management Plan (RMP) for new drugs and biosimilars that are filed for manufacturing and marketing approval on or after April 1, 2013.

As described here, the background to the introduction of the RMP in Japan to strengthen post-marketing safety measures is attributable to efforts to prevent recurrence of drug-induced sufferings.

However, although the RMP has been introduced, it consists of the three conventional pillars of the Japanese PMS system, the "Adverse drug reactions and infections reporting system", "Reexamination system" and "Reevaluation system."

This chapter describes the outline of these core systems, and then discusses the RMP.

4.1 Adverse Drug Reactions and Infections reporting system

After the widespread incidence of thalidomide-induced sufferings in the beginning of 1960s, the spontaneous reporting system was started globally.

It is stipulated in the PMD Act (previous name: PAL) that the MHLW, HCPs such as physicians, dentists and pharmacists, and MAHs should cooperate in collecting and reporting safety information under the ADRs and infection, etc. reporting system in Japan. The number of reports from MAHs and the number of ADRs reported by healthcare professionals in the last 5 years are shown in **Table 4.1**. In addition, in response to the "Review of drug administration, etc. for prevention of recurrence of drug-induced sufferings (final recommendation)" which was released on April 28, 2010, a system for patients directly reporting ADRs was created on a trial basis. After that, Direct ADR reports from patients have been accepted by PMDA from March 26, 2019, either by direct entry to a web system or by mail in paper. (see 4.1.3 in Chapter 4)

84 第4章 わが国の市販後リスク管理の概要

表 4.1 副作用等報告件数

①医薬品

年度	製造販売業者からの報告 (単位：件) [注1]					医薬関係者からの副作用報告[注3] (単位：例)
	副作用報告 [注2]	感染症報告 [注2]	研究報告	外国措置報告	感染症定期報告	
24 年度	41,254	159	884	1,134	1,117	4,147
25 年度	38,329	98	962	1,317	1,138	5,420
26 年度	49,198	78	1,099	1,219	1,098	6,180
27 年度	50,977	88	1,219	1,273	1,102	6,129
28 年度	55,728	89	1,117	1,397	1,140	6,047

注1) 報告受付後，受理した製造販売業者から取り下げ報告（報告後に医薬品を服用していなかったことなどが判明したもの等），対象外報告（報告後に追加情報により，因果関係が否定されたもの等）された報告も数に含む。

注2) 国内症例の報告。

注3) 平成24年度は，インフルエンザワクチン（新型を含む。）の予防接種法上の任意接種，接種事業における副反応及び子宮頸がん予防ワクチン，Hib（ヒブ）ワクチン，小児用肺炎球菌ワクチンのワクチン接種緊急促進事業における副反応について，厚生労働省で一元的に報告を収集したものを含む。また，平成25年度よりすべてのワクチンに係る予防接種後の副反応報告を「医薬関係者からの報告」に含む。

出典：平成29年版厚生労働省白書

4.1.1 企業報告制度

　企業報告制度は副作用自発報告，文献・学会情報や製造販売後調査・試験等からの個別副作用等について企業が収集した副作用・感染症症例を規制当局へ報告するもので，1967年の「医薬品の製造承認等に関する基本方針について」（薬発第645号薬務局長通知：昭和42年9月13日）に基づく行政指導により，新医薬品に対する承認後2年間の副作用報告義務等の対策がとられ，同年10月より開始された。1971年に副作用報告義務期間が3年に延長されたが，当時はこの報告義務期間は新薬の販売独占期間とされた。その後，スモン等の重大な副作用被害の発生を受け1979年10月に薬事法が改正され，副作用報告も当時の薬事法第69条（医薬品医療機器等法第68条の10）として法制化され，具体的な報告基準は薬事法施行規則第62条第2項（医薬品医療機器等法施行規則第228条の20）として定められた。このときの報告期日は，「未知・重篤」副作用のケースでも30日以内であり，報告対象は国内症例に限られていた。1993年の抗ウイルス薬ソリブジンとフルオロウラシル系抗がん薬の併用による重篤な副作用被害の経験から，薬事法施行規則が改正され，1994年4月から「未知・重篤」副作用症例の報告期日は30日以内から15日以内に短縮された。1996年6月には，血液製剤のHIV（Human Immunodeficiency Virus：ヒト免疫不全ウイルス）による汚染などから一層の安全対策強化が図られ，1997年4月より生物由来製品およびその原料や材料由来の感染症症例報告が追加され，副作用・感染症症例報告となった。感染症症例報告における死亡例や重大な

Table 4.1 Number of ADRs, etc. reported.

[1] Drugs

Fiscal year	Reports from MAHs (unit: number of cases)[Note 1]					ADR reports from healthcare professionals[Note 3] (unit: number of subjects)
	ADR reports[Note 2]	Infection reports[Note 2]	Research reports	Reports of measures taken overseas	Periodic reports of infections	
FY 2012	41,254	159	884	1,134	1,117	4,147
FY 2013	38,329	98	962	1,317	1,138	5,420
FY 2014	49,198	78	1,099	1,219	1,098	6,180
FY 2015	50,977	88	1,219	1,273	1,102	6,129
FY 2016	55,728	89	1,117	1,397	1,140	6,047

Note 1) The number includes reports that were withdrawn by MAHs after being accepted (those in which it was found that the drug had not been taken, etc.) and reports that were outside the scope of reporting (those in which the causal relationship was ruled out based on additional information after reporting).

Note 2) Reporting of domestic cases.

Note 3) For FY 2012, the number includes reports centrally collected by the MHLW for adverse reactions in the operation for voluntary vaccination of influenza vaccines (including new types) under the Preventive Vaccination Law and adverse reactions in the operation for emergency promotion of vaccination of HPV vaccine, Hib vaccine and pediatric pneumococcal vaccine. Also, from FY 2013, reports of post-vaccination adverse reactions associated with all vaccines are included in the "Reports from healthcare professionals".

Source: 2017 Annual Report on Health, Labour and Welfare

4.1.1 MAH reporting system

The MAH reporting system is the system for MAHs to report cases of ADRs and infections collected by the company to the regulatory authority, for individual ADRs, etc. from spontaneous reports, literatures/academic conferences, and post-marketing studies. Following the administrative guidance based on the "Basic Policies on Manufacturing Authorization for Drugs" (Notification No. 645 issued by the Director of Pharmaceutical Affairs Bureau, September 13, 1967) in 1967, measures were taken to require reporting of ADRs for 2 years after approval of new drugs. The system was started in October of the same year. In 1971, the period for mandatory reporting of ADRs was extended to 3 years. At that time, this period was regarded as the exclusive marketing period for new drugs. Then, in response to the occurrence of serious ADRs including SMON, the Pharmaceutical Affairs Law (PAL) was revised in October 1979. Reporting of ADRs, etc. was legislated as Article 69 of the old PAL (Article 68-10 of the PMD Act), and the detailed standards for reporting were specified under Article 62, Paragraph 2 of the PAL Enforcement Regulation (Article 228-20 of the PMD Act Enforcement Regulation). At that time, the reporting time frame was within 30 days even for cases of "unexpected/serious" ADRs, and the scope of reporting was limited to domestic cases. Triggered by the occurrence of serious ADRs due to concomitant administration of the anti-viral agent, sorivudine in combination with fluorouracil anti-cancer agents in 1993, the PAL Enforcement Regulation was revised. From April 1994, the reporting time frame for "unexpected/serious" ADRs was shortened from within 30 days to within 15 days. In June 1996, further efforts were made to strengthen the safety measures in response to the contamination of blood products with human

感染症については，15日以内の報告とともに緊急対応の必要性からFAXにより第一報を報告することとされた。また，外国における同一成分医薬品の中止・回収等の重大な措置に関する「外国措置報告」が新設され，15日以内の報告に加え，FAX報告も行うこととなった。さらに2005年の副作用報告基準の見直しにより，製造販売業者等が死亡例，未知・重篤症例や既知・重篤症例をPMDAに緊急報告を行うとともに，未知・非重篤副作用症例については定期報告することになっている（表4.2）。

なお，副作用・感染症症例報告，研究報告や外国措置報告については，現在ICH E2B/M2に基づいた電子報告とされているが，2016年4月1日よりICH E2B（R3）実装ガイドに基づいた電子報告が開始された（2019年3月31日までは猶予期間）。

また，機械器具等と一体的に製造販売するものとして承認を受けた医薬品（いわゆる医薬品たるコンビネーション製品）の機械器具部分の不具合については，医薬品医療機器等法施行規則の改正により，製造販売する医薬品製造販売業者から新たに不具合報告の提出が義務化された（2014年11月25日から施行，報告期限等の基準は医療機器の不具合報告に準じる）。

4.1.2 医療機関報告制度

4.1.1で述べたとおり，日本では1967年9月の基本方針通知を出したが，その前の3月に行政指導に基づく国の医療機関モニター報告制度が開始された。本制度においては，大学病院，国立病院192か所をモニター病院に指定し，医薬品副作用事例を規制当局へ直接報告するよう協力を依頼したもので，その後，1983年ごろを境に企業報告数がモニター報告数を上回るようになったことからモニター病院数が拡大された。しかし，1997年7月からはモニター報告制度を廃止し，医薬品等安全性情報報告制度を発足させ，すべての医療機関および薬局から厚労省が直接医薬品の副作用等の報告を受ける制度を整備し，2002年の薬事法改正により，「薬局開設者，病院，診療所若しくは飼育動物診療施設の開設者又は医師，歯科医師，薬剤師，登録販売者，獣医師その他の医薬関係者は，医薬品又は医療機器について，当該品目の副作用その他の事由によるものと疑われる疾病，障害若しくは死亡の発生又は当該品目の使用によるものと疑われる感染症の発生に関する事項を知った場合において，保健衛生上の危害の発生又は拡大を防止するため必要があると認めたときには，その旨を厚生労働大臣に報告しなければならない。」とされて，2003年より実施されている（医薬品医療機器等法688条の10の2）。さらに後発品シェア80%時代到来とも言われている時代やポリファーマシーによる複合的な副作用の発生などにおいては，医療機関報告の果たす役割はますます重要となっており，「医薬関係者の副作用報告ガイダンス骨子」が公表されている（厚生労働省医薬・生活衛生局総務課・厚生労働省医薬・生活衛生局安全対策課 事務連絡 平成29年7月10日）。この5年間の報告数の推移については，表4.1を参照のこと。

immunodeficiency virus (HIV). Reporting of infections from biological products and their raw materials was added in April 1997 and the system became one for reporting ADRs and infections. For deaths and serious infections in infection case reports, it was specified to send the first report via fax, given the necessity of emergency measures along with a report within 15 days. In addition, "Report of measures taken overseas" was newly established for significant measures taken in foreign countries including discontinuation or recall of drugs with the same ingredient. The report was to be sent via fax, followed by a report within 15 days. Also, based on a review of the ADR reporting criteria in 2005, MAHs etc. are required to submit expedited reports of deaths, unexpected/serious ADRs and expected/serious ADRs to the PMDA as well as submitting unexpected/non-serious ADRs in periodic reports (**Table 4.2**).

Currently, ADR and infection case reports, research reports, and reports of measures taken overseas are made as electronic reports under ICH E2B/M2. Electronic reporting based on the ICH E2B (R3) Implementation Guide was started in April 1, 2016 (to be officially started by March 31, 2019).

An obligation to submit defect reports for medical devices that are approved and marketed as so-called combination products with drugs, came into effect with the revision of the PMD Act Enforcement Regulations (enacted on November 25, 2014, Standards for reporting time frame, etc. conform to defect reports for medical devices).

4.1.2 Medical institution reporting system

As described in section 4.1.1, notification on the basic policy was issued in September 1967 in Japan. In the previous March, the medical institution monitoring report system was started based on administrative guidance. Under this system, 192 university hospitals and national hospitals were designated as monitoring hospitals and were asked to cooperate in direct reporting of ADRs to the regulatory authority. Subsequently, the number of reports from companies exceeded the number of reports from monitoring hospitals in around 1983, and the number of monitoring hospitals was increased. However, the monitoring report system was abolished and the drugs and medical devices safety information reporting system was started in July 1997. A system was established for the Ministry of Health, Labour and Welfare to directly receive reports of ADRs, etc. from all medical institutions and pharmacies. Following the revision of the PAL in 2002, it was specified that "establishers of pharmacies, hospitals, clinics and animal care facilities as well as healthcare professionals such as physicians, dentists, pharmacists, registered sales clerks and veterinarians <u>must report</u> to the Minister of Health, Labour and Welfare the occurrence of disorders, impairments or deaths that are suspected to be caused by reasons such as ADRs associated with pharmaceuticals or medical devices or the occurrence of infections that are suspected to be caused by the use of pharmaceuticals or medical devices when it is deemed necessary to prevent onset or expansion of risks to public health and hygiene." It has been enforced since 2003 (Article 68-10, Paragraph 2 of the PMD Act). Furthermore, reporting from medical institutions has become more and more important now that generic products account for as much as 80% of the share and complex ADRs occur due to polypharmacy, leading to the release of "Outline of the guidance on reporting of ADRs by healthcare professionals (Office memorandum by the General Affairs Division, Pharmaceutical Safety and Environmental Health Bureau

88　第4章　わが国の市販後リスク管理の概要

表 4.2　企業報告制度のタイムフレーム（医薬品）
注：ここで「感染症」とは，医薬品への病原体の混入によると疑われる感染症のことを指す。

	予測性	重篤性	国内	国外
副作用症例の発生	「使用上の注意」から予測できない（未知）	重篤（死亡）	15日 ＋ FAX 等	15日
		重篤（死亡以外）	15日	15日
		重篤でない	医薬品未知・非重篤副作用定期報告：承認後2年間は6か月ごと，それ以降は1年ごと	―
	「使用上の注意」から予測できる（既知）	重篤（死亡）	15日	―
		重篤（死亡以外）	承認2年以内の新有効成分，効能・用法追加等で市販直後調査期間中：15日	―
			上記以外：30日	―
		重篤でない	―	―
重篤な副作用の発生数，発生頻度，発生条件等の発生傾向が「使用上の注意」から予測できないもの，または，発生傾向が著しく変化したもの，発生傾向の変化が保健衛生上の危害の発生または拡大のおそれを示すもの			15日 ＋ FAX 等	15日
感染症症例の発生	「使用上の注意」から予測できない（未知）	重篤（死亡）	15日 ＋ FAX 等	15日 ＋ FAX 等
		重篤（死亡以外）	15日 ＋ FAX 等	15日 ＋ FAX 等
		重篤でない	15日 ＋ FAX 等	―
	「使用上の注意」から予測できる（既知）	重篤（死亡）	15日 ＋ FAX 等	15日 ＋ FAX 等
		重篤（死亡以外）	15日 ＋ FAX 等	15日 ＋ FAX 等
		重篤でない	―	―
研究報告	副作用・感染症により，がんその他の重大な疾病，障害もしくは死亡が発生するおそれがあることを示す研究報告		30日	30日
	副作用症例・感染症の発生数，発生頻度，発生条件等の発生傾向が著しく変化したことを示す研究報告		30日	30日
	承認を受けた効能もしくは効果を有しないことを示す研究報告		30日	30日
外国措置報告	製造，輸入または販売の中止，回収，廃棄その他保健衛生上の危害の発生または拡大を防止する措置の実施		―	15日 ＋ FAX 等

Table4.2　Time frame for MAH reporting system (drugs)

Note) Infections: Infections suspected to be due to contamination of pathogen into drug

	Expectedness	Seriousness	Japan	Overseas
Occurrence of ADRs	Unexpected from "precautions for use" (unknown)	Serious (fatal)	15 days + FAX, etc.	15 days
		Serious (non-fatal)	15 days	15 days
		Not serious	Periodic reports of unknown/non-serious adverse drug reactions: Every 6 months for 2 years after approval, and subsequently once every year	—
	Expected from "precautions for use" (known)	Serious (fatal)	15 days	—
		Serious (non-fatal)	During Early Post-marketing Phase Risk Minimization and Vigilance (EPPV) for new active ingredient, additional indication/dose regimen, etc. within 2 years after approval: 15 days	—
			Other than the above: 30 days	—
		Not serious	—	—
Serious ADRs whose trend of occurrence, such as number of cases, frequency, and conditions for occurrence cannot be expected from "precautions for use" or trend of occurrence has markedly changed or for which a change in trend of occurrence may cause or expand a hazard in terms of health and hygiene			15 days + FAX, etc.	15 days
Occurrence of infections	Unexpected from "precautions for use" (unknown)	Serious (fatal)	15 days + FAX, etc.	15 days + FAX, etc.
		Serious (non-fatal)	15 days + FAX, etc.	15 days + FAX, etc.
		Not serious	15 days + FAX, etc.	—
	Expected from "precautions for use" (known)	Serious (fatal)	15 days + FAX, etc.	15 days + FAX, etc.
		Serious (non-fatal)	15 days + FAX, etc.	15 days + FAX, etc.
		Not serious	—	—
Research reports	Research reports showing that cancer or other significant disease, disability, or death may occur due to ADR and infection		30 days	30 days
	Research reports that the trend of occurrence of ADR and infection such as number of cases, frequency, and conditions for occurrence have markedly changed		30 days	30 days
	Research reports showing failure of the approved indication or effect.		30 days	30 days
Reports of measures taken overseas	Discontinuation of manufacturing, import, or selling, as well as recall, discarding, or other measure to prevent the occurrence or expansion of a hazard in terms of health and hygiene		—	15 days + FAX, etc.

4.1.3　患者副作用報告システム

　欧米各国における患者からの副作用報告制度の導入，ならびに，2010 年 4 月に公表された「薬害再発防止のための医薬品行政等の見直しについて（最終提言）」における「患者からの副作用報告制度の創設」の提言を受けて 2009 年 4 月から厚生労働科学研究事業により「患者から副作用情報を受ける方策に関する調査研究」[1]が実施された。それらの結果を踏まえたうえで，厚労省は 2019 年 3 月 26 日に「患者からの医薬品副作用報告」実施要領（https://www.mhlw.go.jp/content/11126000/000414743.pdf）を公表し，ウェブシステムへの入力または紙媒体の郵送による患者からの医薬品の副作用報告を PMDA にて受け付けることとなった。

この患者副作用報告システムでの必須報告項目は以下のとおりである。

- ・　報告者情報（氏名，年齢，住所など）
- ・　患者情報（報告者と患者の関係，患者性別，患者の副作用発現時の年齢，原疾患，既往歴）
- ・　副作用情報（副作用症状，副作用発現時期，副作用の転帰，医薬品の使用目的）
- ・　医薬品情報（副作用を引き起こしたと思われる医薬品名）
- ・　医療機関情報（副作用症状について詳細を聞くことができる医療機関の有無）

　試行的に開始された 2013 年以降の年次ごとの報告の概要が PMDA のサイト（https://www.pmda.go.jp/safety/reports/patients/0002.html）に掲載されている。

4.1.4　WHO モニタリング制度

　WHO では，1968 年に国際医薬品モニタリング制度を発足させ，2016 年 1 月時点で，123 か国が制度に加入している。WHO は参加国から副作用情報を収集し，現在では 1,400 万もの症例報告を蓄積し，その概要を，参加国にフィードバックしている（図 4.1）。日本は 1972 年より WHO モニタリング制度に参加し，収集した国内における副作用症例を報告している。

4.1.5　ワクチンの副反応報告制度

　ワクチンは，医薬品医療機器等法で定められた医薬品（医薬品医療機器等法第 2条 1 項）である。同時に，予防接種法に定められている「予防接種」に用いるものである。そのため，ワクチン（本節では予防ワクチンを指す）の市販後安全性対策には，通常の医薬品とは異なる点が多い。医薬品としての規制は，他項でも述べられている医薬品医療機器等法第 68 条の 10 であるが，これに加えてワクチン特有の規制である予防接種法が市販後安全性対策においても深くかかわってくる。本節では，ワクチンの副反応報告に焦点を当てて紹介する。

Chapter 4 Summary of post-marketing risk management in Japan **91**

(PSEHB), MHLW, and Safety Division, PSEHB, MHLW, July 10, 2017). See **Table 4.1** for the change in the numbers of reports in the last 5 years.

4.1.3 Patient Adverse Drug Reaction reporting system

In response to the introduction of patient ADR reporting systems in the US and European countries and the recommendation for "Establishment of patient ADR reporting system" in the "Review of drug administration, etc. for prevention of recurrence of drug-induced sufferings (final recommendation)" which was released in April 2010, the "Research on System for Receiving Adverse Reaction Information from Patients"[1] was conducted by the Health, Labour, and Welfare Science Research Operation from April 2009. Based on those results, MHLW published "Guidelines for reporting ADRs from patients directly" on March 26, 2019, and patients can report to PMDA by inputting to the web system or by mailed paper.

[1] Information on reporter (name, age, address, etc.)
[2] Patient information (relationship between reporter and patient, gender of patient, age of patient at the onset of ADR, primary disease, past history)
[3] ADR information (ADR symptom, onset time of ADR, outcome of ADR, reason for using the drug)
[4] Drug information (name of drug suspected to have caused ADR)
[5] Medical institution information (presence/absence of medical institution from which the details of ADR symptom can be inquired)

The outline of the annual report in and after 2013 when the trial operation was started is posted on the PMDA's website (https://www.pmda.go.jp/safety/reports/patients/0002.html).

4.1.4 WHO monitoring system

The World Health Organization (WHO) started the International Drug Monitoring System in 1968 and a total of 123 countries have participated in the system as of January 2016. WHO collects information on ADRs from the participating countries, and has now accumulated 14 million case reports. The WHO sends summaries to the participating countries (**Fig. 4.1**)[18]. Japan joined the WHO monitoring system in 1972 and has been submitting ADR case reports collected in Japan.

4.1.5 Vaccine Adverse Reactions reporting system

Vaccines are drugs specified by the PMD Act (Article 2, Paragraph 1 of the PMD Act). At the same time, they are used for "preventive vaccinations" specified in the Preventive Vaccination Law. As such, post-marketing safety measures for vaccines (preventive vaccines in this section) are different from those for general drugs in many respects. While vaccines as drugs are regulated under the Article 68-10 of the PMD Act as described in other sections, the Preventive Vaccination Law, the law specific to vaccines is also deeply involved in the post-marketing safety measures for vaccines. This section focuses on reporting of adverse reactions to vaccines.

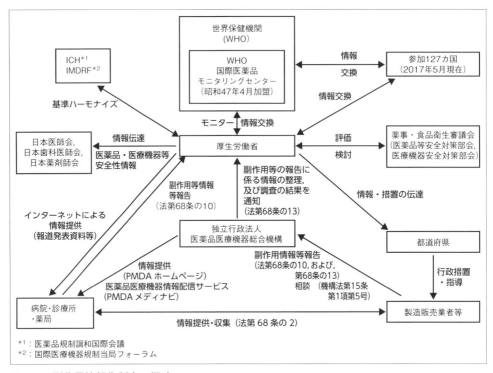

図 4.1 副作用等報告制度の概略 (2012年(平成24年) 厚生労働白書 資料編)

4.1.5.1 ワクチンの副反応報告制度に関する法的根拠

ワクチンの副反応報告は医薬品医療機器等法および予防接種法により規定されている。医薬品医療機器等法第 68 条の 10 で規定されている報告義務の法的根拠については，医薬品で述べられているとおりである。一方，予防接種法上でも副反応報告について規定されている。2013 年 4 月の予防接種法改正では「医療機関から厚生労働大臣への報告」の義務が法律レベルで規定された（予防接種法第 12 条第 1 項）。ここで報告が義務化されているのは「定期の予防接種・臨時の予防接種」の対象となっているワクチンである。つまり，予防接種法上の「義務」の範囲は，「予防接種法で A 類，B 類に規定されている疾病に対するワクチン」のみであり，すべてのワクチンが対象となっていない点には留意が必要である。予防接種法に規定されている報告は医薬品医療機器等法第 68 条 10 第 2 項に規定されている報告としても取り扱うこととされており，当該報告を行った医師は，重ねて医薬品医療機器等法上規定されている報告を行う必要がないことが「定期の予防接種等による副反応の報告等の取扱いについて」（健発 0330 第 3 号，薬食発 033 第 1 号厚生労働省健康局長，厚生労働省医薬食品局長通知：平成 25 年 3 月 30 日）に記載されている。しかしながら，医薬品医療機器等法第 68 条 10 第 1 項の製造販売業者の報告義務を免除するものではない。そのため，同一症例が，製造販売業者が医療機関等より得た情報の製造販売業者から規制当局への報告，および医療機関等からの厚労省への直接

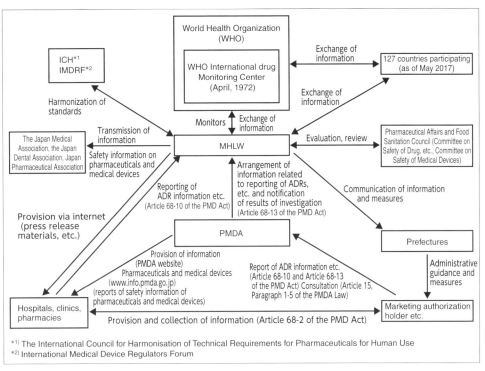

Fig.4.1 Outline of the reporting system of ADRs etc. (From Annual White Paper of the MHLW in 2012)

4.1.5.1 Legal grounds for vaccine adverse reaction reporting system

The reporting of adverse reactions to vaccines is regulated by the PMD Act and the Preventive Vaccination Law. The legal grounds for mandatory reporting specified in the Article 68-10 of the PMD Act are described in the sections of drugs. On the other hand, reporting of adverse reactions is also specified by the Preventive Vaccination Law. In the Preventive Vaccinations Act revised in April 2013, "reporting from medical institutions to the Minister of Health, Labour and Welfare" was mandated by the law (Article 12, Paragraph 1 of the Preventive Vaccination Law). Under this law, reporting is mandated for vaccines that are included in the "routine and provisional preventive vaccinations". Thus, it should be noted that the scope of "mandatory reporting" by the Preventive Vaccination Law only includes "vaccines for diseases that are classified into categories A and B in the Preventive Vaccination Law" and that not all vaccines are subjected to mandatory reporting. The reporting specified by the Preventive Vaccination Law is also regarded as the reporting specified by the Article 68-10, Paragraph 2 of the PMD Act. It is specified in "Handling of reporting of adverse reactions to routine preventive vaccinations" (HSB Notification No. 0330-3, PFSB Notification No. 033-1, March 30, 2013, Director of HSB, MHLW and Director of PFSB, MHLW) that a physician who has filed a report in accordance with the Preventive Vaccination Law is not required to file the same report as specified by the PMD Act. However, this does not exempt MAHs from mandatory reporting under Article 68-10, Paragraph 1 of the PMD Act. Thus, the same case may be reported via two routes: from a MAH reporting the information obtained from a medical institution to the regulatory authority and from a medical

報告，という2つのルートで報告されることがある。

4.1.5.2　報告義務症例の定義と様式

　予防接種法施行規則第5条の規定によると，予防接種法上で医療機関からの報告義務の対象となるのは，「定期の予防接種等を受けたことによるものと疑われる症状として厚生労働省省令で定めるもの」とされている。報告対象発生期間もワクチンごと・事象ごとに細かく設定されている。詳しくは，前述した「定期の予防接種等による副反応の報告等の取扱いについて」の別紙様式1（図4.2）で確認できる。ここで規定されている報告については全例報告対象，つまり実質的には有害事象の収集（因果関係は問わない）となっている。また，規定されているのは「義務」の範囲である。規定に合致しないものを「報告不要」としているわけでない点は留意が必要である。

4.1.5.3　副反応検討部会による収集データの検討

　現在，予防接種政策に対して進言する目的で3つの委員会（予防接種基本方針部会，副反応検討部会，研究開発及び生産・流通部会）が予防接種法で規定されている。このうち副反応検討部会は，ワクチンの副反応を検討する委員会として安全性情報評価の責務を負っている。副反応検討部会は医薬品等安全対策部会安全対策調査会との合同開催として実施され，医薬品医療機器等法に基づき収集された安全性情報と予防接種法に基づいて収集された安全性情報を総合的に検討している。

4.2　市販直後調査

　わが国では1993年，新薬の市販直後に重篤な副作用事例を経験している。すなわち，新薬であるソリブジン（抗ウイルス薬）の添付文書の相互作用の欄にはフルオロウラシル系薬剤について「両剤の併用を避けること」と記載していたにもかかわらず，フルオロウラシル系抗がん薬の使用者での帯状疱疹治療にソリブジンが投与されたことによる重篤な骨髄抑制により，多数の死亡例が報告された。この事件を契機として，新薬の適正使用の徹底と副作用情報収集の徹底を目的とした，新薬に対する市販直後調査が導入された。

4.2.1　目的

　新薬市販直後の安全対策の必要性については，米国食品医薬品局（FDA：Food and Drug Administration）のリスクマネジメントに関するタスクフォースが1999年5月にまとめた報告書 "Managing the Risks from Medical Product Use" でも指摘されていた。

　同報告書は，新薬について，医療機関を限定して販売を開始することや，専門医

Chapter 4　Summary of post-marketing risk management in Japan　95

institution reporting directly to the MHLW.

4.1.5.2 Definitions of cases for mandatory reporting and forms

According to the provisions in Article 5 of the Preventive Vaccination Law Enforcement Regulations, "those specified by the MHLW Ordinance as symptoms that are suspected to be caused by routine preventive vaccinations" are subjected to mandatory reporting by medical institutions under the Preventive Vaccination Law. The relevant time of onset is also specified in details for each vaccine and each event. The details can be checked on the Attached form 1 (**Fig. 4.2**), "Handling of reporting of adverse reactions to routine preventive vaccinations" described above. The reporting specified here targets all cases; therefore, it collects virtually all adverse events (regardless of the causal relationship). In addition, the scope is specified only for "mandatory reporting". It should be noted that those that do not meet the specifications are not "exempted from reporting".

4.1.5.3 Investigation of collected data by Vaccine Adverse Reaction Review Committee

At present, the Preventive Vaccination Law specifies three committees (Committee on Immunization Policy, Vaccine Adverse Reaction Review Committee, and Committee on Vaccine R & D, Manufacturing and Distribution) to provide recommendations on policies related to preventive vaccinations. Among these committees, the Vaccine Adverse Reaction Review Committee has the responsibility to evaluate safety information as the committee which reviews adverse reactions to vaccines. This committee is held together with the Committee on Drug Safety, and conducts a comprehensive review of safety information collected based on the PMD Act and the Preventive Vaccination Law.

4.2 Early post-marketing phase risk minimization and vigilance (EPPV)

In Japan, in 1993, a serious ADR case was experienced immediately after marketing of a new drug. Specifically, in the column of drug interactions in the package insert of the new drug sorivudine (an antiviral drug), fluorouracil drugs were described as "Concomitant use of both agents should be avoided," but there were many reports of deaths from serious bone-marrow suppression due to administration of sorivudine for the treatment of herpes zoster in users of a fluorouracil anticancer agent. In the wake of this incident, the Early post-marketing phase risk minimization and vigilance (EPPV) system was introduced for new drugs with the intention to thoroughly ensure their proper use and collection of their ADR information.

4.2.1 Objective

The necessity for risk minimization measures in the early phase after the launch of a new drug was pointed out in "Managing the Risks from Medical Product Use",[19] a report compiled by a task force related to risk management by the FDA in May of 1999.

The above report proposed that the FDA should determine the conditions for marketing a new drug such as initially restricting the number of medical institutions, restricting sales only to specialized medical institutions and specialists, and requiring

第4章　わが国の市販後リスク管理の概要

図4.2（1）　予防接種後副反応疑い報告書の様式

（別紙様式1）

報告先：（独）医薬品医療機器総合機構
FAX番号：0120－176－146

予防接種後副反応疑い報告書

予防接種法上の定期接種・任意接種の別		□　定期接種		□　任意接種	

患　者 （被接種者）	氏名又は イニシャル	（定期の場合は氏名，任意の場合はイニシャルを記載）	性別　　1 男　2 女	接種時 年齢	歳　　月
	住　所	都　道 府　県	区 市 町　村　　生年月日	T S H	年　月　日生

報　告　者	氏　名	1 接種者　　2 主治医　　3 その他（　　　　　　　　　　　）	
	医療機関名		電話番号
	住　所		

接種場所	医療機関名	
	住　所	

ワクチン	ワクチンの種類 （②〜④は、同時接種したものを記載）	ロット番号	製造販売業者名	接種回数
	①			① 第　期（　回目）
	②			② 第　期（　回目）
	③			③ 第　期（　回目）
	④			④ 第　期（　回目）

接種の状況	接種日　　平成　年　月　日 午前・午後　時　分	出生体重	グラム （患者が乳幼児の場合に記載）
	接種前の体温　　度　分　家族歴		
	予診票での留意点（基礎疾患、アレルギー、最近1か月以内のワクチン接種や病気、服薬中の薬、過去の副作用歴、発育状況等） 1 有 2 無		

症　状 の　概　要	症状	定期接種の場合で次頁の報告基準に該当する場合は、ワクチンごとに該当する症状に○をしてください。 報告基準にない症状の場合又は任意接種の場合（症状名：　　　　　　　）
	発生日時	平成　年　月　日　　午前・午後　時　分
	本剤との 因果関係	1 関連あり　2 関連なし　3 評価不能 ｜ 他要因（他の疾患等）の可能性の有無 ｜ 1 有 2 無
		概要（症状・徴候・臨床経過・診断・検査等）
		○製造販売業者への情報提供 ： 1 有　　2 無

症　状 の　程　度	1 重い	1 死亡　　2 障害　　3 死亡につながるおそれ　　4 障害につながるおそれ 5 入院　病院名：　　　　　　　　　医師名： 　　　　　平成　年　月　日入院 ／ 平成　年　月　日退院 6 上記1〜5に準じて重い　　7 後世代における先天性の疾病又は異常
	2 重くない	

症　状 の　転　帰	転帰日	平成　年　月　日
	1 回復　　2 軽快　　3 未回復　　4 後遺症（症状：　　　　　　）　　5 死亡　　6 不明	

報告者意見	

報告回数	1 第1報　　2 第2報　　3 第3報以後

Chapter 4 Summary of post-marketing risk management in Japan   97

Fig4-2 (1) Form of the Report of Suspected Adverse Reaction following Preventive Vaccination

(Attached form 1)

To be reported to: Pharmaceuticals and Medical
Devices Agency
FAX: 0120－176－146

Report of Suspected Adverse Reaction following Preventive Vaccination

Routine/voluntary vaccination category under the Preventive Vaccination Law				☐ Routine vaccination		☐ Voluntary vaccination		

Patient (person who received the vaccination)	Name or initials	(Enter the name in case of routine vaccination and initials at voluntary vaccination)	Sex	1. Male 2. Female	Age at the vaccination	Years	Months
	Address	Prefecture	City/Town/Village	Birth date	Year Month Day		

Reporter	Name			
		1. Person who provided vaccination 2. attending physician 3. Others ( )		
	Name of the medical institution		Phone number	
	Address			

Place of vaccination	Name of the medical institution	
	Address	

Vaccines	Types of vaccines (indicate concomitant vaccines in 2 to 4)	Lot number	Name of the MAH	Number of vaccinations
	1.			1. Phase XX (XXth)
	2.			2. Phase XX (XXth)
	3.			3. Phase XX (XXth)
	4.			4. Phase XX (XXth)

Circumstances at the vaccination	Date of vaccination	Year Month Day AM/PM Hour Minute	Body weight at birth	grams (indicate if the patient is an infant)
	Body temperature before vaccination	degrees	Family history	
	Considerations based on the pre-interview form (underlying diseases, allergies, vaccinations or diseases within the last one month, ongoing medications, history of adverse reactions, and status of growth, etc.) 1. Present → 2. None			

Summary of the symptoms	Symptoms	Circle the corresponding symptom(s) associated with each vaccine in the case of routine vaccination that meets the reporting criteria on the following page.
		Symptoms that are not stated in the reporting criteria or in the case of voluntary vaccination (Name of the symptom:)
	Date and time of onset	Year Month Day AM/PM Hour Minute
	Causal relationship to this product	1. Related 2. Unrelated 3. not assessable	Presence or absence of potential other factors (other diseases, etc.)	1. Present → 2. None
	Summary (symptoms, signs, clinical course, diagnosis, and tests, etc.)	
	○Provision of information to the MAH: 1. Yes 2. No	

Severity of the symptom	1. Severe →	1. Death 2. Impairment 3. Potentially leading to death 4. Potentially leading to impairment
		5. Hospitalization Name of the hospital: Name of the physician: Admitted on Year Month Day/Discharged on Year Month Day
		6. Severe as 1 to 5 above 7. Congenital disease or abnormality in later generations
	2. Not severe	

Outcome of the symptom	Date of outcome	Year Month Day
	1. Recovered 2. Improved 3. Unresolved 4. Sequelae (symptom:) 5. Death 6. Unknown	

Comment by the reporter	

Number of reports	1. First report 2. Second report 3. Third or later report

98　　第 4 章　わが国の市販後リスク管理の概要

図 4.2（2）

（別紙様式1）

対象疾病	症状		発生までの時間	左記の「その他の反応」を選択した場合の症状
ジフテリア 百日せき 急性灰白髄炎 破傷風	1	アナフィラキシー	4時間	左記の「その他の反応」を選択した場合
	2	脳炎・脳症	28日	
	3	けいれん	7日	a　無呼吸
	4	血小板減少性紫斑病	28日	b　気管支けいれん
	5	その他の反応	－	c　急性散在性脳脊髄炎（ADEM）
麻しん 風しん	1	アナフィラキシー	4時間	d　多発性硬化症
	2	急性散在性脳脊髄炎（ADEM）	28日	e　脳炎・脳症
	3	脳炎・脳症	28日	f　脊髄炎
	4	けいれん	21日	g　けいれん
	5	血小板減少性紫斑病	28日	h　ギラン・バレ症候群
	6	その他の反応	－	i　視神経炎
日本脳炎	1	アナフィラキシー	4時間	j　顔面神経麻痺
	2	急性散在性脳脊髄炎（ADEM）	28日	k　末梢神経障害
	3	脳炎・脳症	28日	l　知覚異常
	4	けいれん	7日	m　血小板減少性紫斑病
	5	血小板減少性紫斑病	28日	n　血管炎
	6	その他の反応	－	o　肝機能障害
結核（BCG）	1	アナフィラキシー	4時間	p　ネフローゼ症候群
	2	全身播種性BCG感染症	1年	q　喘息発作
	3	BCG骨炎（骨髄炎、骨膜炎）	2年	r　間質性肺炎
	4	皮膚結核様病変	3か月	s　皮膚粘膜眼症候群
	5	化膿性リンパ節炎	4か月	t　ぶどう膜炎
	6	その他の反応	－	u　関節炎
Hib感染症 小児の肺炎球菌感染症	1	アナフィラキシー	4時間	v　蜂巣炎
	2	けいれん	7日	w　血管迷走神経反射
	3	血小板減少性紫斑病	28日	x　a〜w以外の場合は前頁の「症状名」に記載
	4	その他の反応	－	
ヒトパピローマウイルス感染症	1	アナフィラキシー	4時間	
	2	急性散在性脳脊髄炎（ADEM）	28日	
	3	ギラン・バレ症候群	28日	
	4	血小板減少性紫斑病	28日	
	5	血管迷走神経反射（失神を伴うもの）	30分	
	6	疼痛又は運動障害を中心とする多様な症状	－	
	7	その他の反応	－	
水痘	1	アナフィラキシー	4時間	
	2	血小板減少性紫斑病	28日	
	3	その他の反応	－	
B型肝炎	1	アナフィラキシー	4時間	
	2	急性散在性脳脊髄炎（ADEM）	28日	
	3	多発性硬化症	28日	
	4	脊髄炎	28日	
	5	ギラン・バレ症候群	28日	
	6	視神経炎	28日	
	7	末梢神経障害	28日	
	8	その他の反応	－	
インフルエンザ	1	アナフィラキシー	4時間	
	2	急性散在性脳脊髄炎（ADEM）	28日	
	3	脳炎・脳症	28日	
	4	けいれん	7日	
	5	脊髄炎	28日	
	6	ギラン・バレ症候群	28日	
	7	視神経炎	28日	
	8	血小板減少性紫斑病	28日	
	9	血管炎	28日	
	10	肝機能障害	28日	
	11	ネフローゼ症候群	28日	
	12	喘息発作	24時間	
	13	間質性肺炎	28日	
	14	皮膚粘膜眼症候群	28日	
	15	その他の反応	－	
高齢者の肺炎球菌感染症	1	アナフィラキシー	4時間	
	2	ギラン・バレ症候群	28日	
	3	血小板減少性紫斑病	28日	
	4	注射部位壊死又は注射部位潰瘍	28日	
	5	蜂巣炎（これに類する症状であって、上腕から前腕に及ぶものを含む。）	7日	
	6	その他の反応	－	

※左端に縦書きで「報告基準（該当するものの番号に「○」を記入）」

注1）　報告受付後，受理した製造販売業者から取り下げ報告（報告後に医薬品を服用していなかったことなどが判明したもの等），対象外報告（報告後に追加情報により，因果関係が否定されたもの等）された報告も数に含む。

注2）　国内症例の報告。

注3）　平成 24 年度は，インフルエンザワクチン（新型を含む。）の予防接種法上の任意接種，接種事業における副反応及び子宮頸がん予防ワクチン，Hib（ヒブ）ワクチン，小児用肺炎球菌ワクチンのワクチン接種緊急促進事業における副反応について，厚生労働省で一元的に報告を収集したものを含む。また，平成 25 年度よりすべてのワクチンに係る予防接種後の副反応報告を「医薬関係者からの報告」に含む。

Chapter 4 Summary of post-marketing risk management in Japan

Fig4-2 (2)

(Attached form 1)

	Target disorders		Symptoms	Time to onset	Symptoms in case "Other reactions" were selected in the left column
Reporting criteria (Circle the corresponding number)	Diphtheria Pertussis Acute poliomyelitis Tetanus	1 2 3 4 5	Anaphylaxis Encephalitis/Encephalopathy Convulsions Thrombocytopenic purpura Other reactions	4 hours 28 days 7 days 28 days —	In case "Other reactions" were selected in the left column a. Apnea b. Bronchospasm c. Acute disseminated encephalomyelitis (ADEM) d. Multiple sclerosis e. Encephalitis/Encephalopathy f. Myelitis g. Convulsions h. Guillain-Barre syndrome i. Optic neuritis j. Facial paralysis k. Peripheral neuropathy l. Paresthesia m. Thrombocytopenic purpura n. Vasculitis o. Hepatic dysfunction p. Nephrotic syndrome q. Asthmatic attack r. Interstitial pneumonia s. Oculomucocutaneous syndrome t. Uveitis u. Arthritis v. Cellulitis w. Vasovagal reaction x. Symptoms other than those in a to w should be described in "Name of the symptom" on the previous page a ~ w
	Measles Rubella	1 2 3 4 5 6	Anaphylaxis Acute disseminated encephalomyelitis (ADEM) Encephalitis/Encephalopathy Convulsions Thrombocytopenic purpura Other reactions	4 hours 28 days 28 days 21 days 28 days —	
	Japanese encephalitis	1 2 3 4 5 6	Anaphylaxis Acute disseminated encephalomyelitis (ADEM) Encephalitis/Encephalopathy Convulsions Thrombocytopenic purpura Other reactions	4 hours 28 days 28 days 7 days 28 days —	
	Tuberculosis (BCG)	1 2 3 4 5 6	Anaphylaxis Systemic disseminated BCG infection BCG osteitis (osteomyelitis, periostitis) Skin tuberculosis-like lesions Suppurative lymphadenitis Other reactions	4 hours 1 year 2 years 3 months 4 months —	
	Hib infection Pediatric Pneumococcal infections	1 2 3 4	Anaphylaxis Convulsions Thrombocytopenic purpura Other reactions	4 hours 7 days 28 days —	
	Human papilloma virus infection	1 2 3 4 5 6 7	Anaphylaxis Acute disseminated encephalomyelitis (ADEM) Guillain-Barre syndrome Thrombocytopenic purpura Vasovagal reaction (with syncope) Various symptoms mainly consisting of pain or movement disorder Other reactions	4 hours 28 days 28 days 28 days 30 minutes —	
	Varicella	1 2 3	Anaphylaxis Thrombocytopenic purpura Other reactions	4 hours 28 days —	
	Hepatitis B	1 2 3 4 5 6 7 8	Anaphylaxis Acute disseminated encephalomyelitis (ADEM) Multiple sclerosis Myelitis Guillain-Barre syndrome Optic neuritis Peripheral neuropathy Other reactions	4 hours 28 days 28 days 28 days 28 days 28 days 28 days —	
	Influenza	1 2 3 4 5 6 7 8 9 10 11 12 13 14 15	Anaphylaxis Acute disseminated encephalomyelitis (ADEM) Encephalitis/Encephalopathy Convulsions Myelitis Guillain-Barre syndrome Optic neuritis Thrombocytopenic purpura Vasculitis Hepatic dysfunction Nephrotic syndrome Asthmatic attack Interstitial pneumonia Oculomucocutaneous syndrome Other reactions	4 hours 28 days 28 days 7 days 28 days 28 days 28 days 28 days 28 days 28 days 28 days 24 hours 28 days 28 days —	
	Pneumococcal infection in the elderly	1 2 3 4 5 6	Anaphylaxis Guillain-Barre syndrome Thrombocytopenic purpura Injection site necrosis or injection site ulcer Cellulitis (or similar symptoms extending from the upper arm to the forearm) Other reactions	4 hours 28 days 28 days 28 days 7 days —	

Note 1) The number includes reports that were withdrawn by MAHs after being accepted (those in which it was found that the drug had not been taken, etc.) and reports that were out of reporting scope (those in which the causal relationship was ruled out based on additional information after reporting).

Note 2) Reporting of domestic cases

Note 3) For FY 2012, the number includes reports centrally collected by the MHLW for adverse reactions in the operation for voluntary vaccination of influenza vaccines (including new types) under the Preventive Vaccination Law and adverse reactions in the operation for emergency promotion of vaccination of HPV vaccine, Hib vaccine and pediatric pneumococcal vaccine. Also, since FY 2013, reports of post-vaccination adverse reactions associated with all vaccines have been included in the "Reports from healthcare professionals".

療機関や専門医に限定して販売すること，販売にあたっては医師に一定の教育を受けさせることを条件とすること等を FDA が検討するよう提言していた。

　海外で開発された新薬等がわが国に導入される場合には，従来は欧米で先行して承認されている場合が大部分であり，欧米での豊富な使用経験があるため，わが国で承認後，まったく新しい未知の副作用が発生する可能性はきわめて低く，市販直後の使用についてもある程度の安心感のようなものが医療関係者にはあったものと思われる。

　しかしながら，ICH の成果として各種ガイドライン等のハーモナイゼーションが進み，外国臨床試験データの相互受け入れも進み，新薬の世界同時開発，同時申請，同時承認，同時発売が現実のものとなり，さらには，欧米での使用経験のない新薬がわが国で初めて使われることも散見されるようになったことから，わが国でも市販直後の安全対策はより一層重要になってきている。

　そのような中で，厚生省は，「医薬品の市販後調査の基準に関する省令の一部を改正する省令（厚生省令第 151 号：平成 12 年 12 月 27 日）」を公布し，翌年の2001 年 10 月 1 日から新医薬品の「市販直後調査」を実施した。この制度は，

- 　新薬販売開始前後の一定期間製造販売業者等が責任をもって新薬の適正使用情報の周知徹底を行うこと
- 　市販直後の期間は安全性情報に特に注意を払うべき期間であり，常に医療機関にその旨をリマインドしながら販売するとともに，重篤な副作用等が発生した場合に遅滞なく報告できるよう一定期間は MR が一定の頻度でフォローアップを行うことにより，適正使用の徹底と，副作用の発生動向を遅れることなく，網羅的に把握できるようにすること

を目的としている。

4.2.2　調査の対象と実施方法

　市販直後調査は新薬を対象とし，期間は通常，販売開始後 6 か月間である。具体的な調査の実施については，「製造販売業者等は，販売開始前に市販直後調査に関する実施方法，訪問の頻度等を定めた実施計画書を作成するとともに，当該医薬品が販売開始後 6 か月間重点的な副作用等の調査対象になっていることを「製品情報概要」，「使用上の注意の解説」等に明示すること」としている（図 4.3）。

　また，製造販売業者等は，当該医薬品を使用する医療機関に対して，原則として納入前に MR により，

- 　当該医薬品が市販直後調査の対象であり，その調査期間中であること
- 　当該医薬品を注意深く使用するとともに，関係が疑われる重篤な副作用等が発現した場合には，速やかに当該製造販売業者等に報告することを説明し，協力依頼を行うこと

としている。

Chapter 4 Summary of post-marketing risk management in Japan

physicians to undertake predetermined training.

When a new drug developed overseas is licensed in Japan, up until now in most cases the drug has already been approved in US and EU countries. Because of the abundant experience of use overseas, it was very unlikely that a completely new, unexpected ADRs would occur in Japan after approval. HCPs therefore felt a certain sense of security concerning the use of new drugs even immediately at the start of marketing.

However, with advances in harmonization of various guidelines as the result of ICH and mutual acceptance of overseas clinical study data, the simultaneous development, filing, and marketing worldwide of new drug are beginning to be realized. Furthermore, under these circumstances, some new drugs without prior experience of use in US and EU are now used in Japan for the first time. As such, risk minimization measures in the early phases of marketing are more important in Japan as well.

Given this background, the MHW promulgated the "Ministerial Ordinance on the Partial Amendment of Good Post-marketing Surveillance Practice Ordinance" (MHW Ordinance No. 151, December 27, 2000) and "Early post-marketing phase risk minimization and vigilance" has been implemented for new drugs since October 1, 2001. This system is intended for the following:

［1］ MAH will be responsible for sufficiently communicating information on the proper use of a new drug for a specified period around the start of marketing of a new drug.

［2］ The early post-marketing phase is a period when special attention should be given to safety information and the marketing of a new drug should regularly be carried out by stressing that MRs should follow up with medical institutions at certain intervals in a predetermined period so that the appearance of serious ADRs, etc. can be reported without delay for the purpose of thoroughly ensuring proper use and comprehensively keeping track of the trend of occurrence of ADRs without delays.

4.2.2 Target and method of EPPV

New drugs are subject to EPPV and the duration is usually 6 months from the start of marketing. With respect to the specific method of vigilance, MAHs, must prepare a plan determining the method of EPPV, frequency of visits, etc. before the start of marketing, and specify in the "Product information brochure" and "Explanations of Precautions", etc. that the concerned drug is subject to intensive monitoring of ADRs, etc. for 6 months after the start of marketing (**Fig. 4.3**).

MAHs should, in principle, provide the following explanation prior to delivery of the concerned drug by MR, to the medical institutions scheduled to use the drug and request their cooperation:

［1］ The concerned drug is subject to EPPV and it is in the vigilance stage.

［2］ The concerned drug should be used carefully and any occurrence of a serious ADR suspected to be causally related to the drug should be reported to the MAH without delay.

In addition, MAHs, should obtain information on serious ADRs from each medical institution to continue investigation and confirmation of (1) and (2) above by visits,

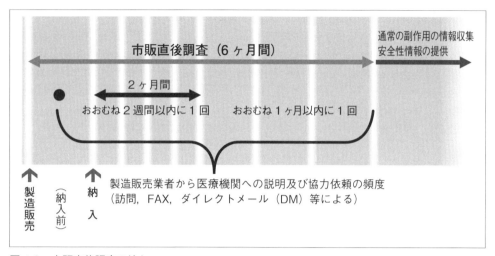

図 4.3　市販直後調査の流れ　　　　　　　　　　　出典：医薬品医療機器等安全性情報 No.315

　さらに，製造販売業者等は，各医療機関に対し重篤な副作用等の情報について，訪問，手紙，FAX，e-mail，卸売一般販売業者等による伝達その他適切な方法により，医療機関への納入開始後2か月間はおおむね2週間以内に1回の頻度で，その後も期間中は適切な頻度（おおむね1か月以内に1回）で上記について調査，確認を継続することとしている。また，製造販売業者等は，医療機関から報告される重篤な副作用等の症例について，迅速に調査できる体制を整備するとともに，重篤な副作用等の発生情報を入手した場合には，速やかな詳細情報の収集に努め，医薬品医療機器等法に規定された報告期限内に速やかに厚労省に症例報告を行うこととしている。

　市販直後調査の結果については，終了後2か月以内に，市販直後調査実施報告書を市販直後調査計画書とともにPMDAへ提出することとされている。

　なお，本章の4.6節で述べるRMPの「追加の医薬品安全性監視活動」および「追加のリスク最小化計画」の中でも市販直後調査は両者に位置付けられている（122ページの図4.9参照）。

4.3　感染症定期報告制度

　血液製剤によるウイルス感染（エイズや肝炎）やvCJD（変異型クロイツフェルト・ヤコブ病）と関連があるといわれる牛海綿状脳症（BSE）等のように，ヒトや動物に由来する医薬品等を介した感染症が社会問題となった。2002年の薬事法改正により，医薬品や医療機器に用いる生物由来製品に関する規制が強化された（医薬品医療機器等法第68条の10）。また従来の感染症症例報告に加えて，生物由来製品の製造販売業者は，当該生物由来製品やその原料や材料による感染症に関する最新

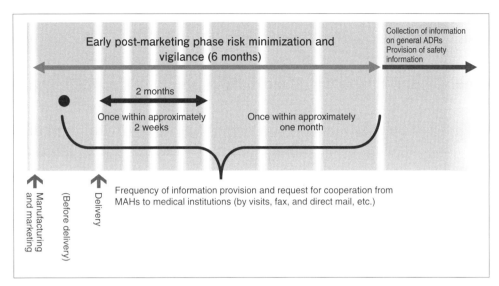

Fig4-3 Flow of EPPV

Source: Pharmaceutical and medical device safety information No. 315

letters, facsimile, E-mail, communication via a wholesaler, etc. or other appropriate methods at intervals of once every two weeks for 2 months after the start of delivery to a medical institution and at appropriate intervals (about once a month) thereafter during the EPPV period. MAHs, should establish a system for promptly investigating cases of serious ADR reported by medical institutions, and promptly collect detailed information upon learning of the appearance of a serious ADR so that a case report is immediately submitted to the MHLW within the time frame stipulated in the PMD Act.

Reporting on the results to the PMDA is required together with the submission of an implementation plan within 2 months after the end of the EPPV period.

In both the "additional pharmacovigilance activities" and "additional risk minimization plans" of the RMP as described in section 4.6 of this Chapter, EPPV is positioned as very important investigation (page 123, **Fig. 4.9**).

4.3 Periodic reporting system for infections

Infections derived from human or animals via drugs, etc. such as viral infections associated with the use of blood products (AIDS and hepatitis) and bovine spongiform encephalopathy (BSE) considered to be related to vCJD (variant Creutzfeldt-Jakob disease) became an issue for society. Revision of the PAL in 2002 strengthened regulation of drugs and medical devices derived from biological materials (Article 68-10 of the PMD Act). Also, in addition to conventional individual infection reports (i.e. reports of adverse events of infections due to contamination of drug product), manufacturers of

の文献等から得られた知見に基づいて評価を行い，2003 年 7 月より 6 か月ごとに感染症定期報告を行うことになった。さらに再生医療等製品についても 2014 年 8 月 12 日付け薬食発 0812 第 7 号局長通知により，感染症定期報告を行うこととなり，2017 年 4 月 28 日付け薬生発 0428 第 1 号の局長通知で，これら 2 つは同じように扱われることとなった。なお，遺伝子組換え製品，抗体医薬品やワクチン等は，原材料や培地等に複数の動物種の原材料を使用していることが多いので，生物由来製品としては 1 製品であっても，その生物由来成分ごとにまとめて感染症定期報告として提出することとされている。

4.4 再審査制度

再審査制度は，承認後一定期間，市販後における医薬品の情報収集を義務付け，期間終了後にその有効性，安全性および品質を再確認する制度であり，1980 年 4 月より開始された。再審査申請資料は，改正 GPSP 施行後では使用成績調査，製造販売後データベース調査，製造販売後臨床試験に関する資料，外国での同一成分を含む副作用・感染症報告および市販後に得られた研究・措置報告等から構成される（医薬品医療機器等法第 14 条の 4 および関連施行規則）。これらの各種調査，臨床試験の詳細は第 7 章 7.2 節を参照されたい。

4.4.1 再審査期間

再審査期間は，表 4.3 に示すように新薬の承認区分に基づいて規定されている。

表 4.3　新医薬品の再審査期間

期　　間	新医薬品の種類
10年	①希少疾病用医薬品（オーファンドラッグ） ②長期の薬剤疫学的調査が必要なもの
8年	③新有効成分含有医薬品
6年	④新医療用配合剤 ⑤新投与経路医薬品
5年10か月	⑥新効能・効果医薬品，新用法・新用量医薬品（既承認薬が，希少疾病用医薬品の効能・効果のみを有するもの）
4年	⑦新効能・効果医薬品（⑥を除く） ⑧新用法・新用量医薬品（⑥を除く）
先行新薬の再審査期間の 残余期間	⑨先行する新医薬品の再審査期間中に承認された追っかけ新薬

注）小児の用量設定のために治療や製造販売後臨床試験を計画する場合には，10 年を超えない範囲で再審査期間を一定期間延長。

Chapter 4 Summary of post-marketing risk management in Japan

these biological products are required to assess them based on findings obtained from the latest, scientific literature and other sources concerning infections induced by the concerned biological materials or their raw materials, and to submit periodic infection reports every 6 months starting in July 2003. Furthermore, periodic infection reports are also required for regenerative medicine products based on the PFSB Notification No. 0812-7 issued by the Director on August 12, 2014. Based on the PSEHB Notification No. 0428-1 issued by the Director on April 28, 2017, these two are handled in the same manner. Because multiple animal-derived materials are often used as raw materials and media for a single genetically-modified product, antibody drug or vaccine, submission of separate periodic infection reports is required for each biological ingredient in the biological product.

4.4 Reexamination system

The purpose of the Reexamination system is to collect post-marketing information on a drug for a predetermined period after approval to reconfirm its efficacy, safety and quality at the end of the period. The system was started in April 1980. After the enforcement of the revised GPSP, the materials for the Reexamination application consist of use-results surveys, post-marketing database studies, and post-marketing clinical trials, overseas reports of ADRs/infections for drugs containing the same ingredients, and research reports and reports of measures taken overseas, etc. obtained after marketing (Article 14-4 of the PMD Act and relevant enforcement regulations). Refer to Chapter 7, Section 7.2 for details of these investigations and clinical trials.

4.4.1 Reexamination period

As shown in **Table 4.3**, the Reexamination period is determined based on the approval category of a new drug.

Table4.3 Reexamination period for new drug

Period	Type of new drug
10 years	[1] Orphan drug [2] Drug requiring long-term pharmacoepidemiological investigation
8 years	[3] Drug containing a new active ingredient
6 years	[4] New ethical combination drug [5] Drug with a new route of administration
5 years 10 months	[6] Drug with new indication (already approved drug which only has an indication as an orphan drug)
4 years	[7] Drug with new indication (excluding [6]) [8] Drug with new dosage and administration (excluding [6])
Remaining period of Reexamination period for the preceding new drug	[9] Separate full application for the same active ingredient as a drug which is still in its Reexamination period.

Note) When planning administration or a post-marketing clinical trial for determining the pediatric dose, the Reexamination period shall be extended for a certain period not exceeding 10 years.

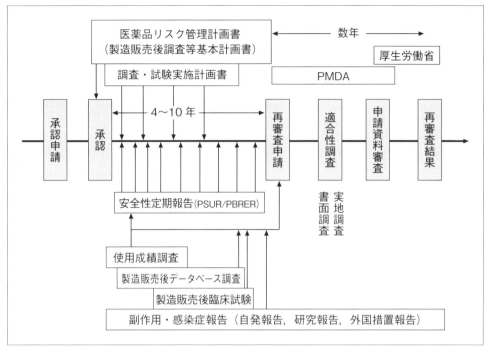

図 4.4 承認申請から再審査結果通知までの流れ

4.4.2 承認申請から再審査結果通知までの流れ

新薬の承認から製造販売後調査の実施や有効性・安全性情報の収集，再審査申請，適合性調査，資料の審査および再審査結果の通知にいたるまでの流れを図 4.4 に示した。

4.4.3 RMP（製造販売後調査等基本計画書）の作成

製造販売後基本計画書は承認申請時の CTD 1.11 に添付しなければならない。なお，2013 年（平成 25 年）4 月 1 日以降に申請された新医薬品（効能追加を含む）では，従前の製造販売後調査等基本計画書案に代わり RMP 案を CTD 1.11 に添付することとなった。また，既承認医薬品であっても製造販売後に，新たなリスクが判明し，追加の措置が必要となった場合，RMP を作成することになる。RMP の詳細については 4.6 参照。

現段階では，RMP が申請資料に添付される以前の品目が再審査申請対象であることより，当面は製造販売後調査等基本計画書に基づき再審査申請および審査が実施されることとなる（2013 年〔平成 25 年〕3 月 31 日までに申請された新医薬品で，製造販売後に RMP を作成する必要がなければ，通常の再審査期間が付与される品目で 2022 年，効能追加品目で 2018 年，希少疾患治療製品の場合，2024 年前後が

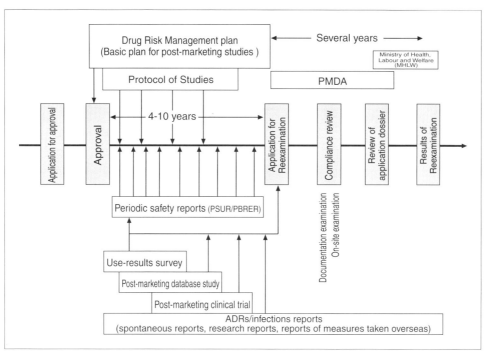

Fig.4.4 Process from application for approval until notification of Reexamination results

4.4.2 Process from application for approval until notification of Reexamination results

Fig. 4.4 shows the process from approval of a new drug, implementation of post-marketing surveillance, collection of efficacy and safety information, application for Reexamination, compliance review, examination (review) of documentation, and notification of Reexamination results.

4.4.3 Preparation of RMP (Basic Plan for post-marketing studies)

The Basic Plan for post-marketing surveillance must be attached to CTD 1.11 of the marketing authorization application. In addition, for new drugs (including additional indications for already approve drugs) for which applications were made on or after April 1, 2013, a draft RMP should be attached to CTD 1.11 in place of the previous draft Basic Plan for post-marketing surveillance. Also for approved drugs, an RMP is to be prepared when a new risk is found after marketing and additional measures are required. See section 4.6 for details of the RMP.

At the present stage, when application for Reexamination is to be made for an item before the RMP is attached to the application dossier, application for Reexamination as well as review will be implemented based on the Basic Plan for post-marketing studies for the time being (if it is a new drug for which application was made by March 31, 2013 and it is not necessary to prepare RMP after marketing, the timing of application for Reexamination may be around 2022 for an item for which the usual Reexamination period is given, 2018 for an item with additional indication, and 2024 for an orphan

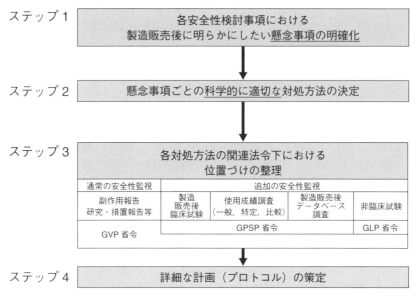

図 4.5 安全性監視計画策定の検討の進め方
出典：PMDA ホームページ https://www.pmda.go.jp/files/000228612.pdf

再審査申請時期と考えられる）。

　追加の安全性監視計画として位置付けられる製造販売後調査・試験については，実施を必要と考えた理由ならびに検討すべきリスク（特に重要な潜在的リスク）を明確にした上で，明確な目的をもって，保健衛生上への影響も考慮しながら計画・実施する必要がある。RMP 指針には，その方法論として医薬品安全性監視計画に関する ICH E2E ガイドラインの考え方を参考にして検討するよう記載されているが，実施には従来の製造販売後調査を定型的に実施されている事例がほとんどである。しかし，2018 年 4 月の GPSP 改正により製造販売後データベース調査が加わったことから，ICH E2E ガイドラインの考え方に基づいた「医薬品の製造販売後調査等の実施計画の策定に関する検討の進め方について」が薬生薬審発 0314 第 4 号，薬生安発 0314 第 4 号，審査管理課長，安全対策課長通知（2019 年 3 月 14 日）として示されている（図 4.5）。

　今後 RMP 指針および ICH E2E ガイドラインに沿った安全性監視計画が発展することが望まれる。

4.4.4　安全性定期報告と PSUR/PBRER

- 安全性定期報告

　　1980 年 4 月に再審査制度が発足して以来，再審査対象医薬品については，再審査期間中は旧薬事法施行規則により 1 年ごとに「新医薬品等の使用の成績等に関する調査及び結果の報告」（いわゆる年次報告）を提出することとされた（医薬品医療機器等法施行規則第 63 条）。企業は 1 年ごとに使用成績

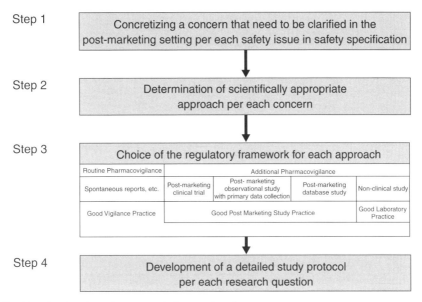

Fig4-5 How to develop pharmacovigilance planning
Source: PMDA website https://www.pmda.go.jp/files/000226080.pdf

drug).

Post-marketing studies performed as additional activities in the pharmacovigilance plan need to be planned/ with clear cut objectives taking into account influences on public health and hygiene after clarifying why they are necessary and the risks (particularly important potential risks) that are being studied. In the RMP guideline, it is described that methodology should be considered with reference to the principles in the ICH E2E guideline regarding pharmacovigilance plans, but conventional post-marketing surveillance is routinely conducted in most cases. However, since post-marketing database studies became available through the revision of GPSP in April 2018, the PMDA presented "Procedures for Developing Post-marketing Study Plan (PSEHB/ELD Notification No 0314-4, PSEHB/SD Notification No 0314-4 dated March 14, 2019)" based on the policies of the ICH E2E guideline (**Fig. 4.5**). It is expected that the pharmacovigilance plan would be developed in accordance with the RMP guideline and ICH E2E guideline.

4.4.4 Periodic safety reports and the PSUR/PBRER

[1] Periodic safety reports

Since the start of the Reexamination system in April 1980, it was stipulated in the old PAL Enforcement Regulations that "Reports of drug use investigations of a new drug and their results" (so-called annual report) should be submitted every year during the Reexamination period for drugs subjected to Reexamination (Article 63 in the Enforcement Regulation of the PMD Act). MAHs are required

調査結果からの副作用発現状況と，厚生省（現 厚労省）に報告した副作用症例報告や研究報告からの情報を併せて検討し，使用上の注意改訂の検討などの今後の安全対策を記載することとされた。

その後，後述のICHにおける定期的安全性最新報告（PSUR：Periodic Safety Update Report）の検討を受けて，年次報告のあり方についても見直しが行われた。年次報告は，安全性定期報告制度と改定され，1997年4月の旧薬事法改正と同時に実施された。再審査期間中，最初の2年間は6か月ごと，その後は1年ごとに報告するように報告頻度を変更し，同一成分に対する国内だけでなく世界各国の情報を収集して評価・検討を行い，PSURを作成していれば，安全性定期報告の添付資料として併せて提出することとなっている。なお，日本でのみ承認されている医薬品の場合には，PSURを作成する必要はない（図4.6）。

なお，医薬品リスク管理計画書が当局に提出されている再審査期間中の新医療用医薬品については，2014年10月1日以降，RMPの実施状況と評価内容を要約して報告する目的で，「医薬品リスク管理計画書の概要の作成及び公表について」（薬生審査発0331第13号，薬生安発0331第13号医薬・生活衛生局審査管理課長・安全対策課長通知：平成28年3月31日）を作成し，添付することとなった。

・PSURからPBRERへ

1990年代半ばから，ICHにおいて市販後における副作用の定期報告，すなわち，PSURについて，それまで欧州で適用されていた制度をもとにして議

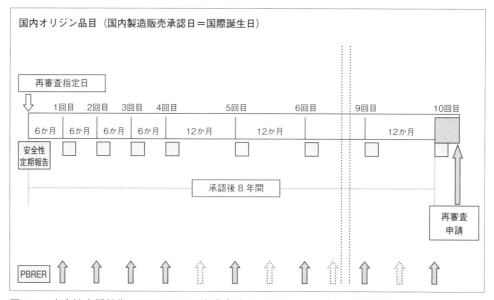

図4.6 安全性定期報告，PBRERと再審査申請のスケジュールより一部改変)

to annually review both the frequency of ADRs in use-results survey and the information in ADR case reports and research reports submitted to the MHLW, and to describe future safety measures such as revision of Precaution for use, etc.

Thereafter, the annual report was also revised in response to deliberations on the ICH PSUR (Periodic Safety Update Report), which will be described below. The annual report was changed to a periodic safety reporting system and implemented at the time of revision of the old PAL in April 1997. A change was made in the frequency of reporting to every 6 months for the first 2 years and every year thereafter during the Reexamination period and the report was required to contain, evaluate and review information collected not only in Japan but also from other countries on drugs with the same active ingredient. If a PSUR is prepared it is to be submitted as an appendix of the Periodic safety report. There is no need to prepare a PSUR for a drug approved only in Japan (**Fig. 4.6**).

On and after October 1, 2014, marketing authorization holders of new prescription drugs which are undergoing re-examination and for which an RMP has been submitted to the regulatory authorities, are required to prepare and submit the "Preparation and Release of the Summary of RMP" (PSEHB/ELD Notification No. 0331-13, PSEHB/PSD Notification No. 0331-13, March 31, 2016) to summarize the status of implementation of the RMP and details of its evaluation.

[2] From PSURs to PBRERs

Periodic reporting of post-marketing ADRs, or the PSUR, was discussed under ICH in the mid-1990s based on the system which had been adopted in Europe. The result was approved in November 1996 by 3 parties Japan, the US and EU as the ICH E2C guideline. This report summarizes global safety information over a predetermined period for drugs containing the same active substance, which is

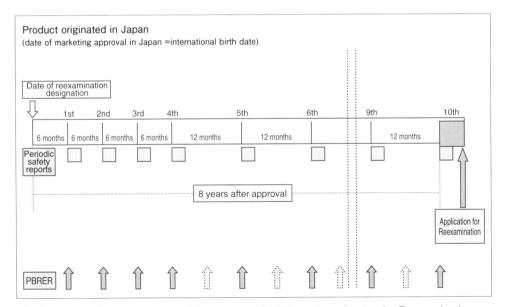

Fig.4.6 Schedule of periodic safety reports, PBRERs and application for Reexamination

論が行われ，1996 年 11 月に ICH E2C ガイドラインとして日米欧三極で合意された。これは同一成分医薬品について一定期間における全世界的な安全性情報をまとめた報告書で，各国で共通の安全対策を講じるときに役立つものであり，日本では 1997 年 10 月より実施された。PSUR は，ICH E2C ガイドラインに従った内容で作成され，原則，成分ごとに 6 か月ごとに作成するもので，1 年ごとの PSUR については，6 か月の PSUR を 2 つ合わせたものでもよい。

この内容については前述のとおり，2013 年（平成 25 年）5 月には ICH E2C（R2）の Step 5 通知が発出されている。

この通知により，「市販医薬品に関する定期的安全性最新報告（PSUR）について（1997 年〔平成 9 年〕3 月 27 日付 薬安第 32 号）および「ICH E2C に対する補遺 臨床安全性データの取扱い：市販医薬品に関する定期的安全性最新報告について」（2003 年〔平成 15 年〕4 月 25 日付医薬審発第 0425001 号・医薬安発第 0425001 号）は廃止された。

これは，医薬品はリスクだけではなくベネフィットについても言及されるべきとの立場から ICH E2C（R2）として検討された結果，個別症例報告よりも集積情報に重きを置き，ベネフィットーリスクバランス評価を取り入れるなど内容的に大幅に更新された定期的ベネフィット・リスク評価報告（Periodic Benefit-Risk Evaluation Report：PBRER）となった（**表 4.4**）。欧米の当局に報告書を提出する企業では，膨大なリソースを費やし PSUR から PBRER へ順次切り替えられ，また，産官学でベネフィットーリスクバランスの評価方法について検討されている。しかしながら，わが国においては，安全性定期報告の内容は PBRER の位置付けとは異なるものであり，記載内容は日本独自の項目となっている。

4.4.5　再審査結果の判定

再審査申請資料は，最終的には下記の 3 区分により判定される。
・　カテゴリー 1：有用性が認められるもの
・　カテゴリー 2：承認事項の一部を変更すれば有用性が認められるもの
・　カテゴリー 3：有用性が認められないもの
これまで大半の品目はカテゴリー 1 と判定され，承認の効能・効果および用法・用量の変更はない。一部の品目についてはカテゴリー 2 と判定され，効能・効果あるいは用法・用量の一部を変更した。カテゴリー 3 と判定され，有用性が否定された品目はない。

Chapter 4 Summary of post-marketing risk management in Japan   **113**

useful for taking the same safety measures in each country. It was enforced in Japan from October 1997. PSURs are prepared in accordance with the ICH E2C Guideline. As a rule, PSURs are prepared every 6 months for each active substance, and two 6-month PSURs may be combined to produce an annual PSUR.

Regarding this matter, as mentioned earlier, the notification of Step 5 under ICH E2C (R2) was issued in May 2013.

Following this notification, "Regarding Periodic Safety Update Reports (PSURs) for Commercially Available Drugs (PAB/SD Notification No. 32 dated March 27, 1997)" and "Regarding Handling of Clinical Safety Data as Supplement for ICH E2C: Periodic Safety Update Reports (PSURs) for Commercially Available Drugs (PFSB/ELD Notification No. 0425001 and PFSB/SD Notification No. 0425001 dated April 25, 2003)" were abolished.

The need to mention not only risks but also benefits of drugs, was considered under ICH E2C (R2), and as a consequence, these reports became the Periodic Benefit-Risk Evaluation Report (PBRER) for which the contents were substantially updated, such as attaching weight to accumulated information rather than individual case reports and incorporating benefit-risk balance evaluations (**Table 4.4**). Companies who submit reports to authorities in the US and Europe have spent a huge amount of resources to switch from the PSUR to the PBRER, and methods of evaluating benefit-risk balance have been considered by industry, regulators and academia. However, in Japan, the contents of periodic safety reports are different from the positioning of the PBRER, and the contents consist of items unique to Japan.

4.4.5 Reexamination results

Applications for Reexamination are finally judged according to the following three categories.

[1] Category 1: Usefulness is confirmed

[2] Category 2: Usefulness is confirmed by a partial change in approval

[3] Category 3: Usefulness is not confirmed

Most of the products have been judged as category 1 and no change was made in their approved indications or dosage and administration. Some products were judged category 2 and a change was made either on indication, or dosage and administration. No products have been judged as category 3 where their usefulness was not confirmed.

表 4.4 「定期的ベネフィット・リスク評価報告（PBRER）について」（薬食審査発 0517 第 1 号，2013 年〔平成 25 年〕5 月 17 日）で示された ICH 調和三極ガイドラインの目次

1. 緒言
   1.1 背景
   1.2 目的
   1.3 PBRER が対象とする範囲
   1.4 PBRER とその他の ICH ガイドラインとの関連
2. 一般原則
   2.1 1 有効成分に 1 つの PBRER
   2.2 配合剤である場合の PBRER
   2.3 複数の企業が製造及び／又は販売する製品
   2.4 参照情報
   2.5 PBRER 内における詳細度
   2.6 有効性／有用性
   2.7 ベネフィット・リスク評価
   2.8 報告頻度と PBRER のデータロックポイント
       2.8.1 国際誕生日とデータロックポイント
       2.8.2 提出頻度の異なる PBRER の扱い
       2.8.3 データロックポイントと提出との期間
   2.9 PBRER の様式と目次
       2.9.1 様式
       2.9.2 目次
3. PBRER の内容に関するガイダンス
   3.1 緒言
   3.2 世界各国における販売承認の状況
   3.3 安全性上の理由で調査対象期間内に実施された措置について
   3.4 安全性参照情報の変更
   3.5 推定使用患者数と使用実態
       3.5.1 臨床試験における累積使用被験者数
       3.5.2 市販後の累積及び調査期間の使用患者数
   3.6 サマリーテーブルのデータ
       3.6.1 参照情報
       3.6.2 臨床試験に基づく重篤有害事象の累積サマリーテーブル
       3.6.3 市販後データの情報源に基づく累積及び調査期間のサマリーテーブル
   3.7 調査期間中の臨床試験で認められた重大な安全性情報の要約
       3.7.1 終了した臨床試験
       3.7.2 継続中の臨床試験
       3.7.3 長期追跡結果
       3.7.4 医薬品の他の治療的使用
       3.7.5 複数成分が関わる治療法に関連する新たな安全性データ
   3.8 非介入試験からの知見
   3.9 他の臨床試験及び情報源からの情報
       3.9.1 その他の臨床試験
       3.9.2 投薬過誤
   3.10 非臨床データ
   3.11 文献
   3.12 他の定期報告
   3.13 比較臨床試験における有効性の欠如
   3.14 データロックポイント後に入手した情報
   3.15 シグナルの概要：新規、評価継続中又は評価確定
   3.16 シグナル及びリスクの評価
       3.16.1 安全性の懸念事項の要約
       3.16.2 シグナルの評価
       3.16.3 リスク及び新しい情報の評価
       3.16.4 リスクの特徴づけ
       3.16.5 リスク最小化策の有用性（該当する場合）
   3.17 ベネフィットの評価
       3.17.1 調査期間開始時における重要な有効性／有用性情報
       3.17.2 有効性／有用性に関して新たに特定された情報
       3.17.3 ベネフィットの特徴づけ
   3.18 承認適応に対する包括的なベネフィット・リスク分析
       3.18.1 ベネフィット・リスクの背景－医学的必要性及びその他の重要な治療選択肢
       3.18.2 ベネフィット・リスク分析の評価
   3.19 結論及び措置
   3.20 PBRER　の添付資料
4. 本ガイドラインの添付資料
添付資料 A - 用語集
添付資料 B - サマリーテーブルの例
添付資料 C - 調査期間に評価が継続中又は評価が確定した安全性シグナルの一覧表の例
添付資料 D - 他の規制関連文書と共用が可能な PBRER の項のリスト
添付資料 E - PBRER 作成時に使用する可能性がある情報源の例
添付資料 F - シグナル及びリスクの PBRER の項へのマッピング

Table4.4 Periodic Benefit-Risk Evaluation Report (PBRER): Table of contents of the ICH guideline harmonized in three regions (PFSB/ELD Notification No. 25-5 issued by the Evaluation and Licensing Division, Pharmaceutical and Food Safety Bureau, MHLW, dated May 2013)

1. Introduction
    1.1   Background
    1.2   Objectives
    1.3   Scope of the PBRER
    1.4   Relation of the PBRER to other ICH guidelines
2. General principles
    2.1   One PBRER for an Active Substance
    2.2   PBRER for a Fixed-Dose Combination Product
    2.3   Product Manufactured and/or Marketed by More than One Company
    2.4   Reference Information
    2.5   Level of Detail within PBRER
    2.6   Efficacy/Effectiveness
    2.7   Benefit-Risk Evaluation
    2.8   Periodicity and PBRER Data Lock Point
        2.8.1   International Birth Date (IBD) and Data Lock Point
        2.8.2   Managing Different Frequencies of PBRER Submission
        2.8.3   Time Interval between Data Lock Point and the Submission
    2.9   Format and Presentation of PBRER
        2.9.1   Format
        2.9.2   Presentation
3. Guidance on Contents of the PBRER
    3.1   Introduction
    3.2   Worldwide Marketing Approval Status
    3.3   Actions Taken in the Reporting Interval for Safety Reasons
    3.4   Changes to Reference Safety Information
    3.5   Estimated Exposure and Use Patterns
        3.5.1   Cumulative Subject Exposure in Clinical Trials
        3.5.2   Cumulative and Interval Patient Exposure from Marketing Experience
    3.6   Data in Summary Tabulations
        3.6.1   Reference Information
        3.6.2   Cumulative Summary Tabulations of Serious Adverse Events from Clinical Trials
        3.6.3   Cumulative and Interval Summary Tabulations from Post-Marketing Data Sources
    3.7   Summaries of Significant Safety Findings i from Clinical Trials during the Reporting Inteval
        3.7.1   Completed Clinical Trials
        3.7.2   Ongoing Clinical Trials
        3.7.3   Long-Term Follow-up
        3.7.4   Other Therapeutic Use of Medicinal Product
        3.7.5   New Safety Data Related to Fixed Combination Therapies
    3.8   Findings from Non-Interventional Studies
    3.9   Information from Other Clinical Trials and Sources
        3.9.1   Other Clinical Trials
        3.9.2   Medication Errors
    3.10 Non-Clinical Data
    3.11 Literature
    3.12 Other Periodic Reports
    3.13 Lack of Efficacy in Controlled Clinical Trials
    3.14 Late-Breaking Information
    3.15 Overview of Signals: New, Ongoing, or Closed
    3.16 Signals and Risk Evaluation
        3.16.1   Summary of Safety Concerns
        3.16.2   Signal Evaluation
        3.16.3   Evaluation of Risks and New Information
        3.16.4   Characterisation of Risks
        3.16.5   Effectiveness of Risk Minimisation (if applicable)
    3.17 Benefit Evaluation
        3.17.1   Important Baseline Efficacy/Effectiveness Information
        3.17.2   Newly Identified information on Efficacy/Effectiveness
        3.17.3   Characterisation of Benefits
    3.18 Integrated Benefit-Risk Analysis for Approved Indications
        3.18.1   Benefit-Risk Context - Medical Need and Important Alternatives
        3.18.2   Benefit-Risk Analysis Evaluation
    3.19 Conclusions and Actions
    3.20 Appendices to PBRER
4. Appendices to this Guideline
Appendix A - Glossary
Appendix B - Example of Summary Tabulations
Appendix C - Example of a Tabular Summary of Safety Signals that were Ongoing or Closed During the Reporting Interval
Appendix D - List of PBRER Sections that May be Shared with Other Regulatory Documents
Appendix E - Examples of Possible Sources of Information that May Be Used in the Preparation of the PBRER
Appendix F - Mapping Signals and Risks to PBRER Sections

4.5 再評価制度

再評価制度は，承認後の医学・薬学の進歩に対応して，医薬品の有効性，安全性あるいは品質等を見直す制度である（医薬品医療機器等法第14条の6）。再評価制度の導入の契機は，サリドマイドの催奇形性やアンプル入り風邪薬のショック死の発生等，医薬品の安全性に対する不信感や活性ビタミン剤や肝臓薬の有効性についての疑問が提示されたことである。1970年9月，当時の厚生大臣の私的諮問委員会として薬効問題懇談会が設置され，1971年7月の答申を受けて，中央薬事審議会（当時）に再評価を担当する特別部会，調査会が設置され，同年12月より，1967年9月までに承認された医療用医薬品について行政指導による再評価（第一次）が開始された。その後，1980年に再評価が法制化されて，1967年10月から1980年3月までに承認された医療用医薬品について第二次再評価が1985年1月から1996年3月まで実施され，現在の再評価（新再評価）に至っている。第二次再評価（薬事法に基づく再評価）では，第1段階で再評価を行う必要があるかどうか文献スクリーニング（基礎調査）が行われ，再評価が必要な成分が選定された。全薬効群の医薬品が対象とされ有効性，安全性について文献スクリーニングにより5年ごとに見直す制度で，1988年から文献スクリーニングが開始され，10年近く続行されてきたものの，現在は中断している。また現在の再評価は，定期的再評価を補完するものとして緊急の問題が発生した場合や薬効群全体として問題になった場合等に再評価を行うものである（図4.7）。

現在の再評価制度においては，「定期的再評価」は中断しており，「臨時の再評価」および「品質再評価」により再評価が必要な品目等を指定し，それらの製造販売業者に資料を提出させて，有効性，安全性あるいは品質について評価を行い，「効能・効果」，「用法・用量」，「配合理由」，「製剤の品質（溶出性）」等について適切な対

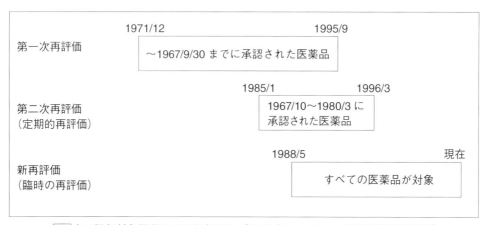

図4.7　各再評価制度における実施期間別の推移

4.5 Reevaluation system

The Reevaluation system is intended to review the efficacy, safety, or quality, etc. of drugs in response to advances in medical/pharmaceutical sciences since their approval (Article 14-6 of the PMD Act). The Reevaluation system was started because of distrust in pharmaceutical safety after teratogenicity induced by thalidomide and deaths from shock due to cold remedies in ampoules, and doubts about the efficacy of activated vitamins and hepatotonics. A conference for discussing drug efficacy as a private advisory committee for the Ministry of Health and Welfare was established in September 1970, and a committee and subcommittee in charge of Reevaluation were established in the Central Pharmaceutical Affairs Council in response to a reply from the Conference in July 1971. The first Reevaluation by administrative guidance was started in December 1971 for ethical drugs that had been approved through September 1967. Reevaluation was legislated in 1980 and the second Reevaluation was performed between January 1985 and March 1996 for ethical drugs approved between October 1967 and March 1980, which led to the current Reevaluation (new Reevaluation) system. In the second Reevaluation (Reevaluation based on the PAL), literature screening (basic investigation) was conducted in the first step to determine whether or not Reevaluation was necessary, and ingredients requiring Reevaluation were selected. The system reviewed the efficacy and safety of drugs of all therapeutic categories every 5 years by literature screening. Literature screening was started in 1988 and had been continued for nearly 10 years, but it is currently suspended. Current Reevaluations are used to supplement periodic Reevaluation and are performed at the onset of an emergency or when an entire therapeutic category becomes problematic (**Fig. 4.7**).

Under the current Reevaluation system, "periodic Reevaluation" has been suspended and efficacy, safety or quality are evaluated by designating those products requiring Reevaluation and obtaining materials from their marketing authorization holders based on the "Ad Hoc Reevaluation" and "Quality Reevaluation" to take appropriate actions for "indications", "dosage and administration", "reason for combination" and "quality

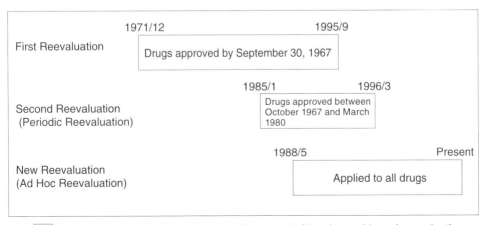

Fig.4.7 Shift of each Reevaluation system by period of implementation

4.5.1 再評価結果の判定

有効性，安全性に関する再評価においては，再審査と同様に最終的には下記の3区分により判定される。

- ・ カテゴリー1：有用性が認められるもの
- ・ カテゴリー2：承認事項の一部を変更すれば有用性が認められるもの
- ・ カテゴリー3：有用性が認められないもの

ただし，再評価では再審査と異なり，カテゴリー3と判定され，有用性が否定され，製品を回収し，承認を整理するものや，カテゴリー2と判定され，「効能・効果」あるいは「用法・用量」の一部を変更したものが多い（**表** 4.5）。

なお，2014年［平成26年］3月25日開催の医薬品再評価部会で議論された漢方エキス製剤7処方（1991年〔平成3年〕2月1日指定），非ステロイド性消炎鎮痛薬（配合剤）7処方（1995年〔平成7年〕5月8日指定）および代謝拮抗薬7成分（1995年〔平成7年〕5月8日指定）については，いずれもカテゴリー1と判定されたが，2016年［平成28年］3月17日開催の医薬品再評価部会で議論されたリゾチーム塩酸塩，プロナーゼといった消炎酵素薬については新たな臨床試験結果よりカテゴリー3と判定された。

4.5.2 品質再評価

1997年2月から開始された品質再評価は，主に後発医薬品の品質確保を目的として，内用固形剤を対象として溶出試験により行われている。

表 4.5　第一次および第二次，新再評価結果について

	第一次再評価 （その1～41： 1973～1995年）	第二次再評価 （その1～14： 1988～1996年）	新再評価 （その1～57： ～2010年5月）
再評価が終了した品目数	19,849	1,860	8,851
有用性が認められるもの	11,098	105	4,606
承認事項の一部変更をすれば有用性が認められるもの	7,330	1,579	3,315
有用性を示す根拠のないもの	1,116	42	66
申請後に承認整理したもの	305	134	864

引用：特定保健食品の表示許可制度専門委員会　平成23年2月28日資料5より

of product (dissolution property)".

4.5.1 Assessment of Reevaluation results

In Reevaluation of efficacy and safety, assessment is made using the following 3 categories in the same manner as for Reexamination:

［1］ Category 1: Usefulness is confirmed
［2］ Category 2: Usefulness is confirmed by a partial change in approval
［3］ Category 3: Usefulness is not confirmed

However, unlike Reexamination, many products have been judged category 3 under Reevaluation where the usefulness is contradicted, the product is recalled and approval is withdrawn, or category 2 where a partial change is made to "indications" or "dosage and administration" (**Table 4.5**).

In addition, 7 formulations of Kampo (traditional herbal medicine) extracts (designated on February 1, 1991), 7 formulations of non-steroidal anti-inflammatory analgesics (combination products) (designated on May 8, 1995) and 7 ingredients of antimetabolites (designated on May 8, 1995) that were discussed in the Reevaluation Committee held on March 25, 2014 were all judged to be category 1. However, anti-inflammatory enzymes such as lysozyme hydrochloride and Pronase that were discussed in the Reevaluation Committee held on March 17, 2016 were judged to be category 3 based on the results of new clinical trials.

4.5.2 Quality Reevaluation

Quality Reevaluations started in February 1997 are performed by dissolution studies of solid formulations for oral use mainly to ensure the quality of generic drugs.

Fig. 4.8 shows an example of the dissolution curve used for a Quality Reevaluation.

Table4.5   First/Second and New Reevaluations[25]

	First Reevaluation (No. 1 - 41: 1973 - 1995)	Second Reevaluation (No. 1 - 14: 1988 - 1996)	New Reevaluation (No. 1 - 57: until May 2010)
Number of products for which reevaluation was completed	19,849	1,860	8,851
Usefulness is confirmed	11,098	105	4,606
Usefulness is confirmed by a partial change in approval	7,330	1,579	3,315
Without grounds for usefulness	1,116	42	66
Approval voluntarily withdrawn after making application	305	134	864

Cited from the document 5 of the Expert Committee on Labeling Approval System for Specified Health Foods, February 28, 2011

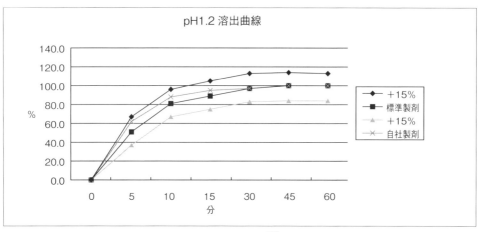

図 4.8　品質再評価における溶出曲線の事例（pH1.2）[26]

　品質再評価については，溶出曲線の事例を図 4.8 に示す。すなわち，最終溶出率が 85％以上の製剤については，標準製剤の溶出曲線に比べて当該製剤の溶出曲線が ±15％以内に収まる場合には，再評価結果において溶出試験で同等とみなされてカテゴリー 1 と判定される。当該製剤の溶出率が規格を満足しない場合にはカテゴリー 3 と判定され，いったん承認を整理するので品質再評価にはカテゴリー 2 はない。その後，溶出規格に合致した製剤を開発して一変申請を行うが，品質再評価の場合においては，市場からの製品回収の必要はない。
　現在，品質再評価は指定された成分については，すでに終了している。

4.6　RMP

4.6.1　RMP の概要

　医薬品は，有効性とともに一定のリスクを伴うものであり，リスクをゼロにすることはできない。しかし，これを可能な限り低減するための方策を講じ，適切に管理していくことが重要である。これまでも，旧薬事法のもと，承認審査の過程を経てリスクを低減するために必要な注意事項が，添付文書に「使用上の注意」として記載されるとともに，副作用・感染症等報告制度，市販直後調査，安全性定期報告制度，未知・非重篤副作用定期報告，再審査・再評価制度により，必要な安全対策が図られてきた。また，製造販売後に新たに判明するようなリスクを検証するためには，従来の医薬品の製造販売後に実施される調査・試験では比較対照群が含まれていないなど，科学的に不十分であった。それを解消すべく参照すべきガイドラインとして，2004 年に日米 EU 医薬品規制調和国際会議（ICH）で整合した「医薬品安全性監視の計画について」（ICH E2E ガイドライン）が示され，対応が行われてきたが，必ずしも十分とはいえなかった。さらに本章の冒頭でも述べた通り，「薬

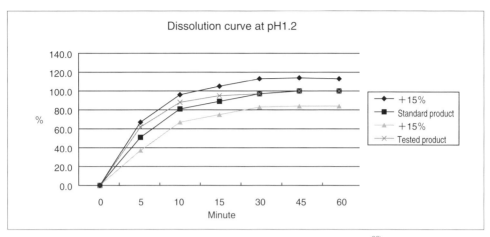

Fig.4.8 Example of dissolution curve for Quality Reevaluation (pH1.2)[26]

Specifically, a formulation with final dissolution rate of 85% or higher is judged to be category 1 if the dissolution curve of the concerned product is within ±15% compared with that of the standard product because they are considered equivalent by Reevaluation of dissolution studies. When the dissolution rate of the product does not comply with the standard, it is judged to be category 3 and approval is withdrawn. No product is judged to be category 2 under the Quality Reevaluation. A partial change application is later filed by developing a product which satisfies the dissolution criteria. Product recall is not necessary for Quality Reevaluations.

Quality Reevaluations have already been terminated for designated ingredients.

4.6 RMP

4.6.1 Summary of the RMP

In addition to their efficacy, drugs involve certain risks, and the risks cannot be reduced to zero. However, it is important to take measures to reduce the risks to the extent possible and manage risk appropriately. Under the old Pharmaceutical Affairs Law (PAL), risk reduction was achieved by identifying issues during the process of marketing application review, describing them in package inserts as "Precautions for use," and implementing necessary safety measures including the ADR / infection reporting system, the Early post-marketing phase risk minimization and vigilance (EPPV), the periodic safety reporting, the unexpected non-serious ADR periodic safety reporting, and the Reexamination/Reevaluation system. However, conventional post-marketing studies of drugs were scientifically insufficient for validating risks that were newly identified during marketing due to lack of a comparative group, etc. In order to address these issues, measures were taken with reference to the "Pharmacovigilance Planning (ICH E2E guideline)" as agreed by the International Conference on Harmonisation of Technical Requirements for Registration of Pharmaceuticals for Human Use (ICH) in 2004. Nevertheless, it cannot be said that these activities have always been sufficient.

害肝炎事件の検証及び再発防止のための医薬品行政のあり方検討委員会」からの最終提言として「開発段階から市販後に懸念される課題を抽出し，市販後において個々の懸念される課題に対応した安全性確保の措置や安全性監視活動が必要かを検討する仕組みが必要であり，欧米における制度を参考に，リスクマネジメントを適切に実施すべきである」とのことから医薬品リスク管理計画（RMP）が実装された。

　RMP は，現在行われている上記の取り組みを医薬品ごとに文書化し，関係者間で共有できるようにすることで，市販後安全対策の一層の充実強化を図ろうとするものである。2012 年 4 月 11 日に「医薬品リスク管理計画指針について」および「医薬品リスク管理計画の策定について」が通知[注1]され，さらに RMP 策定のための指針，様式，提出等の取り扱いが示された。これによって，2013 年 4 月 1 日以降に製造販売承認申請される新医薬品とバイオ後続品から RMP の策定が求められることになった（図 4.9）。

　RMP は，基本的に 3 つの要素（「安全性検討事項」，「医薬品安全性監視計画」，「リスク最小化計画」）から構成される。すなわち，得られた知見に基づいて「安全性検討事項」を特定し，それぞれの安全性検討事項について最適な「医薬品安全性監視計画」および「リスク最小化計画」を策定し，またこれに加え，必要に応じて有効性に関する調査・試験の計画を作成することが求められる。これらの計画の全体

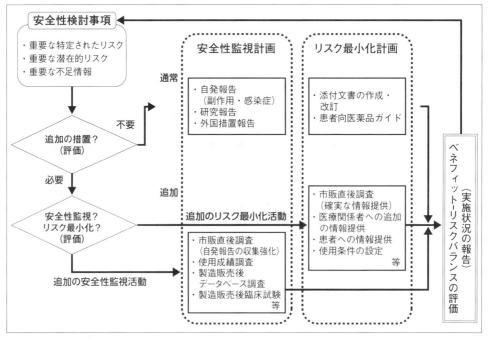

図 4.9　RMP の策定と見直し　　　　　　　　　　　　　　　出典：PMDA ホームページ

注 1　薬食審査発 0426 第 2 号，薬食安発 0426 第 1 号医薬食品局審査管理課長・安全対策課長通知：平成 24 年 4 月 26 日（平成 25 年 3 月 4 日付：薬食審査発 0304 第 1 号・薬食安発 0304 第 1 号，平成 29 年 12 月 5 日付：薬生薬審発 1205 第 1 号・薬生安発 1205 第 1 号により一部改正）

Furthermore, as described in the beginning of this chapter, "It is necessary to have mechanisms to extract issues from the development stage which will be of concern in the post-marketing setting and to consider whether safety assurance measures and pharmacovigilance activities in response to individual issues of concern post-marketing are necessary, and risk management should be appropriately implemented with reference to systems in the US and Europe", which were the final recommendations of the "Review Committee on Drug Administration for Investigation and Prevention of Recurrence of Drug-induced Hepatitis Cases." Thus, Drug Management Plan (RMP) was implemented.

The RMP is intended to further enrich post-marketing safety measures by documenting the currently ongoing above mentioned efforts for a drug in a form that can be shared by the parties concerned. On April 11, 2012, the "Risk Management Plan Guidance" and "Formulation of Drug Risk Management Plan" were issued[Note 1] to provide guidance on the preparation, format, and submission of the RMP. With these notifications, the preparation of an RMP has become required for all new drugs and biosimilar products for which marketing approval application is made on or after April 1, 2013 (**Fig.4.9**).

The RMP is basically composed of three elements the "Safety Specification," "Pharmacovigilance Plan," and "Risk Minimization Plan". Specifically, it is required that, based on the information obtained, the "Safety Specifications" is identified, and for each safety concern an optimum "Pharmacovigilance Plan" and "Risk Minimization

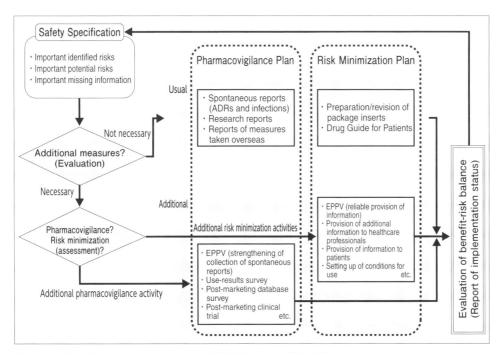

Fig.4.9 Establishment and review of RMP (source: PMDA'S website)

Note 1) PFSB/ELD Notification No. 0426-2 and PFSB/SD Notification No. 0426-1, April 26, 2012 (partially modified by PFSB/ELD Notification No. 0304-1 and PFSB/SD Notification No. 0304-1 dated March 4, 2013, and PSEHB/PED Notification No. 1205-1 and PSEHB/PSD Notification No. 1205-1 dated December 5, 2017)

を取りまとめて文書化したものが，RMP である。

4.6.2 申請時における医薬品リスク管理計画書案の作成と提出

- RMP の策定

  各企業の新医薬品を承認申請するための部門横断的組織において，承認申請資料（CTD：Common Technical Document）が作成され，その一部として RMP 案が作成される。

- 安全性検討事項の特定

  RMP を構成する主な3要素（安全性検討事項，医薬品安全性監視計画，リスク最小化計画）のうち，安全性検討事項の特定を最初に行う。すなわち，開発の進展に応じて蓄積される国内外の臨床データをはじめ，非臨床データ・品質データ等に基づいて安全性検討事項を特定する。

  安全性検討事項は，リスクのうちの「重要」なものである。ICH E2E ガイドラインに基づき，「重要」とは，「その医薬品における特定されたリスク，潜在的リスクおよび不足情報のうち，ヒトにおいて発現した場合に重篤である，又は高頻度に発現する等の理由から，当該医薬品のベネフィット－リスクバランスに影響を及ぼしうる，又は保健衛生上の危害の発生若しくは拡大のおそれがあるような重要なもの」と定義されている。

  当該医薬品が海外ですでに製造販売されている品目の場合，Global RMP，Core RMP，Reference RMP など，全世界で共通の中核となる RMP が策定されている場合があるが，その場合は，国内臨床試験の結果だけでなく，Global RMP や EU RMP，REMS（Risk Evaluation and Mitigation Strategy）等，海外で先行する RMP 関連情報を参考にして安全性検討事項を特定する。この場合，日本版の RMP では，海外で設定された安全性検討事項とは異なる検討事項が選択される場合がある。海外での市販実績が長い場合など Global RMP がない医薬品の場合は，日本の添付文書（適応追加の場合）のほか，海外添付文書（に相当するもの）や定期的ベネフィット－リスク評価報告（PBRER：Periodic Benefit-Risk Evaluation Report）を参考にすることもある。

  このように特定された安全性検討事項の個々に応じて，最適な医薬品安全性監視計画（PvP：Pharmacovigilance Plan）およびリスク最小化計画を策定する。

- 医薬品安全性監視計画の策定

  わが国で市販されるすべての医薬品では，通常，市販後に医療関係者からの自発報告や学会，文献報告などの収集が行われるが，これは「通常の医薬品安全性監視活動」である。これに加えて必要があれば実施されるもの，例えば新医薬品における「市販直後調査」（本章 4.2 節〔94 ページ〕参照），再審

Chapter 4 Summary of post-marketing risk management in Japan **125**

Plan" is formulated, and also that plans are made for an investigation or study on efficacy when necessary. RMP refers to compilation and documentation of these plans.

4.6.2 Preparation and submission of the draft Risk Management Plan at the time of marketing application

［1］ Preparation of the RMP

Each company filing a marketing application will have a cross-functional team which prepares the Common Technical Document (CTD) and the draft RMP should be prepared as a part of the CTD.

［2］ Identification of the Safety Specification

From among the three main elements that make up RMP, i.e. Safety Specification, Pharmacovigilance Plan, and Risk Minimization Plan, the Safety Specification should be prepared first. Specifically, the Safety Specification should be prepared based on domestic and overseas clinical data accumulated according to the progress of development and non-clinical data, quality data, etc.

The Safety Specification should provide a summary of the "important" risks. Under the April 2012 "Risk Management Plan Guidance"[3] , in keeping with the spirit of the ICH E2E Guideline, this is clarified as follows:

"These important identified risks, important potential risks, and important missing information are critical in that they may affect the benefit-risk balance of the drug or may cause or increase public health hazards on grounds such as they may become serious if they occur in humans or frequently occur." If the drug is being marketed overseas, a global common core RMP may have been formulated such as a Global RMP, Core RMP, or Reference RMP, but in such case, the Safety Specification should be identified with reference to not only the results of domestic clinical studies but also preexisting overseas RMP-related information such as the Global RMP, EU RMP, or REMS (Risk Evaluation and Mitigation Strategy). In these cases, the Japanese RMP may include safety concerns within the Safety Specifications different from those established in other countries. On the other hand, if it is a drug for which there is no Global RMP such as where the drug has been commercially available overseas for many years, reference may instead be made to overseas package inserts or Periodic Benefit-Risk Evaluation Report (PBRER) in addition to the Japanese package insert (in case of additional indications).

As described above, an optimal Pharmacovigilance Plan (PvP) and Risk Minimization Plan should be formulated according to individual safety concerns in the safety specification.

［3］ Formulation of Pharmacovigilance Plan

For all drugs marketed in Japan, spontaneous reports from healthcare professionals and information from academic conferences, literature reports, etc. are collected during marketing. These are "routine pharmacovigilance activities." In addition to the above, activities to be conducted if needed, including "EPPV" for new drugs [See section 4.2 of this Chapter (page 95)], and "use-results survey", "post-marketing database survey" and "post-marketing clinical trials" performed for Reexamination/Reevaluation applications are positioned as

査・再評価申請のために実施される「使用成績調査」,「製造販売後データベース調査」「製造販売後臨床試験」などは,「追加の医薬品安全性監視活動」に位置付けられる。医薬品安全性監視活動の手法については, ICH E2E ガイドラインの別添「医薬品安全性監視の方法」を参照する。

- ・ リスク最小化計画の策定

  添付文書の「使用上の注意」による情報提供は, 通常, すべての医薬品に共通して行われる基本的な安全対策であり,「通常のリスク最小化活動」にあたる。また, 医薬品によっては重要なリスクのさらなる低減のために, 市販直後調査で医療関係者への頻繁な注意喚起を行ったり, 重要な注意を要する副作用について適正使用を周知するための資材の配布を行う場合もあるだろう。さらに登録した医師のみ処方を可能とする, 患者にインフォームドコンセントを得た上で投与する, 特定の臨床検査の実施や医療関係者への教育が確認されたといった条件を設定する場合もある。これらは, 通常行われる添付文書による情報提供に加えて実施されるものであり,「追加のリスク最小化活動」に位置付けられる。

  ベネフィット－リスクバランスに影響を与えるようなリスク最小化活動は, 効果があったかどうかをタイムリーに評価することが重要である。リスク最小化活動の評価は, 大きく分けて最小化するための処置（例えば処方や検査など）の実施状況を評価するものと, その処置が最小化するべきアウトカム自体を評価するものがある。

  リスク最小化策の適切な選択とその有効性の評価については, 成川らの研究報告書が有用である[2]。

- ・ RMP の規制当局への提出

  製薬企業は, 承認審査を経て規制当局と内容を合意した RMP を, 販売開始予定の 1 か月前までに独立行政法人医薬品医療機器総合機構（以下, PMDA）に提出しなければならない。この時点で, それまで「（案）」であった RMP が正式版となり, 医薬品医療機器情報提供ホームページに掲載されて公表される。

4.6.3 承認条件の付与, 解除について

　RMP の策定と実施が確実に履行されるように, RMP を承認の条件として義務付け, その策定と実施を GVP の中に位置付けることとされた。このため, GVP 省令および GPSP 省令の改正が 2013 年 3 月 11 日に行われ, 2014 年 10 月 1 日から施行された。これ以降に承認された医薬品については, 追加の措置（医薬品安全性監視活動／リスク最小化活動）が必要な場合, RMP の策定・実施が承認条件として付与される。

　承認条件として付与された RMP を計画どおりに実施し, 必要に応じて見直さな

Chapter 4 Summary of post-marketing risk management in Japan

"additional pharmacovigilance activities." Regarding the methods of pharmacovigilance practices, see the Annex "Pharmacovigilance Methods" to the ICH E2E guideline.

[4] Formulation of Risk Minimization Plan

Provision of information via the "Precautions for use" in package inserts is a basic safety measure taken commonly for all drugs, and corresponds to "routine risk minimization activities." For some drugs, frequent reminders may be performed for healthcare professionals in an EPPV or material may be distributed to make proper use more widely known for ADRs requiring extra attention in order to further reduce significant risks. In addition, conditions such as enabling prescription only by specially registered physicians, administration of a drug after obtaining informed consent from patients, and confirmation of conduct of particular clinical tests and education of healthcare professionals may be necessary. These are to be conducted in addition to the usual provision of information via the package insert, and as such are positioned as "additional risk minimization activities."

For risk minimization activities that may affect the benefit-risk balance, it is important to evaluate in a timely manner whether or not these activities have been effective. Types of evaluation of risk minimization activities are broadly divided into evaluation of the implementation status of a measure for risk minimization (e.g. prescriptions/ laboratory tests) and evaluation of the outcome itself to be minimized by such measure.

For appropriate selection of risk minimization activities and evaluation of their effectiveness, the study report by Narukawa et al. is useful[2].

[5] Submission of the RMP to regulatory authorities

Pharmaceutical companies should submit the RMP, which is agreed upon with the regulatory authorities through approval review, to the Pharmaceuticals and Medical Devices Agency (PMDA) by one month before the scheduled launch. At that point in time, the RMP, which has been "draft" until then, becomes the official version, and it is posted and released on the PMDA website which provides information on pharmaceuticals and medical devices.

4.6.3 Order/removal of conditions for approval

To ensure the production and implementation of an RMP, it was decided that the RMP would be mandated as a condition for approval and that its production and implementation would be positioned under GVP. Such being the situation, revisions of the GVP ministerial ordinance and GPSP ministerial ordinance were made on March 11, 2013, and came into effect on October 1, 2014. For drugs approved after that, if an additional measure (pharmacovigilance activities/risk minimization activities) is necessary, the development and implementation of an RMP will be attached as a condition for approval.

The RMP which is a condition for approval should be implemented as planned and

けれければならない。再審査期間中は，安全性定期報告において進捗状況を報告し，再審査時に審査される。再審査において追加の活動（医薬品安全性監視活動およびリスク最小化活動）が不要と判断されれば RMP の承認条件は解除される。再審査期間終了後の RMP については，本章 4.6.7 項を参照。

4.6.4 RMP の見直し

RMP は一度策定すれば終わりというものではなく，市販後に得られた新たな安全性・有効性の情報に基づき常に見直しを行う必要がある。例えば，新たな副作用が判明した場合など安全性検討事項の内容に変更があったとき，計画に基づき実施した調査または試験が終了して新たな知見が得られたときなどがあげられる。このように，RMP は医薬品の一生にわたって計画の策定，実施，評価，見直しが継続して行われていくことになる。また，見直しの結果は PMDA に報告し，その妥当性の確認が行われる。

4.6.5 製造販売後に新たに RMP を作成する場合

2013 年 4 月時点ですでに市販している医薬品であっても新たな安全性の懸念が判明した場合には，RMP の策定が必要になる場合がある。具体的には，緊急安全性情報（イエローレター）や安全性速報（ブルーレター）による情報提供，注意喚起を行った医薬品等が該当する。ただし，イエローレターやブルーレターなどにより医療関係者へ注意喚起を行う場合，注意喚起によりリスクを最小化することが最優先されるので，RMP の策定はリスク最小化活動が終了した後に速やかに行い，PMDA に届け出た後，公表される。

4.6.6 後発医薬品の RMP

後発医薬品の RMP 作成については，2014 年 8 月 26 日に「医薬品リスク管理計画指針の後発品の適用等について」（薬生審査発 0331 第 3 号・薬生安発 0331 第 13 号医薬・生活衛生局審査管理課長・安全対策課長通知：平成 28 年 3 月 31 日）が通知された。本通知において，RMP が公表されている先発医薬品に対する後発医薬品のうち，「効能又は効果」等が先発医薬品と同一のものの承認申請を行おうとする場合には，申請時に RMP 案を添付することとなった。また先発品と同様，製造販売後に新たな安全性の懸念が判明した時点にも RMP を策定しなければならないこととなった。ただし，複数の企業が一斉に製造販売承認申請を行うことから，各企業から提出された同一成分の内容を，承認審査の間に 1 つに収束させていくことが必要となる。

Chapter 4 Summary of post-marketing risk management in Japan   **129**

readjusted where necessary. During the Reexamination period, the progress status will be reported in periodic safety reports and such measures will be examined at the time of Reexamination. If additional activities (pharmacovigilance activities or risk minimization activities) are judged unnecessary at Reexamination, the RMP will no longer be a condition for approval. Regarding the RMP after the completion of the Reexamination period, refer to section 4.6.7 of this Chapter.

4.6.4 Readjustment of RMP

The RMP is not finished after it has been produced. The RMP will always need readjustment based on new information on safety/efficacy obtained after marketing. Such situations include where there are any changes in the contents of the safety specification, e.g. when a new ADR is found, and when any new knowledge is obtained after the completion of a study implemented based on the plan. In this way, the production, implementation, evaluation, and readjustment of the RMP will be continuously done throughout the life of a drug. Also, the results of readjustment will be reported to the PMDA and its validity will be checked.

4.6.5 New preparation of RMP after marketing

Even for a drug already commercially available as of April 2013, if a new safety concern is found, it may be necessary to create an RMP. Specifically, such cases correspond to drugs, etc. for which information is provided or attention is called via Emergent Safety Communication DHPL (Yellow Letter) or Rapid Safety Communication DHPL (Blue Letter). However, when healthcare professionals are alerted via a Yellow Letter, Blue Letter, or the like, first priority is given to minimization of risks by calling attention, and the formulation of the RMP will be done promptly after the completion of risk minimization activities, and released after submission to the PMDA.

4.6.6 RMP for generic medicines

For the preparation of RMPs for generic medicines, a notification titled "Application of the RMP Guideline to Generic Medicines" was issued on August 26, 2014. It is stated in the notification that applicants need to submit a draft RMP when submitting the marketing authorization application for a generic medicine with "indications" and other details identical to those of a corresponding original medicine for which there is an RMP published on the PMDA website. Apart from this requirement, an RMP needs to be prepared if any new safety concern is revealed after marketing as applied to the original medicine. Since more than one company concurrently can submit a marketing authorization application for a generic medicine, contents of RMPs for the identical ingredient submitted by respective companies need to be harmonized during the authorization review.

4.6.7　再審査期間終了後の RMP 定期報告

　再審査期間終了後の医薬品においては，追加の医薬品安全性活動，追加のリスク最小化活動の内容に応じ，活動の評価結果の報告時期を RMP に規定することとされている。

　報告様式，PMDA への報告方法についての通知「医薬品リスク管理計画の実施に基づく再審査期間終了後の評価報告について」（平成 25 年 12 月 20 日薬食安発 1220 第 14 号）が発出されている。評価報告書の内容は上述の通知に示されている。

文　　　献

1)　望月眞弓他．平成 22 年度厚生労働科学研究費補助金（医薬品・医療機器等レギュラトリーサイエンス総合研究事業）患者から副作用情報を受ける方策に関する調査研究（H22 ―医薬――般― 021）
https://www.mhlw.go.jp/stf/shingi/2r9852000001flxb-att/2r9852000001fm1v.pdf

2)　成川衛，医薬品リスク管理計画制度の効果的な実施と一層の充実のための基盤研究（平成 27 〜 29 年度）国立研究開発法人 日本医療研究開発機構 医薬品等規制調和・評価研究事業　2018 年 3 月

4.6.7 Periodic reporting on RMP following Reexamination period

For drugs after the completion of the Reexamination period, it is stated that the timing of reporting the results of evaluation of activities should be stipulated in the RMP according to the contents of additional pharmacovigilance activities and additional risk minimization activities.

Notification on reporting forms and methods of reporting to the PMDA, "Reports of evaluation after the completion of the Reexamination period based on the implementation of the Risk Management Plan" (PFSB/SD Notification No. 1220-14 dated December 20, 2013) has been issued. Contents of Evaluation reports are shown in the above notification.

References

1) Mayumi Mochizuki, *et al*. 2010 Health, Labor and Welfare Science Research Grant (General Research on Regulatory Science of Pharmaceuticals and Medical Devices), Research on system for receiving adverse reaction information from patients (2010-Medicine-General-021)
https://www.mhlw.go.jp/stf/shingi/2r9852000001flxb-att/2r9852000001fm1v.pdf

2) Mamoru Narukawa. Basic research on effective implementation and further enrichment of risk management plan system (FY 2015–FY 2017). Research on Regulatory Science of Pharmaceuticals and Medical Devices, Japan Agency for Medical Research and Development, National Research and Development Agency, March 2018

第5章

ファーマコビジランス査察と
ファーマコビジランス監査

　製薬企業が遵守すべきルールとして導入された GVP, GQP, GPSP が正しく守られていることを客観的に第三者に示す必要がある。このため，製造販売業者においては自己点検や，（契約に基づく）PV 監査が，規制当局においては GVP 査察や再審査・再評価適合性調査が行われ，信頼性が確保されている。

5.1　GVP および GQP の適合性評価と査察（業査察）

　製造販売業三役の設置，GVP 省令，GQP 省令への適合はわが国において製造販売業の許可要件である。医薬品の製造販売業の許可（業許可）は，総括製造販売責任者が所属する事業所のある都道府県知事により判断される。業許可は，新規に製造販売業を取得してから 5 年ごとに更新される。業許可の取得や維持のため，GVP 省令，GQP 省令への適合性評価が医薬品の場合，都道府県の担当者（例：薬務課）により行われる。したがって，医薬品の製造販売業者は，GVP および GQP に適切に対応するためのシステム（社内体制，手順書等）を策定し，都道府県は，そのシステム（仕組み，ルール）が当該省令に沿っているか，また，普段行われている実務と一致しているかを評価し，製造販売業の許可・更新の可否を判断する。

5.2　再審査・再評価申請資料に対する適合性調査（信頼性保証査察）

　再審査・再評価申請資料の申請者は，申請資料が GLP（Good Laboratory Practice：医薬品の非臨床試験の実施基準），GCP，GPSP および申請資料の信頼性の基準（医薬品医療機器等法施行規則第 61 条：同第 43 条準用）に従って作成されていることの確認を受ける。この基準適合性調査は PMDA 信頼性保証部により行われ，当該申請資料が GLP，GCP および GPSP に従って倫理的，科学的に適切に実施された調査・試験の成績に基づいているかどうか，また，「申請資料の信頼性の基準」に従って，調査・試験結果に基づいて適切かつ正確に作成されているかどうかを実

Chapter 5

Pharmacovigilance inspections and pharmacovigilance audits

It is necessary to objectively show to third parties that GVP, GQP, and GPSP, which were introduced as rules that pharmaceutical companies should comply with, have been followed accurately. Pharmacovigilance (PV) self inspections and PV audits (per PV contracts) are conducted by Marketing Authorization Holders (MAHs), and GVP inspections or Reexamination/Reevaluation compliance audits are conducted by the regulatory authorities in order to secure credibility and reliability.

5.1 GVP and GQP compliance evaluation and inspections (business inspections)

Establishment of the three Supervisors within MAHs and conformity with the GVP ministerial ordinance and GQP ministerial ordinance are license conditions for MAHs in Japan. A medicine marketing authorization (business license) is determined by the governor of the prefecture where the business office of the Pharmaceutical Officer is located. The business license is renewed every 5 years after the marketing license is obtained. To obtain and maintain the business license, evaluation with the GVP and GQP compliance is conducted by the responsible person (e.g. pharmaceutical affairs division) in the prefectural government. or this reason, MAHs develop a system to appropriately deal with GVP and GQP (operational system, written procedures for GVP and GQP, etc.), and prefectural governments evaluate whether such systems (system/rule) follow the relevant ministerial ordinance and are consistent with the actual operations as routinely conducted and determine whether MAH's license can be approved or nenewed.

5.2 Compliance Inspection for Reexamination and Reevaluation dossier (reliability assurance inspections/examinations)

Applicants for Reexamination/Reevaluation undergo inspections to see if the application dossier has been prepared in accordance with GLP (Good Laboratory Practice), GCP, GPSP, and the Standards for the Reliability of Application Data (Article 61 of the Enforcement Regulations of the PMD Act; Article 43 of the regulations applied mutatis mutandis). These inspection is conducted by the Office of Conformity Audit, Pharmaceuticals and Medical Devices Agency (PMDA), where investigations are conducted on site and by documents to review whether the application data are based on results of investigations and studies appropriately implemented in an ethical and scientific manner in accordance with GLP, GCP, and GPSP and whether the data have been appropriately and accurately prepared based on results of investigations and studies in

地および書面で調査が行われる。この基準適合性調査の後に内容の科学的審査を受ける。GPMSP が GVP と GPSP に分離されたことにより，再審査・再評価申請資料に含まれる GVP 由来の情報については「申請資料の信頼性の基準」による適合性が評価される。

PMDA は，再審査適合性調査の円滑・効率的な実施を 5 か年の中期計画に盛り込んでいる。申請資料中の GVP 由来の情報に基づく資料については，これまで

① 手順書等を用いた業務プロセスの確認
② 抽出症例の確認

により適合性調査が行われてきたが，従来の適合性調査手法における問題点として再審査期間内の手順書等の確認にかなりの時間を要し非効率，品目（担当者）ごとに説明内容が異なる場合がある，などの課題があげられていた。

これを解決するために，GVP 由来の安全性情報についてはシステム調査（プロセス調査）の考え方，方法論が最近取り入れられ，試行が行われている。

5.3 自己点検

製造販売業者等は，GVP および GPSP を遵守し，製造販売後の安全性業務が適正かつ円滑に実施されていることを確認するため，市販後安全性業務の自己点検を実施しなければならない。また，必要な場合には，問題点について早急に改善措置をとる。

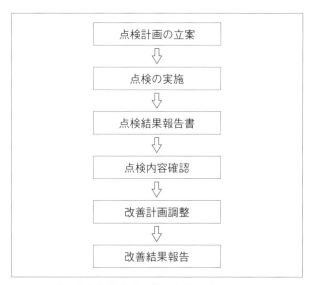

図 5.1　市販後安全性業務の自己点検の手順

accordance with the "Standards for the Reliability of Application Data." After the standards compliance inspection, the contents are scientifically reviewed. As GPMSP was divided into GVP and GPSP, the conformity of information derived from GVP that are included in Reexamination/Reevaluation application data is evaluated according to the "Standards for the Reliability of Application Data."

The PMDA has included smooth and efficient implementation of conformity audits for Reexamination in its 5-year midterm plan. Regarding data based on GVP related information in application data, the following has been done for conformity audits:

[1] Confirmation of operating processes using SOPs, etc., and
[2] Examination of sample cases

However there have been problems with the conventional methods of compliance inspection, such as issues. However there have been problems with the conventional methods of compliance inspection, such as issues "of inefficiency in reviewing SOPs during reexamination and different explanation by different inspectors who are assigned to different medicines".

To solve these problems, the concept and methodology of system inspections (process inspections) have recently been incorporated for GVP related safety information, and have been used on a trial basis.

5.3 Self inspections

MAHs etc. should implement self inspections of post-marketing safety operations, in compliance with GVP and GPSP, in order to confirm that post-marketing safety operations have been implemented properly and smoothly. Also, they should promptly make improvements for problems where necessary.

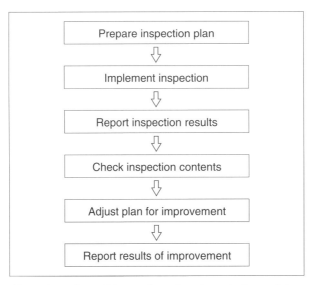

Fig.5.1 Procedures for self inspection of post-marketing safety operations

5.3.1 手順書およびチェックリストの作成

製造販売業者等は製造販売後安全管理手順書等に基づき，また，製造販売業者等は製造販売後調査等業務手順書に基づき，あらかじめ指定する者に定期的に自己点検を実施させる。臨時の自己点検に関する手順も作成し，それら自己点検記録は保存しなければならない。また，改善措置についても記録が保存されなければならない。

自己点検時の点検項目・内容の明確化，また，点検結果の共有化をするために，事前にチェックリストを作成する（図5.1）。

5.3.2 GVP の自己点検

以下について点検を行う。
- 責任者の任命・役割，管理部門体制
- 手順書の作成・配布
- 製造販売業者，総括製造販売責任者・安全管理責任者・品質管理責任者の連携体制
- 情報の収集・評価・措置

5.3.3 GPSP の自己点検

以下について点検を行う。
- 責任者の任命・役割，管理部門体制
- 手順書の作成・配布
- 製造販売業者等，総括製造販売責任者・安全管理責任者・品質管理責任者の連携体制
- 製造販売後調査・臨床試験に関する施設の選定・施設との契約・登録，進捗状況の即時報告・情報共有

5.3.4 自己点検の教育

自己点検について，MR 教育および実施部門への教育を実施する。自己点検の意義（コンプライアンス，医療の安全確保の一員），遵守の確認および改善への取り組みを提案する。コンプライアンスとしては，社内規則，GCP，プロモーションコード等がある。

5.3.5 その他の自己点検の注意点

海外本社からの PV 監査および海外提携先への PV 監査の実施などがこのほかに考えられるが，国内販売提携先については，実施部門選定時の実地調査を必ず行い，依頼後には定期的に自己点検を実施する。また，提携先の自己点検結果の報告が入手できる契約を結ぶ。

5.3.1 Preparation of written procedures and checklist

Designated persons periodically perform self inspections at MAHs based on SOP on post-marketing safety management, SOPs on post-marketing studies, etc. SOP for ad hoc self inspections should be also prepared, and the records of these self inspections should be stored. The record of improvement measures should also be retained.

A checklist should be prepared in advance for clarification of inspection items/contents at the time of self inspections and sharing of inspection results (**Fig. 5.1**).

5.3.2 GVP self inspections

Inspections should be performed for the following:
- Assignment/roles of responsible persons and system at management division
- Preparation/distribution of SOPs
- Collaboration system among MAH and the Pharmaceutical Officer/the Safety Management Officer/the Quality Assurance Officer
- Collection/evaluation/handing of safety information

5.3.3 GPSP self inspections

Inspections should be performed for the following:
- Assignment/roles of responsible persons and system at management division
- Preparation/distribution of written procedures
- Collaboration system among MAH and the Pharmaceutical Officer/the Safety Management Officer/the Quality Assurance Officer
- Selection of institutions for post-marketing investigations/clinical studies; Contract with/registration of institutions; Real-time reporting of progress status and information sharing

5.3.4 Education on self inspections

Regarding self inspections, education for medical representatives (MRs) and division in charge of conducting should be conducted. The education should include significance of self inspections (compliance; safety assurance of medical care), confirmation of compliance, and efforts for improvement. For compliance, there are internal policies, GCP, promotion code, etc.

5.3.5 Other points to consider for self inspections

In addition, there may be PV audits by an overseas business alliance head office and PV audits for overseas partners. For domestic sales partners, an on-site audit for selection of implementing division should be performed, and self inspections should be periodically conducted thereafter. In addition, the contract should include an agreement to review of partners self inspection results.

138   第5章　ファーマコビジランス査察とファーマコビジランス監査

5.4　PV 契約による監査

　国内の医薬品製造販売後安全性に関する規制では自己点検が求められており，PV 監査は言及されていないが，2012 年 7 月に European Union（EU）で施行された EU Directive 2010/84/EU[1] および EU Regulation 1235/2010[2] に規定されており，GVP モジュール IV として EU 圏内の MAH に義務付けられている。

　監査においては，法規制で求められている PV システムが効果的および適切に導入され，かつ稼働していることを客観的証拠の検証および評価により検証する。また，これには PV 活動の品質システムの検証・評価を含む。

5.4.1　EU GVP における PV 監査

①　PV システム

　　PV システムは，GVP モジュール I に定義されている。それには，PV 関連の法規制で義務付けられた事項や市販医薬品の安全性を監視し，また，リスク‒ベネフィットの変化を検知するために設置されたシステムであると定義されている。

　　MAH は，PV システムの一環として品質システムを設置し，それには PV システムの組織・責任・方法・リソースの品質およびリソース管理，遵守管理，記録管理が含まれる。また，PV 業務には，適切に Qualify された，適切な

表 5.1　PV 業務における管理職の責任

・　品質システム業務の文書化がされている
・　品質システム業務に関する文書の作成・改訂・承認・施行に関するコントロールが文書化されている
・　適切な人材が確保され，また，彼らの教育が実施されている
・　業務を行うにあたり，適切な場所，設備が備わっている
・　適切なコンプライアンスの管理がされている
・　記録の管理が適切に行われている
・　定期的に品質システムを含めた PV システム全体がリスクに基づいてレビューされ，効果的に行われているかを確認し，また，必要に応じて CAPA を求める
・　MAH が保持する医薬品の安全性に関する懸念事項について適切，効果的なコミュニケーションが図れる手順が設定されている。これには，問題の管理者へのエスカレーションも含まれる
・　品質および PV システムの要望事項に反する問題があると考えられる場合には，それらを特定し，必要に応じて管理者へのエスカレーションおよび CAPA が設定される
・　監査が実施される
PV システムおよび品質システムのモニタリング
・　モニタリング管理責任者によるシステムの定期的レビュー
・　監査：リスクに基づく定期的監査の実施，監査担当者は，PV 実施部門とは直接に関係しない部門に所属していること，対応の実施，フォローアップ監査
・　遵守状況モニタリング
・　査察
・　リスク最小化対応の評価
・　事業継続計画の設定

Chapter 5 Pharmacovigilance inspections and pharmacovigilance audits 139

5.4 Audits under PV contracts

Under regulations on post-marketing safety regulation of medicines in Japan, self inspection is required. PV audits are not mentioned in those regulations but are specified in EU Directive 2010/84/EU[1] and EU Regulation 1235/2010[2] which came into force in the European Union (EU) in July 2012 and are obligatory for medicine marketing authorization holders (MAHs) in the EU per Good Pharmacovigilance Practices (GVP) Module IV.

Audits examine whether the PV system has been effectively and appropriately implemented and operated and are based on verification and evaluation of objective evidence as required by laws and regulations. This also includes verification and evaluation of the quality system for PV activities.

5.4.1 PV audits under EU GVP

[1] PV system

The PV system is defined in GVP Module I in which the system is defined as a system being place to monitor items that are obligatory under PV-related laws and regulations and the safety of marketed medicines and to detect changes in risk-benefit.

MAHs must place a quality system as a part of the PV system, and this quality system includes the organization, responsibilities, procedures, resource quality, and quality of resource, compliance management, and record management under PV system. PV operations require an appropriate number of staff who are appropriately qualified.

In order to maintain the quality of PV operations in the organization, activities described in **Table 5.1** should be performed as responsibilities of management.

Table5.1   Responsibilities of management level employees in PV operations

- Quality system operations are documented.
- The control of preparation/revision/approval/implementation of documents on quality system operations is documented.
- Appropriate human resources are secured and training is conducted.
- Appropriate places and facilities are available for conducting operations.
- Compliance is controlled appropriately.
- Control of records is performed appropriately.
- The whole PV system including the quality system is periodically reviewed based on risks, whether the system is used effectively is checked, and CAPA is requested as needed.
- Procedures for appropriate and effective communication are specified for any concerns the MAH has about the safety of drugs. These include escalation to managers in question.
- Any apparent problems with the quality or the PV systems, are identified and escalated to managers and CAPA is performed as needed.
- <u>Audits are conducted.</u>

Monitoring of the PV system and quality system
- Periodic review of systems by monitoring manager
- <u>Audits: Implementation of periodic audits based on risks; Persons in charge of audits belong to a division not directly related to the PV implementation division; Implementation of actions; Follow-up audits</u>
- Monitoring of compliance status
- Inspections
- Evaluation of risk minimization actions
- Establishment of business continuity plan

人数のスタッフが必要である。

さらに，PV 業務の品質を組織として維持するには，管理職の責任として**表5.1** のことがあげられる。

また，安全性業務を委託した場合も，同様に MAH は，委託業務に関して有効な品質システムが適用されていることの責任がある。GVP の内容は委託先にも適応される。したがって，委託業務契約書には，それぞれの役割および責任の詳細が規定されているべきである。また，委託業務契約書には，当該契約に合意した内容が着実に実施されているか否かを継続的に確認するプロセスを決める。それには，リスクに基づく監査を定期的に行うことが望ましい。

② リスクに基づく PV 監査

組織の PV システムで最もリスクの高い領域に注目して監査をし，戦略的，戦術的および運用レベルでの監査計画のためのリスク評価を文書化する。

③ 監査結果の報告

監査の指摘事項は監査報告書として文書化し，マネジメント（会社および組織の管理者）にタイムリーに報告する。監査指摘事項は，該当するリスクに沿い，PV システムに対するリスク度合いによって，その重要度に基づき分類する。

④ 監査業務および監査担当者の独立性と客観性

PV 監査は，"independent" に行われるべきであり，会社は PV 監査をする特別な組織を設置する必要がある。また，マネジメントは，監査の「独立性」および「客観性」が明確かつ高度に組織化され，また，それが文書化されていることを保証する義務がある。

監査のスコープ決定，PV 監査業務，監査結果の報告は，常に他からの干渉なしで行われるものである。したがって，監査担当者が独立した客観的な考えを述べることができ，干渉なしで業務を遂行しうるために，監査担当者には会社組織の管理責任があるシニアマネジメントに直接の report-line が設定されることが望ましい。監査担当者は，テクニカルエキスパートや実際のPV 業務担当者等に相談してもよいが，常に偏見のない考え方を維持し，自身の仕事に正直であり，業務の質に妥協を許さないことが大切である。また，「客観性」を維持するために，監査担当者は監査に関する判断をそれ以外のことよりも上位に考えるべきである。

⑤ EU 圏内の MAH の責任

EU の中央承認を受けた医薬品に関する EU 圏外各国の MAH の委託契約は，それらの国々の PV データが入手できるようにしなければならない。

また，MAH は，PV システムに関する監査の Critical および Major 指摘事項について PSMF（Pharmacovigilance System Master File：安全性監視〔PV〕シ

In addition, when safety operations are outsourced, MAHs have responsibility for ensuring that an effective quality system is applied to the outsourced work. The contents of GVP are also applicable to the service providers to which activities are outsourced. A written contract should therefore stipulate the details of the respective parties' roles and responsibilities. Also, for an outsourcing contract, there is a specified process to continuously confirm whether or not contents agreed in the contract have been consistently implemented. For this reason, it is desirable to periodically conduct risk-based audits.

[2] Risk-based PV audits

These audits should be conducted focusing on the high risk area in the PV system in the organization, and there should be documentation of the risk evaluation for audit planning that are strategic, tactical, and performed at the operational level.

[3] Reporting of audit results

Audit findings should be documented in an audit report and reported to management (supervisors of the company and organization) in a timely manner. Audit findings should be classified based on level of importance, in line with corresponding risks and according to the level of risk for the PV system.

[4] Independence and objectivity of audit operations and auditors.

PV audits should be conducted in an "independent" manner, and therefore companies need to establish a special organization which conducts PV audits. Management must guarantee that the "independence" and "objectivity" of audits are clear and highly organized and that this is documented.

Determination of the scope of audits, PV audit procedures, and reporting of audit outcome are to be done at all times without interference from others. For this reason, to ensure that persons in charge of audits can give independent and objective views and execute operations without interference, it is desirable to set up a direct report-line for audit organization to the senior management of the company. The auditors may consult with technical experts or others such as those in charge of actual PV operations, but it is important to always maintain unprejudiced ways of thinking, to be honest about their own work, and to be uncompromising about the quality of the operations. Also, to maintain "objectivity," persons in charge of audits should place a higher priority on their judgment in audits than other things.

[5] Responsibilities of MAHs in the EU

Outsourcing contracts of MAHs in countries outside the EU regarding drugs with central approval by the EU should be made in a way that enables obtaining PV data in these countries.

Also, MAHs have an obligation to describe critical and major PV audit findings in the PSMF (Pharmacovigilance System Master File, GVP Module II) and have an obligation to guarantee that appropriate CAPA (Corrective Action and Preventive Action) for audit findings are considered and implemented. After the completion of the CAPA, records on such findings may be deleted from the PSMF. However, when deleting those records, objective evidence is needed. MAHs have an obligation to keep the audit plan and the list of audits as an

ステムマスターファイル，GVP モジュール II）に記載する責務，ならびに，監査指摘事項への適切な CAPA（Corrective Action and Preventive Action：是正措置および予防措置）が検討され，施行されることを保証する責務がある。CAPA の完了後には，当該指摘事項に関する記録を PSMF から削除できる。ただし，記録を削除する場合には，客観的な証拠が必要である。MAH は，監査計画および完了した監査のリストを PSMF の Annex に残す責務がある。また，当該規制，GVP ガイダンスおよび内部報告手順等に従い，監査報告をする。監査日程，監査結果およびフォローアップ監査について記載されていることも必要である。

5.4.2　PV 契約の役割

　PV 業務の国内外の提携会社あるいはベンダーへの委託については，PV 契約を結ぶ必要があるが，それには互いの委託業務，相互関係およびデータ交換を詳細に記載することが大切である。さらに，PV 契約で合意された内容が着実に実行されているか否かを継続的に確認するプロセスを示すことが求められる。例えば，EU の MAH である国内企業に海外に提携先がある場合，PV 契約に監査に関する条項を入れ，当該委託業務を監視するための手段とすることができる。

　国内企業が EU の MAH である場合には，委託先に対して監査を実施することになる。また，国内企業が EU の MAH と業務提携している場合には，MAH による PV 監査を受けることになる。

　PV 業務を委託している場合でも，EU の MAH が，PSMF の完結度および正確な内容の保持について責任をもたなければならない。

文　　献

1）　Directive 2010/84/EU of the European Parliament and of the Council of 15 December 2010, amending, as regards pharmacovigilance, Directive 2001/83/EC on the Community code relating to medicinal products for human use:
　　https://ec.europa.eu/health//sites/health/files/files/eudralex/vol-1/dir_2010_84/dir_2010_84_en.pdf

2）　Regulation (EU) No 1235/2010 of the European Parliament and of the Council of 15 December 2010, amending, as regards pharmacovigilance of medicinal products for human use, Regulation (EC) No 726/2004 laying down Community procedures for the authorisation and supervision of medicinal products for human and veterinary use and establishing a European Medicines Agency, and Regulation (EC) No 1394/2007 on advanced therapy medicinal products:
　　https://eur-lex.europa.eu/LexUriServ/LexUriServ.do?uri=OJ:L:2010:348:0001:0016:EN:PDF

Chapter 5 Pharmacovigilance inspections and pharmacovigilance audits

Annex to the PSMF. Also, audit reports should be made in accordance with these regulations, the GVP guidance, and internal reporting procedures, etc. It is also necessary that the audit schedule, audit results, and follow-up audits should be described.

5.4.2 Roles of PV contracts

When outsourcing PV work to a domestic/overseas partner company or vendor, it is necessary to make a PV contract, but it is important to describe in the contract the details of the outsourced work, mutual relationship, and data exchange procedure between the parties. In addition, a process to continuously check whether or not contents agreed upon in the PV contract have been consistently executed should be demonstrated. For example, if a domestic company as an MAH in the EU has an overseas partner, putting terms related to audits in the PV contract can be used as a means to monitor these outsourced work.

If a domestic company is an MAH in the EU, audits of outsourced vender are supposed to be conducted. Also, if a domestic company has a partnership with an MAH in the EU, the company is supposed to undergo PV audits by the MAH.

Even when PV work are outsourced, the MAH in the EU has the responsibility for maintaining complete and accurate contents of the PSMF.

References

1) Directive 2010/84/EU of the European Parliament and of the Council of 15 December 2010, amending, as regards pharmacovigilance, Directive 2001/83/EC on the Community code relating to medicinal products for human use:
https://ec.europa.eu/health//sites/health/files/files/eudralex/vol-1/dir_2010_84/dir_2010_84_en.pdf

2) Regulation (EU) No 1235/2010 of the European Parliament and of the Council of 15 December 2010, amending, as regards pharmacovigilance of medicinal products for human use, Regulation (EC) No 726/2004 laying down Community procedures for the authorisation and supervision of medicinal products for human and veterinary use and establishing a European Medicines Agency, and Regulation (EC) No 1394/2007 on advanced therapy medicinal products:
https://eur-lex.europa.eu/LexUriServ/LexUriServ.do?uri=OJ:L:2010:348:0001:0016:EN:PDF

第6章

医薬品等による健康被害救済制度

　1979年10月，サリドマイド事件やスモン事件をきっかけとして医薬品副作用被害救済基金法が制定され，医薬品副作用被害救済基金が設立された。同法第1条の目的は，「医薬品副作用被害救済基金は，医薬品の副作用による疾病，廃疾又は死亡に関して，医療費，障害年金，遺族年金等の給付を行うこと等により，医薬品の副作用による健康被害の迅速な救済を図ることを目的とする。」とされている。医薬品が適正に使用されたにもかかわらず，防ぎえなかった一定以上の健康被害について，負担の大きい裁判によらず救済するための医薬品副作用被害救済制度が，世界に先駆けて定められ，翌1980年5月から実際の業務が開始された。

　医薬品においては「有効性」と「副作用」とは不可分の関係にある。本制度は，医薬品の使用に伴い生じる副作用被害について，民事責任とは切り離し，医薬品の製造販売業者の社会的責任に基づく共同事業として，迅速かつ簡便な救済給付を行うという一種の保険システムである。救済給付に必要な費用は，製造販売業者から納付される拠出金が原資となっている。

　さらに，2004年4月には新たに，生物に由来する原料や材料を使ってつくられた医薬品と医療機器による感染等の健康被害について救済する「生物由来製品感染等被害救済制度」が創設された。また，2013年11月に医薬品医療機器総合機構法が改正され，再生医療等製品による健康被害についても，副作用被害救済制度および感染等被害救済制度の対象となった（適用は2014年11月25日以降）。

　これらの救済制度に基づく健康被害救済業務は，医学薬学的判断を除いて，PMDAが行っている。

6.1　医薬品副作用被害救済制度の概要

6.1.1　救済の対象

　救済は，医療用および一般用の医薬品が適正な目的で適正に使用されたにもかかわらず，1980年5月1日以降に発生した副作用被害で，「入院相当の治療が必要な被害」，「1・2級程度の障害」，「死亡」の場合を対象にしている。ただし，以下の

Chapter 6

Relief Services System for Adverse Health Effects

The Law for the Adverse Drug Reaction Relief Service Fund was promulgated in October 1979 after the thalidomide and SMON incidents, and the Adverse Drug Reaction Relief Service Fund was established. The Article 1 of this law says "the purpose of the Fund is to provides prompt relief of health damage caused by ADRs by paying medical fees, disability pensions, survivor pensions, etc. for diseases, disabilities or death caused by ADRs." Japan was an international pioneer in establishing the Relief Service for Adverse Drug Reactions to provide redress for health damage exceeding a certain level that could not be prevented in spite of proper use of a drug without the burden of going to court. The system started operation from May 1980.

For drugs, "efficacy" and "adverse drug reactions" are inextricably linked. This system is a kind of insurance system to provide relief and benefits promptly and simply as a joint project based on the social responsibilities of drug Marketing Authorization Holders (MAHs) whereby compensation for injuries from adverse drug reactions is separated from civil responsibility. Contributions (general, additional) paid by MAHs provide the funding for relief and benefits.

In April 2004, a new "relief service system for infections derived from biological products" was established to provide relief for infections caused by drugs and medical devices made from ingredients or raw materials of biological origin. Since the Act on the Pharmaceuticals and Medical Devices Agency was revised in November 2013, health damages due to regenerative medicine products became covered under the Adverse Drug Reaction Relief Service System and the Relief Service System for Infections. Since the Act on the Pharmaceuticals and Medical Devices Agency was revised in November 2013, health damages due to regenerative medicine products became covered under the Adverse Drug Reaction Relief Service System and the Relief Service System for Infections (applied after November 25, 2014).

Health damage relief operations based on these relief systems are conducted by PMDA with the exception of the medico-pharmaceutical judgments.

6.1 Summary of the Relief Service for Adverse Drug Reactions

6.1.1 Scope of relief

This relief system applies to damages due to ADRs occurring on or after May 1, 1980 irrespective of whether caused by prescription or OTC drugs as long as they were used properly for an approved indication. The system covers "Damage requiring treatment equivalent to hospitalization," "Level 1 or 2 physical disability" and "Death." However,

場合には給付の対象にはならないとされている。
① 医薬品の使用目的・方法が適正であったとは認められない場合
② 医薬品の副作用において，健康被害が入院治療を要する程度ではなかった場合などや請求期限が経過した場合
③ 対象除外医薬品（抗がん剤，免疫抑制剤など）による健康被害の場合
④ 医薬品の製造販売業者などに明らかに損害賠償責任がある場合
⑤ 救命のためにやむをえず通常の使用量を超えて医薬品を使用し，健康被害の発生があらかじめ認識されていたなどの場合
⑥ 法定予防接種を受けたことによるものである場合（予防接種健康被害救済制度がある。なお，任意に予防接種を受けた場合は本制度の対象となる）

※文献1）より一部改変。

6.1.2 給付の請求から給付の決定まで

図6.1に医薬品副作用被害救済制度の概要を示した。まず，健康被害に遭った患者本人またはその遺族が，給付申請をPMDAに対して行う。このとき，発症した症状，経過とそれが医薬品などを使用したことによるものだという関係を証明する必要がある。そのためには，副作用の治療を行った医師の診断書や投薬証明書が必要となるので，請求者は，それらの書類の作成を医師に依頼し，請求者が記入した請求書とともにPMDAに提出する。請求書，診断書などの用紙はPMDAに備えて

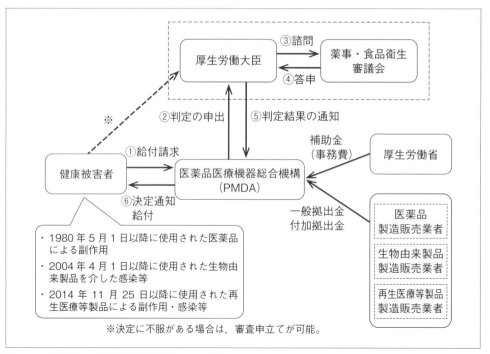

図6.1 副作用・感染救済給付業務の流れ[2]

the following cases are not covered for benefits:
[1] Purpose and method of use of the drug are not considered proper.
[2] The health damage caused by the Adverse Drug Reaction did not require inpatient treatment, or the claim period has ended.
[3] Health damages due to excluded drugs (anticancer drugs, immunosuppressive agents, etc.)
[4] The MAH, etc. of the drug obviously has liability for the damage.
[5] The drug was used in an amount higher than the normal dosage, out of necessity for life saving, where the occurrence of health damage was expected in advance.
[6] The damage was due to receiving a mandatory preventive vaccination (There is a separate Relief Services System for Adverse Health Effects with Vaccination. If receiving preventive vaccination voluntarily, such damage is covered by this system.)

* Partially modified from Reference [1].

6.1.2 Process from application through decision on benefits

A summary of the Relief Service for Adverse Drug Reactions is shown in **Fig. 6.1**. First, the patient suffering health damage or his/her bereaved family makes a request for benefits to the PMDA. At such time, it is necessary to demonstrate a relationship between the symptom(s) that occurred and its course, and that it was caused by use of the drug, etc. Therefore, since it is necessary to obtain a diagnostic report from the physician who treated the ADR and drug treatment certificate, the applicant requests their physicians to prepare these papers, fills in the request form and submits them to the PMDA. The PMDA prepares the request form, diagnostic form and other materials and

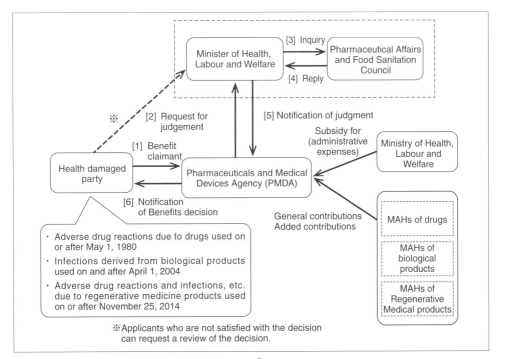

Fig.6.1 Flow of operations for relief & benefits[2]

148　　第 6 章　医薬品等による健康被害救済制度

あり，健康被害を受けた本人や家族からの申し出により無料で送付されている。また，PMDA の Web サイトから必要な書類をダウンロードすることもできる。

　　PMDA では，給付の請求があった健康被害について，その健康被害が医薬品の副作用によるものかどうか，医薬品が適正に使用されたかどうかなどの医学的薬学的判断について，厚生労働大臣に判定の申し出を行い，厚生労働大臣は，PMDA からの判定の申し出に応じ，薬事・食品衛生審議会（副作用被害判定部会）に意見を聴いて判定を行うこととされている。そして，PMDA は，厚生労働大臣による判定に基づいて給付の支給の可否を決定する。なお，この決定に対して不服がある請求者は，厚生労働大臣に対して審査を申し立てることができる。

　　支給される給付には以下の種類がある。

① 　疾病（入院を必要とする程度）について医療を受けた場合
　　　→ 　医療費，医療手当
② 　一定程度の障害（日常生活が著しく制限される程度以上のもの）の場合
　　　→ 　障害年金，障害児養育年金
③ 　死亡した場合
　　　→ 　遺族年金，遺族一時金，葬祭料

6.1.3　統計

　　医薬品副作用被害救済制度は，PMDA 等の広報の強化により，請求件数・支給決定件数は年々増加傾向にあるが（2017 年度は減少した），さらなる広報の努力が期待されている。2013 ～ 2017 年度の請求・決定件数等は**表 6.1** に示したとおりである。また，表 6.1 よりわかるとおり，年々，事務処理の迅速化も引き続き進んでいる。

　　2013 ～ 2017 年度の副作用による健康被害の器官別大分類別の内訳は，**図 6.2** に

表 6.1　副作用被害救済の実績 [3]

年　　度	2013 年度	2014 年度	2015 年度	2016 年度	2017 年度
請求件数	1,371 件	1,412 件	1,566 件	1,843 件	1,491 件
決定件数	1,240 件	1,400 件	1,510 件	1,754 件	1,607 件
支給決定 不支給決定 取り下げ	1,007 件 232 件 1 件	1,204 件 192 件 4 件	1,279 件 221 件 10 件	1,340 件 411 件 3 件	1,305 件 298 件 4 件
6 か月 以内　件数 　達成率[*1]	754 件 60.8%	867 件 61.9%	915 件 60.6%	1,182 件 67.4%	1,113 件 69.3%
処理中件数[*2]	910 件	922 件	978 件	1,067 件	951 件
処理期間（中央値）	5.8 月	5.7 月	5.6 月	5.3 月	5.3 月

[*1] 　当該年度中に決定されたもののうち，6 か月以内に処理できたものの割合
[*2] 　各年度末時点の数値

forwards them free of charge in accordance with the requests of the person who suffered the damage or his or her family. The necessary documents can be downloaded from the PMDA website (http://www.pmda.go.jp).

The PMDA requests the Minister of Health, Labour and Welfare to make a medical and pharmacological judgement on whether or not the health damage is due to an adverse reaction of the drug and on whether or not the drug was correctly used related to the injury for which a request for benefits was made. The Minister, in response to the request for judgement from the PMDA, requests the opinion of the Pharmaceutical Affairs and Food Sanitation Council (Committee on Judgement of Sufferers from Adverse Drug Reactions). The PMDA decides on whether or not to pay the benefits on the basis of the judgment made by the Minister. Applicants who are not satisfied with this decision can request the Minister to review the decision.

The following types of benefits are paid

[1] Cases where treatment was received for a disease (severity requiring hospitalization)
→ Medical expenses, medical allowances
[2] Cases of disability to a certain degree (degree that markedly hinders activities of daily living or greater)
→ Disability pension, disabled child support pension
[3] Cases leading to death
→ Survivor pensions, survivor lump sum payments, funeral expenses

6.1.3 Statistics

In the ADR Relief Service System, the number of requests and number of decisions on benefits tend to increase every year with the strengthening of publicity by PMDA, etc. (it was reduced in the FY 2017), but there are expectations for further publicity efforts. The number of requests and decisions in FY 2013-2017 are shown in **Table 6.1**. As shown in Table 6.1, administrative processing times have been continuously shortening dramatically year over year.

Table6.1   Performance in Adverse Reaction Relief Service[3]

Fiscal Year		2013	2014	2015	2016	2017
No. of applications		1,371	1,412	1,566	1,843	1,491
No. of decisions		1,240	1,400	1,510	1,754	1,607
	Decisions to pay Decisions not to pay No. of withdrawals	1,007 232 1	1,204 192 4	1,279 221 10	1,340 411 3	1,305 298 4
No. for 6 months	Achievement rate[*1]	754 60.8%	867 61.9%	915 60.6%	1,182 67.4%	1,113 69.3%
No. in process[*2]		910	922	978	1,067	951
Processing time (median value)		5.8 mos	5.7 mos	5.6 mos	5.3 mos	5.3 mos

[*1] Percentage of processing completed within 6 months among decisions made in the fiscal year concerned.
[*2] Numerical value as of the end of each fiscal year

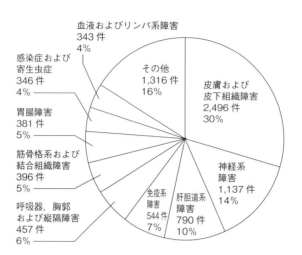

皮膚および皮下組織障害

内訳	比率
多形紅斑	31.2%
過敏症症候群	22.5%
皮膚粘膜眼症候群	11.2%
紅斑丘疹型薬疹	11.1%
その他	24.0%

原因薬の薬効小分類	比率
抗てんかん剤	18.2%
解熱鎮痛消炎剤	15.4%
主としてグラム陽性・陰性菌に作用するもの	11.8%
消化性潰瘍用剤	7.3%
総合感冒剤	3.5%
合成抗菌剤	3.5%
その他	40.3%

神経系障害

内訳	比率
低酸素脳症	16.9%
悪性症候群	7.4%
運動機能障害	6.9%
ジストニア	6.6%
その他	62.2%

原因薬の薬効小分類	比率
精神神経用剤	46.8%
ワクチン類	4.7%
血液凝固阻止剤	3.6%
局所麻酔剤	3.4%
催眠鎮静剤，抗不安剤	2.7%
その他	38.9%

肝胆道系障害

内訳	比率
肝機能障害	95.6%
劇症肝炎	3.0%
肝不全	0.5%
その他	0.9%

原因薬の薬効小分類	比率
解熱鎮痛消炎剤	13.1%
漢方製剤	12.1%
消化性潰瘍用剤	9.2%
主としてグラム陽性・陰性菌に作用するもの	5.8%
その他	59.9%

免疫系障害

内訳	比率
アナフィラキシーショック	65.6%
アナフィラキシー	26.3%
その他	8.1%

原因薬の薬効小分類	比率
X線造影剤	16.9%
主としてグラム陽性・陰性菌に作用するもの	16.0%
解熱鎮痛消炎剤	11.4%
合成抗菌剤	8.6%
その他	47.0%

呼吸器，胸郭および縦隔障害

内訳	比率
間質性肺炎	62.6%
肺塞栓症	17.7%
その他	19.7%

原因薬の薬効小分類	比率
解熱鎮痛消炎剤	13.1%
漢方製剤	11.2%
他に分類されない代謝性医薬品	7.9%
精神神経用剤	6.7%
その他	61.2%

注）上記の件数は，一般的な副作用の傾向を示した内訳ではなく，救済事例に対する解析結果である。また，上記の件数は，疾病，障害その他認められた健康被害の延べ件数である。

図 6.2　副作用による健康被害の器官別大分類別の内訳（文献 4）より一部改変）
2013 年（平成 25 年度）〜 2017 年（平成 29 年度）に給付された請求事例（6,135 件）の副作用による健康被害を MedDRA/J の器官別大分類で集計した延べ 8,206 件を対象とした。

Chapter 6 Relief Services System for Adverse Health Effects

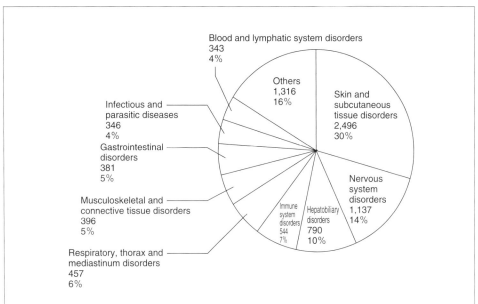

Skin and Subcutaneous tissue disorders

Breakdown	Percentage
Erythema multiforme	31.2%
Hypersensitivity syndrome	22.5%
Muco-cutaneo-ocular syndrome	11.2%
Papuloerythematous drug eruption	11.1%
Others	24.0%

Therapeutic subcategories of drugs causing ADRs	Percentage
Anti-epileptic agents	18.2%
Antipyretic, analgesic and anti-inflammatory agents	15.4%
Agents that mainly act on Gram-positive and Gram-negative bacteria	11.8%
Agents for peptic ulcers	7.3%
Combined cold medicine	3.5%
Synthetic antimicrobial agents	3.5%
Others	40.3%

Nervous system disorders

Breakdown	Percentage
Hypoxic encephalopathia	16.9%
Malignant syndrome	7.4%
Motor dysfunction	6.9%
Dystonias	6.6%
Others	62.2%

Therapeutic subcategories of drugs causing ADRs	Percentage
Antipsychotics and agents for nervous systems	46.8%
Vaccines	4.7%
Anti-coagulant agents	3.6%
Local analgesic agents	3.4%
Sedative-hypnotic agents, anti-anxiety agents	2.7%
Others	38.9%

Hepatobiliary disorders

Breakdown	Percentage
Hepatic function disorder	95.6%
Fulminant hepatitis	3.0%
Hepatic failure	0.5%
Others	0.9%

Therapeutic subcategories of drugs causing ADRs	Percentage
Antipyretic, analgesic and anti-inflammatory agents	13.1%
Herbal preparations	12.1%
Agents for peptic ulcer	9.2%
Agents that mainly act on Gram-positive and Gram-negative bacteria	5.8%
Others	59.9%

Immune system disorders

Breakdown	Percentage
Anaphylactic shock	65.6%
Anaphylaxis	26.3%
Others	8.1%

Therapeutic subcategories of drugs causing ADRs	Percentage
X-ray contrast media	16.9%
Agents that mainly act on Gram-positive and Gram-negative bacteria	16.0%
Antipyretic, analgesic and anti-inflammatory agents	11.4%
Synthetic antimicrobial agents	8.6%
Others	47.0%

Respiratory, thorax and mediastinum disorders

Breakdown	Percentage
Interstitial pneumonia	62.6%
Pulmonary embolism	17.7%
Others	19.7%

Therapeutic subcategories of drugs causing ADRs	Percentage
Antipyretic, analgesic and anti-inflammatory agents	13.1%
Herbal preparations	11.2%
Other metabolic drugs	7.9%
Antipsychotics and agents for nervous systems	6.7%
Others	61.2%

Note) the above numbers of cases are not a breakdown of trends of general ADRs, but are results of analysis for relief cases. Furthermore, the above numbers of cases are total number of cases of disease, disability, or confirmed health damage.

Fig.6.2 Health damage caused by ADRs classified by system organ class (partially modified from Reference[4])

The investigation was done in a total of 6,135 reports summarized by system organ class of MedDRA/J for health damages due to ADRs in claim cases (8,206 cases) to which benefits were provided between 2013 and 2017.

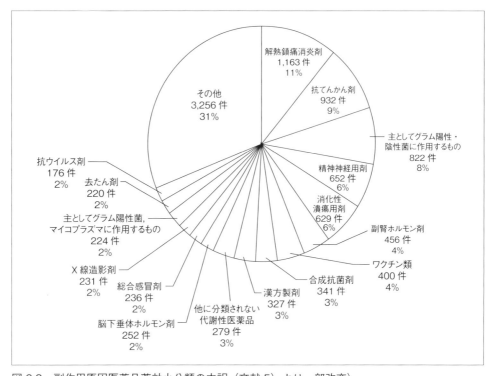

図 6.3　副作用原因医薬品薬効小分類の内訳（文献 5）より一部改変）
平成 25 年度〜平成 29 年度に給付された請求事例（6,135 件）の原因薬延べ 10,596 品目の薬効別分類（小分類）を対象とした。

示したとおりであり，多い順から，皮膚および皮下組織障害，神経系障害，肝胆道系障害となっている。

また，副作用の原因医薬品を薬効小分類の内訳で表せば，図 6.3 のとおりとなる。多い順から，解熱鎮痛消炎剤，抗てんかん剤，主としてグラム陽性・陰性菌に作用するものの順となっている。

6.2　生物由来製品感染等被害救済制度の概要

6.2.1　救済の対象

　ヒトや動物などの生物に由来するものを原料や材料とした医薬品や医療機器（生物由来製品）については，ウイルスなどが入り込むおそれがあるため，さまざまな措置が講じられているが，生物由来製品による感染被害のおそれを完全になくすことはできない。

　このような背景から，2004 年 4 月に新たに生物由来製品感染等被害救済制度が創設された。これは，2004 年 4 月 1 日以降に生物由来製品を適正に使用したにもかかわらず，その製品を介した感染により生じた，入院が必要な程度の疾病や障害などの健康被害について救済を行う制度である。また，感染後の発症を予防するた

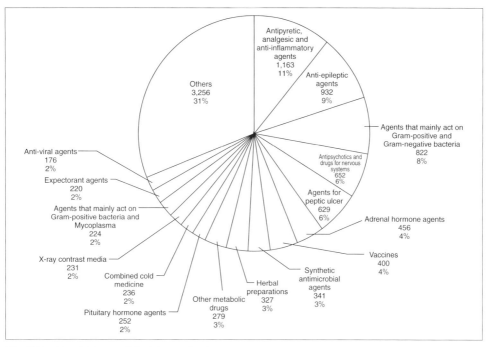

Fig.6.3 Partially modified from the breakdown of therapeutic subcategories of drugs causing ADRs (Reference 5)

The investigation was done in therapeutic categories (subcategories) of suspected drugs (a total of 10,596 products) for claims (6,135 cases) for which benefits were provided between 2013 and 2017.

Fig. 6.2 shows the health damage caused by ADRs in FY 2013-2017 classified by system organ class. The classes showing the highest values were skin and subcutaneous tissue disorders, nervous system disorders and hepatobiliary in that order.

Fig. 6.3 shows the therapeutic subcategories of drugs causing ADRs. The most common were antipyretic analgesic anti-inflammatory agents, antiepileptic agents, and agents that mainly act on Gram-positive and Gram-negative bacteria.

6.2 Summary of the Relief Service for Infections derived from Biological Products

6.2.1 Scope of relief

Drugs and medical devices with raw materials or ingredients derived from living organisms such as humans and animals (biological products) can contain viruses and other organisms, and as such, various precautionary measures have been taken, but the possibility of infectious hazards caused by biological products cannot be completely eliminated.

With this background, a new Relief Service System for Infections derived from Biological Products was established in April 2004. This system provides relief for health damage such as diseases and disorders of sufficient severity to require hospitalization or the equivalent when infections occur via the product in spite of its proper use on or after April 1, 2004, and treatment to prevent onset after infection and patients with secondary

154 第6章 医薬品等による健康被害救済制度

表 6.2 感染等被害救済の実績 [6)]

年　　度	2013 年度	2014 年度	2015 年度	2016 年度	2017 年度
請求件数	7 件	3 件	6 件	1 件	3 件
決定件数	4 件	7 件	2 件	5 件	2 件
支 給 決 定	4 件	6 件	1 件	3 件	2 件
不支給決定	0 件	1 件	1 件	2 件	0 件
取 り 下 げ	0 件	0 件	0 件	0 件	0 件
処理中件数[*1]	5 件	1 件	5 件	1 件	2 件
達成率[*2]	100.0%	42.9%	50.0%	20.0%	50.0%
処理期間（中央値）	4.3 月	6.3 月	7.5 月	10.0 月	10.2 月

[*1]　各年度末時点において決定にいたらなかったもの
[*2]　当該年度中に決定されたもののうち，6 か月以内に処理できたものの割合

めの治療や二次感染者なども救済の対象となる。

6.2.2　給付の請求から給付の決定まで

これは医薬品副作用被害救済制度と同じである（146 ページの図 6.1 参照）。

6.2.3　統計

表 6.2 に示すように，まだ請求・決定件数とも 1 年間に 10 件以下（ほぼ年々減少）で推移している。制度創設から 2017 年度までの健康被害の内訳は，ウイルス感染による健康被害が計 46 件，細菌感染による健康被害が計 12 件である。なお，感染の原因となった生物由来製品は，すべて輸血用血液製剤である。

6.3　予防接種健康被害救済制度

予防接種を受けた人の中には，実施にあたった医師等の関係者に過失がない場合にもきわめて稀にではあるが，不可避的に重篤な副反応がみられ，そのための医療を要し，障害を残し，ときには死亡する場合がある。本制度は，予防接種法に基づく予防接種により，無過失の健康被害を受けた人の迅速な救済を図るための措置として設けられている。予防接種は公共の目的のために行われるもので，この結果，健康被害を生ずるにいたった被害者に対しては，国家補償的精神に基づき救済を行い，社会的公正を図ることが必要との考えに基づいている。

救済の対象となる健康被害の範囲は，予防接種法に基づく予防接種による異常な副反応に起因する疾病により，被接種者が現に医療を要し，または後遺症として一定の被害を有し，あるいは死亡した場合である。

予防接種健康被害救済制度による救済措置の給付を申請する場合には，申請者は，予防接種を実施した市町村の担当部署に届け出て，市町村長に申請することになっ

Table6.2　Performance of Infectious Diseases Relief Service (fiscal year 2013)[6]

Fiscal Year	2013 年度	2014 年度	2015 年度	2016 年度	2017 年度
No. of applications	7	3	6	1	3
No. of decisions	4	7	2	5	2
Decisions to pay	4	6	1	3	2
Decisions not to pay	0	1	1	2	0
No. of withdrawals	0	0	0	0	0
No. in process [*1]	5	1	5	1	2
Achievement rate [*2]	100.0%	42.9%	50.0%	20.0%	50.0%
Processing time (median value)	4.3 mos	6.3 mos	7.5 mos	10.0 mos	10.2 mos

[*1] Not decided as of the end of each fiscal year
[*2] Percentages of processing completed within 6 months among decisions made in the applicable fiscal year

infections are also covered.

6.2.2　Process from application through decision on benefits

This is the same as for the ADR Relief Service System (Refer to Fig. 6.1, page 147).

6.2.3　Statistics

As shown in **Table 6.2**, there are 10 or less applications and decisions every year (usually decreasing year by year). Since the establishment of the system to fiscal year 2017, there have been a total of 46 incidents of health damage due to virus infections and 12 incidents of health damage due to bacterial infections. In all cases the biological products causing the infections were blood products for transfusion.

6.3　Relief Services System for Adverse Health Effects following Vaccination

In some people who get a preventive vaccination, even if the parties concerned including the doctor who implement it are not at fault, there is a very rare but inevitable serious adverse reaction which requires medical care, leaves them seriously disabled, and sometimes leads to death. This system was set up as a measure for prompt relief for people who suffer no-fault health damage due to a mandatory preventive vaccination based on Preventive Vaccination Act. The system is based on the concept that preventive vaccinations are conducted for public purposes, and therefore people who develop health damage as a result of such vaccinations need to be helped based on the spirit of national compensation for social justice.

Health damages covered for relief are cases where the vaccine recipient actually needs medical care, has certain damage as sequela, or died due to a disease caused by an abnormal adverse reaction to such a preventive vaccination.

When an application for benefits as a relief measure under the Relief Services System for Adverse Health Effects with Vaccination is to be made, the applicant is required to

ている。申請内容は厚労省に届けられ，その健康被害が予防接種によって引き起こされたものか，別の要因によるものなのかの因果関係を，疾病・障害認定審査会で審議し，予防接種によるものと認定された場合には，規定に定められた給付を受けることができる。厚生労働省の Web サイト[7]によると，1977 年 2 月から 2017 年 12 月末までの予防接種健康被害認定者総数は 3,233 人で，そのうち 1,041 人が MMR ワクチンによる健康被害者である。

　ただし，予防接種健康被害救済制度による定期接種の場合に対する給付内容と，他の予防接種の場合の給付内容（医薬品副作用被害救済制度による）に大きな違いがある等の問題が指摘されている。

文　　献

1) 独立行政法人 医薬品医療機器総合機構，誰よりも知ってほしい。伝えてほしい。医薬品副作用被害救済制度：

   https://www.pmda.go.jp/kenkouhigai/file/higaikyusai.pdf

2) 独立行政法人 医薬品医療機器総合機構，健康被害救済業務 - 救済給付業務の流れ：

   https://www.pmda.go.jp/relief-services/adr-sufferers/0001.html および https://www.pmda.go.jp/relief-services/infections/0001.html

3) 独立行政法人 医薬品医療機器総合機構，平成 30 事業年度 第 1 回救済業務委員会（2018 年〔平成 30 年〕6 月 18 日開催）資料 1-2，p.48

4) 独立行政法人 医薬品医療機器総合機構，平成 30 事業年度 第 1 回救済業務委員会（2018 年〔平成 30 年〕6 月 18 日開催）資料 1-2，p.70

5) 独立行政法人 医薬品医療機器総合機構，平成 30 事業年度 第 1 回救済業務委員会（2018 年〔平成 30 年〕6 月 18 日開催）資料 1-2，p.76

6) 独立行政法人 医薬品医療機器総合機構，平成 30 事業年度 第 1 回救済業務委員会（2018 年〔平成 30 年〕6 月 18 日開催）資料 1-2，p.55

7) 厚生労働省 Web サイト，予防接種健康被害救済制度 認定者数：

   https://www.mhlw.go.jp/topics/bcg/other/6.html

Chapter 6 Relief Services System for Adverse Health Effects **157**

make the application to the need of the municipal government by notifying it to the responsible division at the municipal government that conducted the preventive vaccination. The contents of the application are notified to the MHLW and the causal relationship as to whether such health damage was caused by the preventive vaccination or other factors is deliberated at the Examination Committee for Certification of Sickness and Disability. If the damage is certified as one due to the preventive vaccination, benefits specified in the regulations can be received. According to the website of the MHLW,[7] the total number of people certified as having health damage caused by a preventive vaccination from February 1977 to the end of December 2017 is 3,233, among whom 1,041 are people with health damage caused by the MMR vaccine.

However, problems have been raised, such as that there are major differences between the benefits in vaccinations under the Relief Services System for Adverse Health Effects with Vaccination and the benefits for other types of preventive vaccination (under the Relief Service for Adverse Drug Reactions).

References

1) You should know more than anyone. Please tell them about it. The Relief Service for Adverse Drug Reactions, p.2, PMDA:
   https://www.pmda.go.jp/kenkouhigai/file/higaikyusai.pdf

2) Health Damage Relief Operation-Flow of Operation for Relief & Benefits, PMDA:
   https://www.pmda.go.jp/relief-services/adr-sufferers/0001.html and https://www.pmda.go.jp/relief-services/infections/0001.html

3) First Meeting of the Committee on Relief Operations for Fiscal Year 2018 (held on June 18, 2018), Material 1-2, p.48, PMDA

4) First Meeting of the Committee on Relief Operations for Fiscal Year 2018 (held on June 18, 2018), Material 1-2, p.70, PMDA

5) First Meeting of the Committee on Relief Operations for Fiscal Year 2018 (held on June 18, 2018), Material 1-2, p.76, PMDA

6) First Meeting of the Committee on Relief Operations for Fiscal Year 2018 (held on June 18, 2018), Material 1-2, p.55, PMDA

7) MHLW website: Number of people certified under the Relief Services System for Adverse Health Effects with Vaccination:
   https://www.mhlw.go.jp/topics/bcg/other/6.html

第 7 章

市販後安全対策各論

　医薬品医療機器等法の改正，ならびに医薬品リスク管理計画の導入に伴う GVP/GPSP 省令の改正などにより，医薬品の市販後安全対策に関わる業務に変更がなされている。本章では，企業および行政における安全管理情報の取り扱いなど，流れに沿って個々に解説する。

7.1　企業が担う安全管理情報の収集

　わが国における安全管理情報の根幹を成すのはサリドマイド事件に端を発した世界各国における自発報告制度（日本では現在は「副作用・感染症報告制度」）であるが，本制度自身の歴史的な発展については第 4 章 1 節を参照願いたい。副作用・感染症報告制度以外にも，国内外の研究者によって主に安全性に関する研究結果（主には文献）について，企業の意見と今後の対策を報告する「研究報告」や，外国での重要な安全性に関する規制措置について報告する「措置報告」などがある。

7.1.1　副作用・感染症報告の情報源
　上述した 3 つの報告に供される情報源については，大別すると以下のとおりである。

1.　自発的情報源：いわゆる「依頼に基づかない」（unsolicited）情報源
　これら情報は極めてまれに発現する事象を検出できる長所がある反面，使用された患者数が不明であることがほとんどであることから，発現頻度を求めることは困難である。
　　・自発報告
　　　製薬企業や規制当局等に対する医師，薬剤師等の医療専門家や一般使用者からの自発的な意思に基づく報告（社内関連部門，顧客相談窓口，広報等含む）。
　　・市販直後調査
　　　新薬発売後 6 か月間，新薬納入施設に適正使用を呼びかけるとともに，重篤な副作用等の自発報告を積極的に収集する短期間の積極的な集中モニタリングで，ICH E2E 別添における「自発報告の強化」に該当する。

Chapter 7

General discussion on post-marketing pharmacovigilance

Operations related to post-marketing safety measures for drugs have been modified in response to events such as the revision of the Pharmaceutical and Medical Device Act and the amendment of the GVP/GPSP ministerial ordinances in association with the introduction of Risk Management Plans. Topics such as handling of safety management information by MAHs and governments are explained individually in this chapter along with the process for each.

7.1 Collection of safety management information by MAHs

Safety management information in Japan is based on the spontaneous-report system in many countries that was started after the thalidomide incidents (at present, "the reporting system for ADRs and infections" in Japan). Refer to Chapter 4-1 for the historical development of the system. In addition to the reporting system for ADRs and infections, there are "research reports" in which domestic/overseas researchers provide the company's comment and future measures for research results (mainly, scientific literature) regarding mainly safety and "measures-taken report" to provide important regulatory measures regarding safety overseas, etc.

7.1.1 Information sources of adverse drug reaction and infection reports

The information sources for the above three reports are mainly divided into the following:

1. Spontaneous information sources: so-called "not dependent on a request" (unsolicited)

Such information can help detect events that rarely occur, but cannot show the incidence because the number of patients who used the drug is unknown in most cases. Therefore, it is difficult to detect incidence.

- Spontaneous reports

  Reports based on a voluntary act of health care professionals (HCPs) such as physicians and pharmacists and from ordinary patients to pharmaceutical companies or the regulatory authorities (including in-house relevant departments, customer service department, public relations, etc.)

- Early post-marketing phase risk minimization and vigilance (EPPV)

  EPPV is classified as "stimulated reporting" in the annex of ICH E2E and refers to active intensive monitoring during a short period by actively collecting spontaneous reports on serious ADRs together with calls for proper use at medical institutions

・文献・学会情報

文献・学会情報から検索した副作用・感染症症例報告や相互作用に関する報告，さらには安全性評価を目的とした薬剤疫学研究や毒性に関する動物実験等がある。これらについては副作用・感染症報告や研究報告として規制当局へ提出する。研究報告については，別途述べる。

・提携企業，規制当局

・インターネットからの情報

自社が管理する Web サイトを定期的に検索して得た報告（自発報告として扱われる）

・その他

一般紙やテレビ等のマスコミからの副作用情報

これらは収集対象が不特定多数であることから，ごくまれにしか発現しない有害事象も検知することができる反面，真贋を見極めることも重要である。

2. 製造販売後調査・試験等からの情報：いわゆる依頼に基づく（solicited）情報源

GPSP に規定された全例調査を含む使用成績調査，特定使用成績調査および製造販売後臨床試験等（GCP 下で実施される適応拡大等の治験）の調査票からの個別副作用情報で，使用患者数が判明していることから発現頻度がわかる反面，きわめてまれな事象を検出することは困難である。

7.1.2　安全管理情報の収集から報告まで

副作用・感染症報告制度の主要部分である医療関係者等からの自発的情報源からの報告について，収集から報告までの流れを記す。

副作用・感染症報告について，情報の収集から報告までの流れを図 7.1 に示した。

医師，歯科医師，薬剤師等の医療関係者から自社製品に関する副作用・感染症報告を企業が受ける（主に担当 MR であるが，顧客情報窓口等さまざまである）と，受け取った者はその内容を報告書に記載して本社の安全管理統括部門に第一報報告を行う。安全管理統括部門では，副作用のうち未知あるいは重篤な副作用であれば，医薬品医療機器等法に基づいて期限内に独立行政法人医薬品医療機器総合機構（以下，PMDA）へ「完了報告」または「未完了報告」として報告しなければならない。報告に際しては，安全管理統括部門では副作用感染症症例の評価（因果関係，予測性，重篤性，措置の要否など）を行い，医薬品医療機器等法で報告を求められている副作用等についてその期限内に PMDA に電子報告する。評価に必要な情報が不足している場合，安全性管理統括部門は担当 MR に追跡（詳細）調査を指示し，MR は報告医師に追跡（詳細）調査を依頼し，追跡（詳細）調査票を受領した後，安全管理統括部門に送付する。その後，安全管理統括部門は再調査の情報に基づき必要に応

that purchased new drugs for a period of 6 months after marketing of the drugs.

- Literature/academic conference information

  This includes case reports of ADR or infections and interactions screened from information in the published literature and from presentations at academic conferences, and toxicity studies in animals and pharmacoepidemiology research for the purpose of safety assessment, etc. Such information is submitted to the regulatory authority as an adverse drug reaction and infection report or research report. Research report is stated separately.

- Affiliated companies, regulatory authorities
- Information from the Internet

  Reports obtained by periodic screening of company websites (handled as spontaneous reports)

- Others

  ADR information from media such as general newspapers or television

Because there are so many, unspecified people who may be the sources of this information, it may be possible to detect adverse events that rarely occur but it is also important to identify which cases are really true or not.

2. Information from post-marketing studies, etc.: so-called dependent on a request (solicited)

Includes ADR information from case report forms (CRFs) during use-results survey, specified use-results survey and post-marketing clinical trials including all-patient survey performed under GPSP (clinical trials for additional indication, etc. performed under GCP) The number of patients who used the drug is known and the incidence can be determined. On the other hand, it can hardly detect rare events.

7.1.2 From collection of safety management information to its submission

The process from collection to submission of spontaneous reports from health care professionals (HCP), etc., which is the main part of the reporting system for ADRs and infections.

Fig. 7.1 shows the process from collection of information to submission of adverse drug reaction and infection reports.

When adverse drug reaction and infection reports on their company's products are received from healthcare professionals such as physicians, dentists, and pharmacists, (mainly by the MR in charge, or customer-service counters, etc.) the person who received them enters the contents in a report form and forwards a preliminary report to the General Safety Management Division of the company. If the ADR is unexpected or serious, the General Safety Management Division must report it as a "final report" or "incomplete report" to the Pharmaceuticals and Medical Devices Agency (PMDA) within a certain time frame based on the PMD Act. When filing reports, the ADR and infection cases are evaluated by the General Safety Management Division (in terms of causality, expectedness, seriousness, taking a measure or not, etc.). When the ADR, or infection requires reporting based on the PMD Act, an electronic report is sent to the PMDA within the time limit. If there is a lack of information necessary for assessment, the General Safety Management Division requests the MR for a (detailed) follow-up

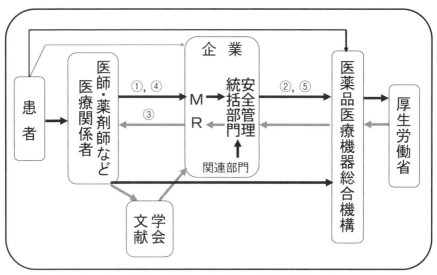

①第一報 ②未完了報告 ③追跡調査 ④詳細情報 ⑤完了報告
図 7.1 副作用・感染症報告の収集から報告までの流れ
出典：2018 年度 安全管理・調査エキスパート研修 上野茂樹 第 4 講 副作用・感染症報告，研究報告及び外国措置報告と安全管理業務で使用される用語について 2018 年 5 月 28 日

じて PMDA に電子報告する。

7.1.3 研究報告の情報源

　文献・学会情報について 7.1.1 で言及したが，医薬品医療機器等法施行規則第 228 条の 20 には「当該医薬品若しくは外国医薬品の副作用若しくはそれらの使用による感染症によりがんその他の重大な疾病，障害若しくは死亡が発生するおそれがあること，当該医薬品若しくは外国医薬品の副作用による症例等若しくはそれらの使用による感染症の発生傾向が著しく変化したこと又は当該医薬品が承認を受けた効能若しくは効果を有しないことを示す研究報告」とある。これらは文献・学会情報から得られるような当該薬と他剤を比較した安全性に関する薬剤疫学研究や臨床試験結果など公衆衛生に及ぼす影響がある場合が多く，内容を理解するためには科学的・批判的吟味能力が必要である。なお，研究報告書中には，その内容ばかりではなく，その研究に関する企業としての意見や，とるべき今後の対策について，述べておくことが求められている。

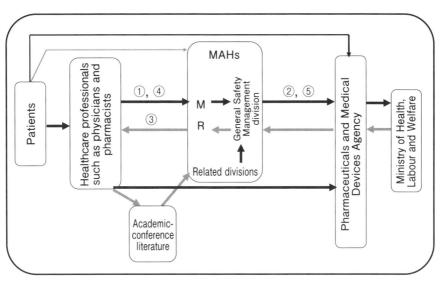

[1] Preliminary report [2] Incompleted report [3] Follow-up [4] Detailed information [5] Final report

Fig.7-1　Flow from collection to reporting of Adverse Drug Reaction and Infection reports
Source: FY2018 Safety Management/Investigation Expert Training, Shigeki Ueno, Lecture 4: Adverse Drug Reaction and Infection reports, research reports and reports on measures taken overseas and the terms used in safety management activities, May 28, 2018

report. The MR requests the reporting physician to complete this (detailed) follow-up report. When the (detailed) follow-up CRF is received by the MR, it is forwarded to the General Safety Management Division. Thereafter, an electronic report is sent to the PMDA by the General Safety Management Division based on the additional information if necessary.

7.1.3. Information source of research reports

As mentioned in 7.1.1, Article 228-20 of the Enforcement Regulations of the PMD Act specifies literature/academic conference information as research reports correspond to those of a cancer or other significant disease/disorder or death that may occur due to an ADR to a relevant test drug, etc. or infection associated with the use of such drug, those of a substantial change in tendency of occurrence such as the number/frequency of cases, occurrence conditions, etc. of a disease suspected to be associated with an ADR to a relevant test drug or infection suspected to be associated with the use of such drug, or those showing that a relevant test drug, etc. has no effect for a disease that is the target for the clinical trial. As it includes the results of pharmacoepidemiology research or clinical studies where the applicable drug is compared with other drugs for safety as acquired from literature/academic conference information, which often affects public hygiene, it is necessary to examine the details from scientific and critical viewpoints for further understanding. Of note, the research report needs to include not only the details but also company's opinions regarding the research or future actions to be taken.

7.1.4 措置報告の情報源

1. 海外規制当局や提携企業からの情報

海外規制当局が公表した回収や販売中止等の重大な安全性に関わる情報や安全確保措置に関する情報（DHPL〔Dear Healthcare Professional Letters：医薬関係者へのお知らせ〕の配布や，CCDS〔Company Core Data Sheet：企業中核データシート〕の変更など）がある。これらについては，医薬品医療機器等法施行規則第228条の20「外国医薬品に係る製造，輸入又は販売の中止，回収，廃棄その他保健衛生上の危害の発生又は拡大を防止するための措置の実施」とあり，外国での重大な措置として報告するとともに，企業としての意見や今後の対策を述べておくことが求められている。

7.2 製造販売後調査・試験

調査や試験はそれぞれ観察研究と介入研究に相当する（図7.2）。観察研究とは，日常診療下の使用実態どおりにデータを集めて，仮説の検出や確認を行うものである。多様な患者集団からリスクとしての副作用等を収集するには，多数の症例を必要とするので，観察研究が適している。これは日本では使用成績調査，製造販売後データベース調査が該当する。

一方，介入研究とは，研究目的に応じて特定の検査や治療を実施して仮説を検証するもので，実験的研究ともいわれる。一定の条件の患者集団を無作為に被験薬投与群と非投与群に割り付けて有効性を確認する比較臨床試験は介入研究の代表例であり，製造販売後臨床試験も介入研究に位置付けられる。

改正GPSP省令（2018年）では，観察研究のうち医療機関から収集した情報を用いた調査を使用成績調査，医療情報データベースを用いた調査を製造販売後デー

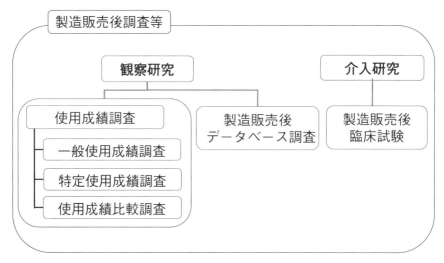

図7.2　観察研究と介入研究について（改正GPSP省令下での範囲における）

7.1.4 Information source of measures-taken reports

1. Information from foreign regulatory authorities and affiliated companies

This includes significant information on safety such as recalls or discontinuation of marketing and information on safety assurance measures which have been disclosed by overseas regulatory authorities (such as distribution of DHPL [Dear Healthcare Professional Letters] and a revision in the CCDS [Company Core Data Sheet]). With regard to this, Article 228-20 of the Enforcement Regulations of the PMD Act states, "discontinuation of manufacturing, import, or selling, recall, disposal due to a product used in a foreign country with the same ingredient or implementation of other measure to prevent the occurrence or spread of a hazard in health and hygiene", requiring not only to report it as an overseas significant measure but to present the company's opinions and future measures.

7.2 Post marketing studies

Investigations (surveys) and studies correspond to observational studies and interventional studies, respectively (**Fig. 7.2**). An observational study consists of collection of data under conditions of use in routine medical practices, and is used for hypothesis generation or confirmation. To collect ADRs, etc. as risks from various patient populations, many cases are needed, and therefore an observational study is appropriate. In Japan, this corresponds to use-results survey and post-marketing database studies.

In contrast, an interventional study is an experimental study that involves testing a hypothesis by performing specific examinations and treatment in accordance with the objective of the study. One example of an interventional study is a comparative clinical trial to confirm efficacy by assigning the patient population under fixed conditions randomly to a group treated with the test drug or an untreated group. Post-marketing clinical trials are also a form of interventional study.

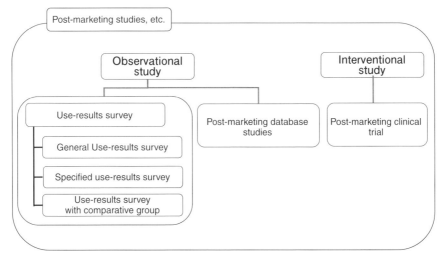

Fig7-2 Observational study and interventional study (under the range of the revised GPSP Ministerial Ordinance)

166　　第 7 章　市販後安全対策各論

タベース調査としている。さらに使用成績調査のうち，改正 GPSP 省令前の狭義の使用成績調査を一般使用成績調査とし，小児・高齢者・妊産婦・腎機能障害または肝機能障害を有する者，医薬品を長期に使用する者その他医薬品を使用する者の条件を定めて行う調査を特定使用成績調査としている。使用成績調査の中で，当該医薬品を使用しない比較群を設定した調査の場合は使用成績比較調査と区分している。

7.2.1　使用成績調査（改正 GPSP 省令では一般使用成績調査に該当）

　改正 GPSP 省令では使用成績調査とは，従来の①一般使用成績調査，②特定使用成績調査，③使用成績比較調査の 3 つに分類される。

①　一般使用成績調査は，医薬品の使用実態下において，未知の副作用，副作用の発生状況の変化や安全性または有効性に影響を与える要因を把握するために行うものである。調査症例数は製品特性に応じて設定する。また，中央登録方式，連続調査方式あるいは全例調査方式により，症例の抽出に偏りのないように症例を登録する（「医療用医薬品の製造販売後調査等の実施方法に関するガイドラインについて」（平成 17 年 10 月 27 日：薬食審査発第 1027001 号）より）。また全例調査方式による全例調査とは，近年，いわゆるブリッジングにより外国臨床試験を外挿して承認申請する場合や，抗がん薬のように国際共同治験を用いて申請するような国内での臨床症例が少ないままで承認される医薬品が増加している。また，生物学的製剤等，既存薬に比べて新規の作用機序を有するなど，有効性に優れた新薬が増加する一方で，重篤な副作用のリスクを併せもつ医薬品が増加している。このため，従来，全例調査は希少疾病用医薬品のみに課せられてきたが，それ以外の重篤な副作用の発現が危惧される医薬品についても，調査への協力が得られ，なおかつ，施設・医師の要件を満たすことを条件として製品を納入・処方することによる，リスク最小化策の一環として全例調査が課されるようになってきている。

②　特定使用成績調査は，承認時の治験では組み込まれることの少ない対象患者（小児，高齢者，妊産婦，腎または肝機能障害患者等），あるいは長期使用時における有効性または安全性に関する情報の把握のために行われる調査である。使用成績調査と同様に，中央登録方式，連続調査方式あるいは全例調査方式により症例を登録する。（「医療用医薬品の製造販売後調査等の実施方法に関するガイドラインについて」（平成 17 年 10 月 27 日：薬食審査発第 1027001 号）より）

　以下に主な事例を示す。

Chapter 7 General discussion on post-marketing pharmacovigilance 167

The revised GPSP ordinance (2018) regards an observational study using information collected from medical institutions as a use-results survey, and an investigation using electronic healthcare data as a post-marketing database study. Moreover, the use-results survey defined in a narrow sense prior to the revised GPSP ordinance among use-results survey is regarded as a general use-results survey while a survey which focuses on some specific condition(s) of those taking the drug, such as children, the elderly, pregnant women, patients with renal or hepatic dysfunction, patients on long-term administration or patients using other drugs is regarded as a specified use-results survey. If a use-results survey has comparative group of patients who do not use the drug, it is classified as a use-results survey with comparative group.

7.2.1 Use-results survey(regarded as General Drug Use Investigations in the revised GPSP ordinance)

Use-results survey is divided into the following three categories in the revised GPSP ordinance: the conventional [1] general use-results survey, [2] specified use-results survey, [3] use-results survey with comparative group.

[1] General use-results survey are performed to obtain information on the factors that affect unexpected ADR, changes in the circumstances under which an ADR occurs, and the efficacy or safety in clinical settings. The number of patients investigated is set based on the characteristics of the product. The patients are enrolled using a central registration system, continuous investigation system or all-patient survey system in order to avoid any bias in selection of patients ("Guideline on the Implementation Procedures of Post-Marketing Surveillance, etc. for Prescription Drugs" Evaluation and Licensing Division, Notification No. 1027001 PFSB MHLW dated October 27, 2005). As for all-patient survey using the all-patient survey system, in recent years, drugs approved with few clinical trial subjects from Japan are increasing in cases where the marketing application is filed by extrapolation from overseas clinical trials using bridging studies or the application is filed using global clinical trials like those for anticancer agents, etc. In addition, there is an increase in new drugs such as biological products with excellent efficacy and features such as new mechanisms of action compared with existing drugs, but on the other hand, these drugs may involve a risk of serious ADRs. For this reason, while in the past, all-patient survey were performed only for orphan drugs, now other drugs showing a risk of onset of serious ADRs are also undergoing all-patient survey where the concerned products are delivered and prescribed on condition that cooperation is provided for the investigation and requirements for institutions and prescribing physicians are met.

[2] Specified use-results survey are performed to obtain information on efficacy and safety in patients whose number is limited (children, the elderly, pregnant women or patients with renal or hepatic dysfunction) in pre-approval clinical trials or patients on long-term administration. Similar to use-results survey, the patients are enrolled using a central registration system, continuous investigation system or all-patient investigation system. ("Guideline on the Implementation Procedures of Post-Marketing Surveillance, etc. for Prescription Drugs" (Evaluation and Licensing Division, Notification No. 1027001 PFSB MHLW dated October 27,

168 第7章 市販後安全対策各論

- 小児，高齢者，妊産婦，腎または肝機能障害を有する患者等の特別な背景を有する患者，医薬品を長期に使用する患者での調査
 特別な背景を有する患者での調査については，通常，治験に組み込まれることが少なく，元来，対象症例が少ない。そこで，通常の使用成績調査では収集困難な小児，高齢者，妊産婦や特定の合併症（肝疾患，腎疾患など）の対象について，特定使用成績調査として，安全性主体の調査が行われることが多い。

- 長期使用に関する調査
 長期使用に関する調査においては，承認前を上回る投与期間の調査を実施し，長期（例えば 24 週以上）使用した患者での有効性，安全性について確認する。参考として新薬の臨床評価ガイドラインにおいては，長期投与試験の実施が求められている薬効群（経口避妊薬，脳循環・代謝改善薬，脂質異常症治療薬，抗不安薬，睡眠薬，抗心不全薬，降圧薬，骨粗鬆症薬，抗不整脈薬，抗狭心症薬）があり，降圧薬や抗不整脈薬であれば，投与期間 6 か月間では 300 〜 600 例，1 年間では 100 例を収集すべきとされている。

③ 使用成績比較調査とは，特定の医薬品を使用する者の情報と当該医薬品を使用しない者の情報とを比較することによって行う「使用成績調査」のことであり，薬剤疫学研究でいうところのコホート研究にほぼ該当すると推定されるが，これまでの日本における実績もごくわずかで，例えば症例対照研究がこれに含まれるかは不明である。

7.2.2 製造販売後臨床試験

以下に主な事例を示す。

- 腎機能障害患者等の特別な背景を有する患者での適正使用の確立のための薬物動態試験
 腎排泄型の薬剤においては，腎障害の程度に応じて腎からの薬物の排泄が遅延することがある。クレアチニンクリアランス値により腎障害患者を軽度・中等度・重度に層別して，健康成人との比較で薬物動態試験を行い，血中濃度や尿中排泄率の推移を確認する。

- 長期使用による延命効果，QOL 改善等に関する臨床試験
 抗がん薬，降圧薬等の有効性評価は，一般に承認時の治験では，その薬理作用に基づく腫瘍縮小効果，降圧作用等の代替のエンドポイントを用いて比較

2005))

The following are the main examples.

- Survey on special populations such as children, the elderly, pregnant women, patients with renal or hepatic dysfunction, and patients on long-term administration Patients with special characteristics are infrequently included in clinical trials and so the number of such cases is low. For children, elderly subjects, pregnant or parturient women, and those with particular concomitant diseases (hepatic disease, renal disease, etc.) which are difficult to collect in typical use-results survey, safety is mainly studied using specified use-results survey.

- Survey of long-term administration In investigations of long-term administration, the exposure periods in the study exceed those studied before approval and efficacy and safety are confirmed in patients during long-term administration (e.g. 24 weeks or longer). For reference, in the new drug clinical evaluation guidelines given under reference, the following therapeutic categories (oral contraceptives, drugs to improve cerebral circulation and metabolism, anti-hyperlipidemic drugs, anti-anxiety drugs, hypnotics, drugs to treat heart failure, antihypertensive agents, drugs to treat osteoporosis, antiarrhythmic drugs and anti-anginal drugs) are specified. For antihypertensive agents and antiarrhythmic drugs, 300 to 600 cases of administration of 6 months or 100 cases of administration of one year should be collected.

[3] Use-results survey with comparative group is a "use-results survey" that compares the information on the users of a specific drug to non-users, which is believed to be almost the same as a cohort study in pharmacoepidemiological research. To date there are very few examples of such studies in Japan, and it is unclear whether case-control studies are included in this category, for instance.

7.2.2 Post-marketing clinical trials

The following are the main examples.

- Pharmacokinetic studies to establish proper use in patients with special characteristics such as renal dysfunction For drugs excreted via the kidney, drug excretion may be delayed according to the severity of the renal disorder. Pharmacokinetic studies of renally impaired patients in comparison with healthy adults are performed by stratifying the level of renal disorder into mild, moderate or severe according to creatinine clearance values and confirming profiles of blood concentrations and urinary excretion rates.

- Clinical trials on survival, QOL (quality of life) improvements, etc. by long-term use Efficacy evaluation of anticancer agents, antihypertensive agents, etc. in clinical trials at the time of approval is generally conducted over a relatively short period with the use of surrogate endpoints such as tumor-shrinking effect, antihypertensive effect, etc. based on the drug's pharmacological actions. However, the original reasons for

的短期間で行われる。しかし，薬剤を使用する本来の目的は，延命効果，脳卒中や心筋梗塞等の心血管イベントの予防やQOL（quality of life）の改善等であり，そのための指標を真のエンドポイントという。薬剤を長期に使用しないと真の評価指標の把握が困難であり，また予防効果をみる場合には投与全症例でイベント（死亡，脳卒中や心筋梗塞等の心血管イベント等）が起きるわけではないので，数百例から数千例以上の規模となるために，大規模臨床試験として市販後に実施されることがある。

- 臨床評価ガイドライン（厚労省）に基づく有効性や安全性の検証のための臨床試験
  有効性再評価のために二重盲検比較試験において，プラセボに対する優越性を証明するために行われるもので，過去には再評価制度の一環として脳循環代謝改善薬等で実施されている。
- 検出された安全性，有効性に影響を及ぼす要因の検証のための臨床試験
  使用成績調査（特定使用成績調査）等から，安全性，有効性に影響を及ぼす要因が検出された場合には，それを検証するために臨床試験を実施する。

7.2.3　製造販売後データベース調査

　改正 GPSP 省令（2018 年）で製造販売後データベース調査は「医療情報データベース取扱事業者が提供する医療情報データベースを用い，医薬品の副作用による疾病等の種類別の発現状況並びに品質，有効性及び安全性に関する情報の検出又は確認のために行う調査」と定義された。また，通知で「製造販売後の医薬品安全性監視における医療情報データベースの利用に関する基本的考え方について」（平成 29 年6 月 9 日：薬生薬審発 0609 第 8 号，薬生安発 0609 第 4 号）が示された。

　基本的考え方の中では，調査する事例として下記が示されている。
- 副作用等報告情報から懸念される事象が認められた際に，特定集団における当該事象の発現頻度，発現傾向またはそれに関連する要因を探索する場合
- 適正使用に関する情報提供の方法および内容を検討するにあたって処方実態を調査する場合
- 評価に必要とされる症例数や調査期間を考慮すると，製造販売業者等がデータを自ら医療機関から収集する調査の実施が適当ではないと考えられる場合
- 医薬品使用の有無に関わらず発生しうる有害事象について，その原因が特定の医薬品に基づくものであるのか否か等を，対照群をおいて評価する場合
- リスク最小化活動が実施された結果としてリスク最小化活動の実施前と比較してリスクが軽減されているか等の，安全対策の実施や効果を定量的または経時的に評価する場合

また，データベース利用に際してはデータベース選定で注意する点，実施計画書

Chapter 7 General discussion on post-marketing pharmacovigilance 171

using drugs include extending life, preventing cardiovascular events such as stroke and myocardial infarction, and improving QOL. Indexes for those purposes are called true endpoints. It is difficult to assess true endpoints when drugs are not used for long periods and when the desired efficacy is preventative because the target events (death and cardiovascular events such as strokes and myocardial infarction) do not occur in all treated patients. Therefore, it is necessary to increase the scale from several hundred to several thousand subjects. Such large scale clinical trials are sometimes performed after marketing.

- Clinical trials to verify efficacy and safety based on clinical evaluation guidelines (MHLW)
  To verify superiority over placebo, the drug is tested in double-blind comparative studies during reevaluation of efficacy. In the past, such studies were performed for reevaluation of drugs such as those used to improve cerebral circulation and metabolism as a part of the Reevaluation system.
- Clinical trials to verify factors influencing safety and efficacy
  When factors that affect safety and efficacy are detected in use-results survey (specified use-results survey) etc., clinical trials are performed to confirm the finding.

7.2.3 Post-marketing database studies

In the revised GPSP ordinance (2018), post-marketing database studies are defined as "an investigation that is performed to detect or confirm information on quality, efficacy and safety as well as the onset status of diseases, etc. caused by ADR per type using the electronic healthcare data provided by electronic healthcare data suppliers." In addition, a notification was issued on "Basic Principles on the Use of Medical Information Databases in Post-marketing Pharmacovigilance (June 9, 2017: PSEHB/ELD Notification No. 0609-8, PSEHB/SD Notification No. 0609-4)".

The basic concept is illustrated below.

- When exploring the incidence, trends, or factors relating to an event in a specified group if an event that can be expected from ADR report information was observed
- When investigating actual prescription status to discuss the method and contents of information provision regarding proper use
- When it is considered inappropriate for MAHs to conduct an investigation by collecting data by themselves from medical institutions in view of the sample size and investigation period required for assessment
- When making an assessment of whether an adverse event which may occur irrespective of the use of the drug is caused by a specific drug by comparing with a control group
- When making a quantitative or time-course assessment for the implementation and effects of safety measures, such as whether risks have been reduced compared to before risk minimization activities were initiated, etc., as a result of the activities.

The concept also shows what needs to be focused on when selecting a database, and the comparative-group, in principle, as well as the clinical significance of data items when protocols are prepared. Because data have already been available and various trials

作成の際には，データ項目の臨床的意義とともに，原則として対照群の設定が示された。データベース研究では，データがすでに存在し多くの試行錯誤が可能であることから，フィジビリティー調査実施時には対象となる医薬品が意図的に有利な調査計画の策定にならないよう留意することも示されている。アウトカムの定義を慎重に検討するとともに，バリデーション研究の結果に基づいて，評価の対象となるアウトカムを高い確度で特定できることをあらかじめ確認しておく必要がある。

さらに，再審査提出時の信頼性担保に関する留意点が「医薬品の製造販売後データベース調査における信頼性担保に関する留意点について」（平成30年2月21日：薬生薬審発0221第1号）にて通知された。その中で「医療情報データベース」の具体例として，病院情報システムデータ（電子カルテデータ，診断群分類別包括評価（DPC）データ等），診療報酬および調剤報酬明細書（健康保険組合レセプトデータ等），疾患登録データ等の電子的な医療情報を体系的に集積したデータベースを想定しており，今後は疾患レジストリも対象となるであろう。

信頼性担保のために，製薬企業が確認すべきデータベース事業者の医療情報データベースに係る手順書等の例として，「構築・管理に関する規定」「データクリーニングに関する基準・手順」「コード化に関する基準・手順」「セキュリティに関する規程・手順」「データバックアップ及びリカバリーに関する規程・手順」「情報源から収集した医療データの品質管理に関する規程」「構築・管理に関わる者への教育訓練に関する規程」等が示された。

製造販売後データベース研究の実施計画書の詳細は，PMDA のホームページで実施計画書の記載要項が示されている[1]。記載内容は EU GVP の PASS（Post-authorisation Safety Studies）のプロトコールテンプレートとほぼ同じであるが，日本独自の項目として「調査の結果に基づいて実施される可能性のある追加の措置及びその開始の決定基準」等，独自の項目があり，PASS のテンプレートを社内 SOP で利用しているときは注意が必要である。

7.2.4 製造販売後調査等の実施計画に関する策定の進め方

製造販売後調査等の手法として医療情報データベースを用いた製造販売後の調査の位置付けが明確になったことから，個々の調査目的に応じて科学的に最適な手法を選択して効率的，効果的な調査を実施することが，より重要になった。そこで「医薬品の製造販売後調査等の実施計画の策定に関する検討の進め方について」（平成31年3月14日：薬生審発0314第4号, 薬生安発0314第4号）にて通知された（「第4章4.3 製造販売後調査等基本計画書の作成」参照）。

この中では製造販売後調査を実施する場合，リサーチ・クエスチョンを明確にした上で，過不足なく適正に実施することが重要であること，またそれと同時に，目的が不明瞭な調査を漫然と実施することがないよう留意し，あらかじめ調査目的や必要性について十分に検討する必要が示されている。

Chapter 7 General discussion on post-marketing pharmacovigilance   173

and errors are possible in database research. The notification also shows a reminder that target drug should not intentionally placed to gain the upper hand over comparators after feasibility investigations. It is necessary to discuss the definition of the outcome carefully and to ensure in advance the ability to specify the outcome subjected to the assessment with high accuracy based on the results of a validation research.

Furthermore, the cautions regarding reliability assurance when submitting re-examination documents were notified in "Points to Consider for ensuring Reliability in conducting post-marketing database study" (PSEHB/ELD Notification No. 0221-1 dated February 21, 2018). Some concrete examples of the assumed "electronic health record data" in the notification are databases in which electronic medical information has been systematically collected, such as hospital-information system data (electronic medical records, diagnosis procedure combination (DPC) data, etc.), medical-fee bills and dispensing-fee bills (prescription data from health insurance programs, etc.) and disease registration data, etc. In the future, disease registries will be included.

To ensure reliability, some examples of the procedures that pharmaceutical companies need to confirm regarding electronic healthcare data from data suppliers were presented: "provisions regarding establishment/management", "standards/procedures for data cleaning", "standards/procedures for encoding", "provisions/procedures for security", "provisions/procedures for data backup and recovery", "provisions for quality control of medical data collected from the source", "provisions for education/trainings of people who are involved in establishment/management", etc.

For details on the protocols on post-marketing database study, the PMDA website provides a summary of protocols[1]. The contents are almost the same as the protocol template of PASS (Post-authorisation Safety Studies) of EU-GVP. However, they include some Japan-specific items, such as "Decision criteria for additional actions that may be taken based on the study results and their initiation". Therefore, be mindful when the PASS template is being used for company SOPs.

7.2.4 How to create an implementation plan for post-marketing studies

As the position has been clarified for post-marketing studies using electronic healthcare data as a means of post-marketing studies, etc., it has become more important to conduct efficient and effective investigations by selecting scientifically optimal methods according to each investigation objective. In this regard, "Procedures for Developing Post-marketing Study Plan" is notified (PSEHB/ELD Notification No. 0314-4, PSEHB/SD Notification No. 0314-4 dated March 14, 2019) (See Chapter 4, 4.3 Preparation of the basic protocol of post-marketing studies").

It states that when conducting post-marketing studies, it is important to clarify research questions first and conduct them properly with no excesses or deficienies. At the same time, it also note that aimless research without clear objectives should be avoided and the research objectives and their necessity should be fully discussed in advance.

The research questions shown here refer to concrete and clear investigation issues,

174 第7章 市販後安全対策各論

ここで示されたリサーチ・クエスチョンは，具体的かつ明確な調査の課題のことであり，対象集団，当該薬剤，比較対照，対象とする有効性・安全性検討事項，対象期間の要素が含まれる。

RMP の中で安全性監視計画の具体化については，科学的な観点および現行の承認審査の過程を考慮すると，1) 各安全性検討事項における製造販売後に明らかにしたい懸念事項の明確化，2) 懸念事項ごとの科学的に適切な対処方法の決定，3) 各対処方法の関連法令下における位置付けの整理，4) 詳細な調査計画（プロトコル）の策定，の大きく4ステップ（第4章の図 4.5 参照）に分けることができる。原則として承認時までにステップ3までは PMDA と申請者間で合意される必要がある。

7.2.5 製造販売後調査・試験ガイドライン

本ガイドラインは，「医療用医薬品の製造販売後調査等の実施方法に関するガイドラインについて」（平成 17 年 10 月 27 日：薬食審査発第 1027001 号）として製造販売後に実施する使用成績調査，特定使用成績調査および製造販売後臨床試験の標準的な実施方法が示されたものであり，改正 GPSP（2018 年）前の旧来の調査・試験の要点を示すものである。

すでに 7.2.1 から 7.2.3 で各種調査・試験の要点は言及済みであるため，ここでは症例登録方式と調査方式について述べる。

ア）症例登録方法

調査開始に先立ち症例を登録するが，次のように症例の抽出に偏りを生じない方法で行う必要がある。結果的に観察期間内で最後まで残った症例，いいかえれば副作用がなく，効果がみられて投与継続された症例のみを評価対象とすることがないように，投与開始した調査全症例を追跡する必要がある。

ⅰ）中央登録方式

調査担当医師に当該医薬品の投与を開始した時点で，企業の製造販売後調査管理部門やあらかじめ定めた登録センター等へ登録してもらい，登録したすべての症例を調査票に記載する方法。

→ 通常の経口・外用剤等の調査に適用

ⅱ）連続調査方式

調査担当医師に当該医薬品を開始する（または開始した）症例を依頼症例数に達するまで連続して（もれなく）調査票に記載してもらう方法。

→ 急性期治療のための抗菌薬注射剤や救急用注射剤等の調査に適用

ⅲ）全例調査方式

調査担当医師に一定の依頼調査期間中に当該医薬品を使用する（または使用した）全症例について（もれなく）調査票に記載してもらう方法。

→ 対象症例が少ない希少疾病用医薬品や安全性の観点から製造販売後，一定数の症例に係るデータが集積されるまでの間は，流通管理を実施

Chapter 7 General discussion on post-marketing pharmacovigilance

including factors like the target population, the drug, the comparator for control, the applicable efficacy/safety endpoints, and the period.

Considering the scientific viewpoints and the current process for approval, the concrete actions of a pharmacovigilance plan in RMP can be roughly divided into the following 4 steps (see **Fig. 4.5** in Chapter 4): 1) Concretizing a concern that need to be clarified in the post-marketing setting per each safety issue in safety specification, 2) Determination of scientifically appropriate approach per each concern, 3) Choice of the regulatory framework for each approach, 4) Development of a detailed study protocol per each research question. In principle, the PMDA and the applicant must agree upon the contents to step 3 by the approval.

7.2.5 Guidelines for post-marketing studies

These guidelines show standard methods for use-results survey, specified use-results survey and post-marketing clinical trials performed during marketing as the "Guideline on the Implementation Procedures of Post-Marketing Surveillance, etc. for Prescription Drugs" (Evaluation and Licensing Division, Notification No. 1027001 PFSB MHLW dated October 27, 2005), also providing an outline of the former investigations/studies prior to the revised GPSP (2018).

As the outline of each former post-marketing study has been mentioned in 7.2.1. through 7.2.3., patient enrollment methods and study methods are provided here.

A) Patient enrollment methods

Patients are enrolled before the start of the investigation, but it is necessary to use the following methods to avoid bias in the selection of patients. It is necessary to follow effectively all patients who started treatment through the end of the investigation period so as to avoid evaluating only those patients remaining on therapy at the completion of the observation period, (i.e. not just evaluate only those patients who completed treatment because efficacy was found with no ADRs).

i) Central registration system

With this method, registration is performed in the sponsoring company's post-marketing study management division or the registration center designated in advance, at the start of administration of the test drug by the physician in charge of the investigation and all enrolled patients are entered in the case record forms (CRF).

→Applied in investigations of ordinary oral or topical agents etc.

ii) Continuous investigation system

Under this system, the physician in charge of the investigation enters the patients who will start (or have started) receiving the test drug on case report forms (CRF) continuously (without exception) until the requested number of patients is reached.

→Applied in investigations on antibacterial injections for acute phase treatment or injections for emergencies

iii) All-patient survey system

Under this system, all patients (without exception) who use (or have used) the test drug during the specified investigation period are entered on the CRFs by the

する必要のある医薬品等の調査に適用

イ）プロスペクティブな調査とレトロスペクティブな調査
　ⅰ）プロスペクティブな調査
　　　これから薬剤が使用される患者について，有効性・安全性を調査するプロスペクティブな調査（前向き調査）においては，症例の抽出にバイアスがかからないようにするために調査の開始前に症例の抽出方法や症例の登録方法をあらかじめ決定しておく。これを，中央登録方式という。臨床試験や通常の使用成績調査は，プロスペクティブな手法で行われる。
　ⅱ）レトロスペクティブな調査
　　　過去に薬剤が使用された患者について有効性・安全性を調査するレトロスペクティブな調査（後ろ向き調査）においては，症例の抽出が恣意的にならないような工夫が必要である。これには症例をもれなく登録する連続調査方式，あるいは全例調査方式などが採用される。特別な背景を有する患者の特定使用成績調査の場合には，症例収集が困難なケースもあり，プロスペクティブな手法だけでなく，レトロスペクティブな手法も用いられる。

7.3　安全管理情報の評価

7.3.1　シグナル検出と評価

　当該医薬品に関し，新たなリスクがないか，すでに特定されているリスクについてもその発生状況に変化がないかについて監視し，発見していく活動がシグナル検出といわれている。

　通常は個別症例や集積情報等の検討から，リスクのサイン（シグナル）を発見し，そのシグナルを検証・評価していく。

　シグナルとしては，重要な個別症例や個別症例の集積，製造販売後調査等の結果，副作用データベース（例えばJADERやAERS）を用いたデータマイニングの結果，文献・学会情報，各規制当局からの照会，措置等が考えられる。

　市販直後の重篤な副作用（個別症例）の発現や文献・学会情報，規制当局からの照会などは情報入手時に随時検討すべきシグナルと考えられるのに対し，個別症例の集積状況，副作用データベースを用いたデータマイニング（不均衡分析）の結果の検討等は定期的に検討すべきシグナルと考えられる。企業は製品ごとにこれらシグナル検出・評価の実施計画を立案，実施し，その結果を記録していくことが望まれるため，手順についてもあらかじめ定めておく必要がある。いわば積極的な安全管理活動である。ただし，データマイニングの結果が陽性であってもリスクを意味するものではなく，あくまで検討する優先順位が高いというだけの意味であり，その後の評価がより重要である。

physician in charge of the investigation.

→Applied in investigations on orphan drugs for which there are few target cases and drugs, etc. for which distribution management needs to be performed during marketing until the accumulation of data from a certain number of cases from the viewpoint of safety.

B) Prospective investigations and retrospective investigations

　i) Prospective investigations

In prospective investigations (forward-looking investigations) to examine efficacy and safety in patients who will use the test drug, the patient sampling method and patient enrollment method are decided before the start of the investigation to prevent bias in patient selection. This is called the central registration system. Clinical trials and typical Use-results survey use the prospective method.

　ii) Retrospective investigations

In retrospective investigations (backward-looking investigations) to examine efficacy and safety in patients who used the test drug in the past, it is necessary to devise a patient sampling method that will avoid arbitrary selection. The continuous investigation system or all-patient investigation system to register all of cases is employed. In Specified use-results survey of patients with special characteristics, both prospective and retrospective methods may be used when collection of patients is difficult.

7.3 Assessment of safety management information

7.3.1 Signal detection and assessment

Signal detection usually refers to an action to be vigilant for and find not only the presence/absence of new risks regarding a drug but also any changes in the occurrence of already-identified risks.

In general, a sign (signal) of a risk is found as a result of consideration of individual cases and collected information, etc. and verified/assessed.

Signals may include important individual cases, multiple cases, results from post-marketing studies, etc., data-mining results using an ADR database (e.g. JADER and AERS), literature/academic conference information, inquiries from regulatory authorities, actions, etc.

The occurrence of early post-marketing serious ADRs (individual cases), literature/academic conference information, inquiries from each regulatory authority, etc. are considered to be signals that should be considered every time information is available. On the other hand, the collection status of individual cases and data-mining (disproportionality analysis) results using an ADR database are considered to be signals that should be periodically considered. As MAHs are required to make an implementation plan for the above signal detection/assessment, implement it and record the results for each product, the procedures need to be provided in advance. It is a so-called active safety management activity. Of note, even if a data-mining result is positive, it does not mean a risk has been confirmed: the result just means a higher priority for consideration. Therefore, the subsequent assessment is more important.

7.3.2 個別症例の評価

　企業による日常的な個別症例の評価で重要なことは，報告された医薬品と有害事象との因果関係，予測性，重篤性等を検討することである。

- ・　予測性の評価

　市販薬の予測性は，添付文書の「使用上の注意」の記載の有無で判断する。また，新たに「使用上の注意」を改訂した場合は，医療関係者への伝達通知完了まで未知（予測できない）と評価する。なお，予測性の判断に用いる「使用上の注意」の項目は次のとおりである。「警告」，「禁忌」，「原則禁忌」，「効能又は効果に関連する使用上の注意」，「用法及び用量に関連する使用上の注意」，「慎重投与」，「重要な基本的注意」，「相互作用」，「副作用」，「高齢者への投与」，「妊婦，産婦，授乳婦等への投与」，「小児等への投与」，「臨床検査結果に及ぼす影響」，「過量投与」，「適用上の注意」

　なお，現在新記載要領に移行中であるが，「慎重投与」，「高齢者への投与」，「妊婦，産婦，授乳婦等への投与」，「小児等への投与」などは「特定の背景を有する患者に関する注意」へ集約される。

- ・　重篤性の評価

2005年4月1日から ICH E2D ガイドライン（承認後の安全性情報の取扱い：緊急報告のための用語の定義と報告の基準について）が施行されているので，以下の基準が報告された副作用の重篤性の評価に用いられている。

（ア）死に至るもの

（イ）生命を脅かすもの

（ウ）治療のための入院又は入院期間の延長が必要となるもの

（エ）永続的又は顕著な障害・機能不全に陥るもの

（オ）先天異常・先天性欠損を来すもの

（カ）その他の医学的に重要な状態と判断される事象又は反応

　なお，上記（ウ）の判断は ICH E2D ガイドラインの記載と一部解釈が異なっているため，外国企業と情報交換をする際には確認が必要である。上記（カ）の判断は，臨床医を交えて臨床的に判断されるが，以下を参考にしている企業もある。

- ・　重篤副作用疾患別対応マニュアル[2]：厚労省が作成したマニュアルで，スティーヴンス・ジョンソン症候群，間質性肺炎など77疾患が医薬品医療機器情報提供ホームページに掲載されているが，順次改訂中である。元来は重篤副作用の早期発見・対応のポイント，判別基準や治療法等を紹介したものであるが，重篤な副作用の評価の参考にもなる。
- ・　重篤度分類基準：「医薬品等の副作用の重篤度分類基準について」（平成4年6月29日付け薬安第80号厚生省薬務局安全課長通知）に示されている。主要な副作用の症状や臨床検査値を組織器官別にまとめて，グレード1から3

Chapter 7 General discussion on post-marketing pharmacovigilance   **179**

7.3.2 Assessment of individual cases

What is important in the MAH's daily assessment of individual cases is to examine the causal relationship between the reported drug and adverse events, expectedness, seriousness.

- Expectedness assessment

  The expectedness of reported ADRs to marketed drugs is evaluated based on whether or not there is an entry in the "Precautions" section of the package insert. Also, when the "Precautions" are revised, the reaction is considered "unexpected" (cannot be predicted) until HCPs are notified. The sections under Precautions used in the assessment of expectedness are as follows: "Warning", "Contraindications", "Relative contraindications", "Precautions related to indications", "Precautions related to dosage and administration", "Careful administration", "Important precautions", "Interactions", "Adverse reactions", "Use in the elderly", "Use during pregnancy and lactation", "Pediatric use", "Effects on laboratory test results", "Overdosage", and "Precautions for administration"

  Of note, these descriptions and categories are now being shifted to a new description format. "Careful administration", "Use in the elderly", "Use during pregnancy and lactation", and "Pediatrics Use" are consolidated into "Precautions concerning patients with specific backgrounds".

- Seriousness assessment

  Since the publication of the ICH E2D guideline (Post-approval Safety Data Management: Definitions and Standards for Expedited Reporting) on April 1, 2005, the following standards are used for assessment of the seriousness of ADRs.

  (A) Results in death

  (B) Is life-threatening

  (C) Requires inpatient hospitalization or prolongation of existing hospitalization (for ADR treatment)

  (D) Results in persistent or significant disability or incapacity

  (E) Is a congenital anomaly or birth defect

  (F) Is a medically important event or reaction

  The clinical judgment in (C) above is differently interpreted in part from the description in the ICH E2D guideline, and therefore confirmation is needed when exchanging information with foreign MAHs. The clinical judgment in (F) above is entrusted to a physician, but some MAHs also use the following for reference.

- Manuals for management of individual serious ADRs[2]: Manuals published by the MHLW, covering 77 diseases including Stevens-Johnson syndrome and interstitial pneumonia have been posted on the PMDA website. Updates are ongoing. These manuals are intended to introduce points related to early detection of and measures for serious ADRs, criteria for differential diagnosis and treatment methods, and also serve as a reference for evaluation of serious ADRs.

- Seriousness classification criteria: It is described in "the Standards for Seriousness Classification of Adverse Drug Reactions" (Safety Division, Notification No. 80, Pharmaceutical Affairs Bureau (PAB) MHW dated June 29, 1992). The symptoms and laboratory values associated with major ADRs are compiled by system organ class and graded from 1 to 3. These criteria were previously used in evaluation of

に分けて示したもので元来は重篤性の判定基準に用いられていたが，ICH E2A ガイドラインで重篤性の定義が示されたため，現在では重症度の基準として用いられている。

- ・ 因果関係の評価（個別症例）

投与された医薬品と報告された有害事象との因果関係は，以下の観点から検討し，できれば臨床医を交えて評価される[3]。あくまでこれは 1 つの例である。

- ・ 時間的関連性：治療開始とイベントの始まりとの時間的な関係，治療中止後にイベントは軽快したか，治療再開後に再発したか
- ・ 別の要因：イベント発生を説明するような合併症，併用薬，薬以外の曝露
- ・ イベントの性質：あるイベントにはしばしば薬が原因になるものがあり，それ自体，薬との関係を示唆する（例：ある種の皮膚反応）
- ・ 尤もらしさ：すでにこの薬（または類似薬）による反応であることが認識されているか。あるいは薬理学的に生物学的メカニズムを考えることができるか

7.3.3　集積情報の評価・分析

　個別症例における因果関係評価の結果のみならず，原則的にすべての有害事象が集積情報の評価・分析のステップの検討対象となるべきである。さらに当該医薬品のみならず，比較群を有した研究結果も集積情報の有用な情報源である。このような集積情報の評価については，CIOMS Ⅵの Appendix 7 [4] に記述のある "Evidence from Multiple Cases" を参考にするとよい。

　複数の症例に基づくエビデンス（Evidence from Multiple Cases）とは，

1. 安全性に的を絞った研究でのポジティブな結果
2. 発現割合がプラセボや対照薬に対して一貫して高い（統計的に有意であるかは問わない）
3. 用量反応関係が認められる（固定用量あるいは漸増法の研究）
4. その事象による中止症例の割合が対照群より高い
5. 対照群に比較して，より早期に発現している，あるいは重症度が高い
6. 関連する症状のパターンに一貫性がある
7. 発現までの時間に一貫性がある
8. 異なる研究間で一貫した傾向が観察される
9. 臨床的状態や潜伏のパターンが一貫している

7.3.4　医療情報データベース等の利用による評価・分析

　GPSP 省令が 2018 年 4 月に改正されたことにより，製造販売後データベース調

seriousness, but since the definition of seriousness in the ICH E2A guideline was specified. They are now used as a severity grading.

· Causality assessment (individual cases)

The causality between the administered drug and reported adverse event is examined based on the following points by consultation with physicians if possible[3]. The following is just an example.

- · Temporal relationship: Temporal relationship between start of the treatment and onset of the event, whether the event resolved after discontinuation of the treatment or relapsed after re-start of the treatment.
- · Alternative cases: concomitant diseases, concomitant drugs, or exposure to anything other than drugs that may explain the occurrence of the event.
- · Nature of event: Certain events are often caused by a drug, and those events per se suggest a relationship with the drug (e.g.: certain skin reactions).
- · Biological plausibility: Whether it is already recognized that the reaction was caused by the drug (or a similar drug). Whether it is possible to consider the mechanism of the occurrence based on pharmacology.

7.3.3 Assessment and analysis of multiple cases

In principle, all adverse events as well as the results of causality assessment in individual cases should be considered during assessment and analysis of collected information. Moreover, research results from a study with a comparative group in addition to the drug are a useful source of collected information. "Evidence from Multiple Cases" should be read for reference, which is described in Appendix 7[4] of CIOMS VI for assessment of such collected information.

What is the evidence based on multiple cases (Evidence from Multiple Cases)?

1. Positive outcome in targeted safety study (ies)
2. Consistently higher incidence vs placebo or active comparator (whether statistically significant or not)
3. Positive dose-response (fixed or escalating dose studies)
4. Higher incidence vs comparator (s) of event-specific patient discontinuations.
5. Earlier onset and/or greater severity in active vs comparator group (s).
6. Consistency of pattern of presenting symptoms.
7. Consistency of time to onset the occurrence.
8. Consistent trends across studies.
9. Consistent pattern of clinical presentation and latency.

7.3.4 Assessment and analysis by use of electronic healthcare database

A research design has been legally available using electronic healthcare data, etc., since the GPSP ordinance was revised in April, 2018 and post-marketing database studies was

査が追加され，医療情報データベース等を用いた研究デザインが法的に利用可能となった。データベースを用いて行うことのできる可能性のある調査の代表的なものとしては，現時点では患者背景の調査，背景発生率，医薬品使用実態の調査などが主である。なお，日本で利用可能な医療情報データベースについては，PMDA が運営管理している MID-NET® をはじめ，民間のメディカル・データ・ビジョン株式会社が保有する診療データベース，株式会社 JMDC が保有するレセプトデータベースをはじめとしていくつか知られている。詳細は一般財団法人日本薬剤疫学会のまとめを参照されたい [5]。

7.4　措置の立案

　個別症例報告，集積報告，海外との提携先や海外本社による総合的な評価，さらには海外規制当局からの情報に基づき，患者をリスクからできるだけ守るための措置の立案が行われる。措置の種類としては，以下のとおりである。
- ・　添付文書，主には使用上の注意の改訂とそれに伴う情報提供
- ・　緊急安全性情報
- ・　安全性速報
- ・　医薬・生活衛生局（旧医薬食品局）安全対策課長通知に基づく使用上の注意等改訂の情報提供
- ・　企業の自主的な使用上の注意等改訂の情報提供
- ・　再審査・再評価に基づく情報伝達，効能・効果などの承認事項の変更に伴う情報提供

さらには，
- ・　市場における販売制限
- ・　市場からの撤退（承認取り消し，取り下げ等）

などがある。

　なお，これら措置をとり行うための中心となるのは適正使用のための資材作成と提供が重要であるが，それらの詳細については第8章を参照のこと。

　措置の立案を行う閾値のようなものは存在しないが一般的には証拠の強さ，公衆衛生への影響，および国民の認識などを参考として行政当局が最終的な措置を決定する。

　「重大な副作用」への追記に関しては，ごくまれにしか生じないような副作用や主に薬剤性として知られている副作用については，因果関係を十分に吟味した上で数例（海外症例も含む）の関連性が高い症例が蓄積された場合に追記されることが多いが，最近では特に海外において背景発現率の高い，心血管系疾患や自殺，発がんなどについて注意喚起される場合がかなり増えつつある。この場合は，単に蓄積例数だけで決まることはありえず，比較研究（試験も含む）が決め手となる。「その他の副作用」への追記に関しても，記載閾値はなく，あくまで科学的な評価が必

Chapter 7 General discussion on post-marketing pharmacovigilance　183

added. The typical researches that can be conducted today with databases mainly include investigations on patient demographics, background incidence, drug utilization surveys. Among healthcare databases available in Japan, several databases are known as the sources included in MID-NET®, which is under the operation and management of PMDA, an administrative database owned by a private company, Medical Data Vision Co., Ltd. (MDV) and a claim database owned by JMDC Inc. See the summary by the Japanese Society for Pharmacoepidemiology for details[5].

7.4 Measures to be taken

Actions to protect patients from as many risks as possible are planned based on information from individual case reports, aggregate reports, comprehensive assessment by overseas affiliated companies/headquarters and overseas regulatory authorities. Types of actions are as follows:
- Revision of package inserts, mainly in the "Precautions" section, and Accompanying information provision
- Emergent Safety Communication DHPL (The Yellow Letter)
- Rapid Safety Communication DHPL (The Blue Letter)
- Information provision of revision in the Precautions, etc. based on notifications issued by Director of Safety Division, Pharmaceutical Safety and Environmental Health Bureau (the former Pharmaceutical and Food Safety Bureau).
- MAHs' voluntary provision of information on revision in the "Precautions" section.
- Information communication based on reexaminations/reevaluation, information provision accompanied by amendment of approved items such as indications

In addition,
- Marketing restrictions
- Withdrawal from the market (approval cancellation/nullification etc.)

are also included as actions.

In addition, preparation and provision of materials for proper use would be important for implementing these actions. See Chapter 8 for details.

The administrative authorities make the final decision on actions, generally taking into account the robustness of evidence, impact on public health and awareness by the public.

As for additional descriptions on "Clinically significant adverse reactions", very rare ADRs or ADRs known to be mainly induced by drugs are usually added following full examination of the causality if several cases (including overseas cases) which are highly related to the event have been accumulated. More warnings have been recently presented regarding cardiovascular diseases, suicide, cancer development, etc. with a high background incidence, especially from overseas. In the above case, the accumulated number of cases alone cannot determine the decision: comparative study (including trials) will be the decisive factor. Additional descriptions for "Other adverse reactions" do not have any written threshold. Scientific assessment is required for them.

要であろう．

7.5 行政における安全性情報の評価・分析

企業ならびに医薬関係者から報告された情報は，図 7.3 に示すような流れの中で評価・分析が行われている．

7.6 行政が行う安全性情報関連の実施事業・調査

わが国の医薬品等の安全対策に資する PMDA を中心として積極的な取組みが図られており，PMDA ホームページで紹介されている「医薬品安全対策の新たな事業・調査」[6] の「PMDA の実施事業・調査」に詳細が記載されている．現在も進行中のものを中心に簡単に述べる．

- MIHARI Project：PMDA における，第二期中期計画（平成 21 年度〜25 年度）において，医薬品処方後の有害事象発現リスクの定量的評価や，安全対策措

安全対策業務の流れ

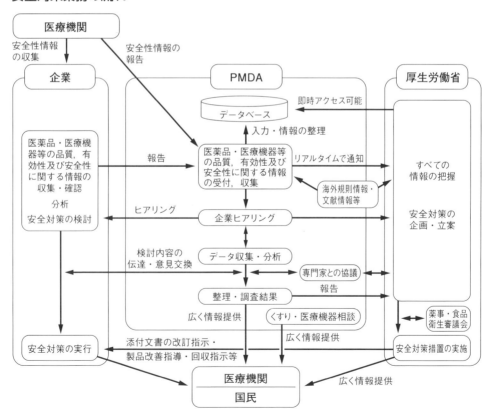

図 7.3 行政における安全対策業務の流れ

7.5 Evaluation and analysis of safety information by MHLW and PMDA

Information reported by MAHs and HCPs is evaluated and analyzed by the process shown in **Fig. 7.3**.

7.6 Implementation business/research relating to safety information by MHLW and PMDA

Proactive initiatives that contribute to Japanese drug safety measures have been taken mainly by PMDA and their details have been introduced in "Business/research conducted by PMDA" of "New business/research for drug safety measures"[6] on the PMDA website. Here is an outline mainly of the business/research that are ongoing today.

- MIHARI Project: After establishment of the system whereby a quantitative assessment of the occurrence risks of adverse events after drug prescription, impact assessment of safety measures, prescription actual surveys, etc. can be performed in the second interim period plan (FY2009 to FY2013) at PMDA, actions have been taken to utilize this system for the safety measures of each item in the third

Process of safety measure operation

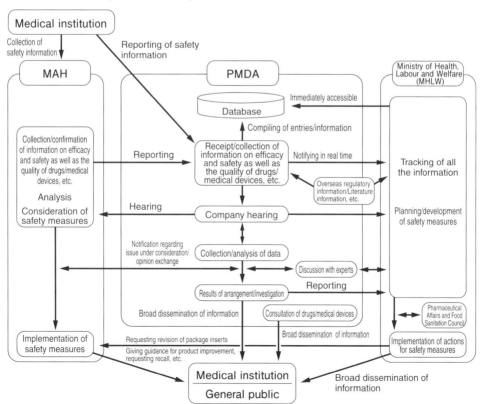

Fig7-3　Process of safety measure operation in MHLW and PMDA

置の影響評価，処方実態調査等が行える体制を構築したのちに第三期中期計画（平成26年度〜平成30年度）では，この体制を個別品目の安全対策措置に活用する活動を行っている。また，並行して新規データソースや，新規手法については引き続き各種試行調査を通じて，その利用可能性について検討を重ねている。

- MIHARI Communication：MIHARI Project で実施した各種薬剤疫学調査の結果を比較的平易な言葉で要約したもので，薬剤疫学を専門としていない医療従事者にも理解可能なコミュニケーションツールとして，平成26年度より開始している。

- MIHARI Archive：これまで MIHARI Project で実施した調査について，報告書，MIHARI Communication，学会発表，論文等の関連する情報を集約して提供している。さらに関連するガイドラインおよび関連通知として，医薬品GPSP省令関連，薬剤疫学調査関連，医薬品リスク管理計画関連通知などが掲載されている。

- 医療情報データベース基盤整備事業：MID-NET 構築に関する事業のことである。

- データベース分析手法高度化事業：成果として「医療情報データベース等を用いた医薬品の安全性評価における薬剤疫学研究の実施に関するガイドライン」が公表されている。

- 医療機関における安全性情報の伝達・活用状況に関する調査：医療機関（病院，薬局，診療所）から無作為抽出で選定された調査対象施設に調査票等を郵送し，管理薬剤師または DI 担当者に回答を依頼した。ウェブ調査票への入力，または紙面調査票の返送により回答を得ることにより，伝達・活用状況を継続して毎年調査している。またその成果もその都度公表されている。

- 医薬品の安全管理審査に関する調査事業（TERMS に関する調査：その1）：厳格なリスク管理方策（TERMS：Thalidomide Education and Risk Management System）を条件に承認されたサリドマイドについて，そのリスク管理方策の実施状況に係る患者調査を行い，その改善点の抽出などを行うことにより，今後の未承認薬の審査迅速化に資することを目的として調査が行われた。

- 未承認薬審査迅速化のためのリスク管理体制構築に資する調査事業（TERMSに関する調査：その2）：上述の TERMS に関する調査その1に引き続き，サレドカプセル服用患者を対象に服用状況等の実態調査を実施した。この調査結果は，サリドマイドのように使用方法や管理方法を誤ると，重篤な副作用などをもたらすような，取扱いに注意が必要な医薬品を将来承認する際の参考にすることができる。

- 電子保存された診療録等を用いた医薬品の安全性に関する調査：PMDA の第一期中期計画（2004年4月〜2009年3月）において，市販後の安全対策

interim period plan (FY2014 to FY2018). Moreover, for new data sources and new methods, their availability has been continuously discussed at the same time through various trial surveys.

· MIHARI Communication: Is a summary described in relatively plain language regarding the results of various pharmacoepidemiological study conducted in the MIHARI project, and was started in FY2014 as a communication tool that allows healthcare professionals who are not pharmacoepidemiologists to understand them.

· MIHARI Archive: A summary format of information related to reports, MIHARI Communications, academic conference presentations, literature, etc. is provided regarding the surveys that have been conducted in the MIHARI project.
The archive also provides notifications related to the drug GPSP ministerial ordinance, pharmacoepidemiology, and RMP as the relevant guideline and notifications.

· Infrastructure Development Project for Medical Information Database: refers to a project for MID-NET establishment.

· Advanced Database Analysis Method Project: "Guidance on Conduct of Pharmacoepidemiological study utilizing medical record database for drug safety assessment" has been disclosed as a result.

· Surveys for communication/utilization status of safety information at medical institutions: A survey form, etc. was sent by post to target institutions that were randomly selected among medical institutions (hospitals, pharmacies and clinics) to ask the supervising pharmacist or the person in charge of DI to reply to the survey. The survey for the communication/utilization status has been continuously conducted every year by acquiring replies from entries on the web or in paper survey form. The results have been made public each time.

· Survey project for drug safety management review (Survey for TERMS: No. 1): For thalidomide approved under the conditions of strict risk management measures (TERMS: Thalidomide Education and Risk Management System), a patient survey was conducted on the implementation status of the risk management measures, the points to be improved were extracted in order to help promote a shorter-period of review for unapproved drugs in the future.

· Survey project to help establish a risk management system to promote a shorter-review period for unapproved drugs (Survey for TERMS: No. 2): A utilization survey on the oral administration status in patients who receive Thaled capsules subsequently after the above Survey for TERMS: No. 1 was conducted. These survey results may be useful in future approval of drugs whose handling needs careful attention, such as a drug that can induce serious ADRs if its methods of use or management are wrong as seen in thalidomide.

· Investigations regarding pharmaceutical safety using electronic medical records, etc.: In the PMDA midterm plan for the first term (April 2004 - March 2009), a new system for post-marketing safety, the network of sentinel sites for collecting information (organization of medical institutions for specified therapeutic categories, products and diseases to improve the precision of analysis of ADR information and form a network to collect information intensively within a certain period) was established to place more emphasis on post-marketing safety measures.

の重点化を図るため，市販後安全体制に関する新規システムとして，情報収集拠点医療機関ネットワーク（副作用情報の解析精度を高めるため，特定の薬効群，品目および疾患ごとに医療機関を組織化したもので，一定期間内に集中的に情報を収集することを目的とする医療機関のネットワーク）を設置し，小児薬物療法に関する安全性確認のための調査として小児における「維持液投与後の低 Na 血症発生に関する電子媒体を用いた遡及的調査（拠点医療機関ネットワーク構築のための試行調査）」を行っている。さらに特定の「拠点医療機関」に限らず，多数の医療機関から得た診療に関する大規模なデータから分析・解析を行うために電子的な診療情報データを用いた医薬品の副作用に関する分析・解析の方法についても試行調査を行うこととし，(1) 電子カルテデータを基にした，「Medical Informatics System（MIS）調査」と (2) DPC データを基にした，「DPC 調査」の両データソースの特性比較，副作用データ抽出条件の検討，抽出データを利用した試行的解析により，電子診療情報の二次利用の可能性について評価している。

- 抗がん剤併用療法実態把握調査：上述の「電子保存された診療録等を用いた医薬品の安全性に関する調査」に基づき，2004 年 4 月から，厚労省の検討会で検討された抗がん薬の併用療法に関する実態把握調査（使用実績や副作用等について）を 22 療法について検討（「抗がん剤併用療法実態把握調査」）し，2005 年 6 月から調査を実施している。

- 市販直後の定点観測：企業が行う市販直後調査とは別に，新規性が高く，国内の治験症例数が少ない新医薬品または重点監視医薬品（緊急安全性情報等の発出を指示するなど，安全性について注意喚起を行った医薬品）について，行政が市販直後の定点観測を実施した。市販後の一定期間（原則 6 か月間），医薬品の副作用発生状況，臨床現場の企業の活動状況，情報の活用状況等の情報を直接収集・評価の上，必要な対応を図るものである。現在では実施されていない。

- 妊娠と薬情報センター：厚労省は 2005 年 10 月，国立成育医療研究センターに「妊娠と薬情報センター」を設置した。その目的は，次の 2 つである。
  - 妊婦またはこれから妊娠を希望する女性からの相談に応じ，正確な情報を伝えることで不安を取り除き，最善の医療が行えるようにすること，出産後の方を対象に，服薬の授乳に対する影響に関する相談など（相談業務）
  - 妊娠の結果情報を収集・評価し，将来の相談者への貴重な情報として役立てること（調査業務）

  国立成育医療研究センターや拠点病院等における外来相談に対応し，出産後，出生児の状況に関する情報を収集している。また，妊娠と薬に関する活動で広く知られているカナダのトロント大学病院とも連携し，小児科病院で

Chapter 7 General discussion on post-marketing pharmacovigilance

A "retrospective survey using electronic media on onset of hyponatremia after fluid maintenance therapy (trial survey on establishment of a network of sentinel sites)" in children has been performed to confirm the safety of pediatric drug treatment. A trial survey for the analysis methods for ADRs using electronical medical counselling information data was conducted to analyze a large data on medical counselling in not only specified sentinel medical institutions but also many other institutions. The possibility of secondary use of electronical medical information is assessed (1) in "Medical Informatics System (MIS) survey" based on electronic medical-record data and (2) by comparison of the characteristics in both data sources of "DPC Survey", which is based on DPC data, consideration of extract criteria to extract ADR data, and a trial analysis using extract data.

· The survey on the current status of combination therapy with anticancer agents: Based on the above "Investigations regarding the pharmaceutical safety using electronically saved medical records, etc.", the study group on current status of combination therapy with anticancer agents (results of use and ADRs etc.), an MHLW study group examined 22 treatment methods (the survey on current status of combination therapy with anticancer agents) from April 2004 and started the survey on the current status of anticancer agent combination therapy from June 2005.

· Fixed-point observations of pharmacovigilance activities in medical institutions at an early post-marketing stage: In addition to Early Post-marketing Phase Risk Minimization and Vigilance (EPPV) performed by the MAH, the MHLW implemented early post-marketing fixed-point observations (of PV activities) for highly innovative new drugs with few Japanese patients in clinical trials or priority monitoring drugs (drugs requiring special cautions concerning safety such as instructions to distribute a "Yellow Letter"). Information on the occurrence of ADRs, MAH's activities in medical practices and status of use of information for a fixed period after marketing (six months, in principle) are collected directly and evaluated, and necessary measures are taken. It is not implemented today.

  · Pregnancy and Medicine Information Center: the MHLW established the "Pregnancy and Medicine Information Center" in the National Center of Child Health and Development in October, 2005. The objectives are the following two:

   · Anxiety is eliminated by providing correct information in consultation with women who are pregnant or women who wish to become pregnant so that the best treatments are provided and for women after delivery, the effect on breastfeeding by medication is advised (consultation work)

   · Information on the outcomes of pregnancies is collected and evaluated to serve as valuable information for future consultations (survey work)

Information is collected on the status of neonates after delivery via outpatient consultations in the National Center or core hospitals. The program is also affiliated with Toronto University Hospital in Canada, which is widely known for its activities related to pregnancy and drugs, and utilizes information, etc. accumulated at pediatric hospitals. As of today, at least 1 sentinel site has been registered in every prefecture. Based on information, etc., accumulated since 2016, a business has been started to promote including them in package inserts. As a result, the statement for

蓄積された情報等を活用している。現在ではすべての都道府県に1か所以上の拠点医療機関が登録されている。2016年から集積された情報等を踏まえ，添付文書への反映を推進する事業を開始しており，2018年7月にはその成果として，免疫抑制剤3剤について，従来妊婦への投与は禁忌であったが，「治療上の有益性が危険性を上回ると判断される場合にのみ投与する」と緩和された。

文　　献

1) 独立行政法人医薬品医療機器総合機構，製造販売後データベース調査実施計画書の記載要領（2018年1月23日）．PMDAホームページ：
www.pmda.go.jp/files/000222302.pdf

2) 厚生労働省，重篤副作用疾患別対応マニュアル（医療従事者向け）．PMDAホームページ：
https://www.pmda.go.jp/safety/info-services/drugs/adr-info/manuals-for-hc-pro/0001.html

3) Patrick Waller 著，久保田潔監訳：医薬品安全性監視入門　第2版—ファーマコビジランスの基本原理，じほう，2018，p.38-39

4) Management of safety information from clinical trials. Report of CIOMS Working Group VI より，Appendix 7

5) 日本薬剤疫学会，日本における臨床疫学・薬剤疫学に応用可能なデータベース調査結果（日本語版）：http://www.jspe.jp/mt-static/FileUpload/files/JSPE_DB_TF_J.pdf

6) 独立行政法人医薬品医療機器総合機構，医薬品安全対策の新たな事業・調査．PMDAホームページ：https://www.pmda.go.jp/safety/surveillance-analysis/0020.html

Chapter 7 General discussion on post-marketing pharmacovigilance 191

3 immunosuppressive drugs became less strict in July, 2018: the administration to pregnant patients used to be contraindicated but it was changed to "administered only if the expected therapeutic benefits outweigh the possible risks associated with treatment".

Literature

1) Guidance on development of post-marketing database protocol, PMDA (January 23, 2018), PMDA website
www.pmda.go.jp/files/000222302.pdf

2) Manuals for handling disorders due to adverse drug reactions (for healthcare professionals), MHLW, PMDA website
https://www.pmda.go.jp/safety/info-services/drugs/adr-info/manuals-for-hc-pro/0001.html

3) Introduction to Pharmacovigilance Second Edition – The Basic Pharmacovigilance Principles, by Patrick Waller (author), Kiyoshi Kubota (translation supervisor), Jiho, 2018 p.38-39

4) Management of safety information from clinical trials. Report of CIOMS Working Group VI, Appendix 7

5) Japanese Society for Pharmacoepidemiology, Results of survey of database applicable to clinical epidemiology/pharmacoepidemiology in Japan (Japanese version): http://www.jspe.jp/mt-static/FileUpload/files/JSPE_DB_TF_J.pdf

6) New projects/investigations for drug safety measures, PMDA, PMDA website. https://www.pmda.go.jp/safety/surveillance-analysis/0020.html

第8章

製品基本情報と適正使用情報（の内容と伝達）

わが国では，医薬品医療機器等法第68条の2（旧 薬事法第77条の3）「情報の提供等」の第1項においては，「医薬品，医療機器若しくは再生医療等製品の製造販売業者（中略）は，医薬品，医療機器又は再生医療等製品の有効性及び安全性に関する事項その他医薬品，医療機器又は再生医療等製品の適正な使用のために必要な情報を収集し，及び検討するとともに，（中略）医薬関係者に対し，これを提供するように努めなければならない。」（抜粋）と規定されている。また，第2項で「（中略）医師，歯科医師，薬剤師，獣医師その他の医薬関係者は医薬品，医療機器若しくは再生医療等製品の製造販売業者（中略）が行う医薬品，医療機器又は再生医療等製品の適正な使用のために必要な情報の収集に協力するよう努めなければならない。」（抜粋）と規定されている。

さらに，2005年4月以降，製造販売業者等の許可要件となった「医薬品，医薬部外品，化粧品及び医療機器及び再生医療等製品の製造販売後安全管理の基準に関する省令」（GVP省令）の第5条において，安全管理情報の収集・検討ならびに安全確保措置の立案・実施等に関する製造販売後安全管理業務手順書等の作成が義務付けられている。

また，2014年10月に施行された改正GVP省令では，医薬品リスク管理を行う場合の「医薬品リスク管理に関する手順書」の作成，ならびに「製造販売後調査等管理責任者との相互の連携に関する手順書」の作成が義務付けられた（第2章参照）。

8.1 製品基本情報

8.1.1 企業中核データシート（CCDS：Company Core Data Sheet）

ICH E2C（R1）の提案事項に従い，販売承認取得者（わが国の製造販売業者等）が医薬品ごとにグローバルでひとつのCCDSを作成することが一般的に行われており，安全性，承認適応，用法・用量，薬理その他医薬品に係る情報が記載されている。CCDSに含まれる中核的な安全性情報は，CCSI（Company Core Safety Information）と呼ばれる。

CCDSは企業内文書として作成されるものであり，規制当局による規制を直接受けることはなく，また一般に公表されるものでもないため，「製品基本情報」とは

Chapter 8

(The Contents and Communication of) Basic Product Information and Information on Proper Use

I n Article 68-2, Paragraph 1 (Provision of information, etc.) of the PMD Act (Article 77-3 of the old PAL) in Japan, it is specified that "MAHs ... of drugs and medical devices, etc. must make efforts to collect and examine information related to efficacy and safety of drugs and medical devices, etc. and other required information for their proper use, and provide it to HCPs ... (excerpt)". Moreover, in Paragraph 2, it is specified that "... physicians, dentists, pharmacists, veterinarians and other healthcare professionals must make efforts to cooperate in collecting information required for the proper use of drugs, medical devices or regenerative and cellular therapy products, etc. ... done by MAHs of drugs, medical devices or regenerative and cellular therapy products, etc. ..." (excerpt).

In addition, in Article 5 of the Ordinance on standards for post-marketing safety management of drugs, quasi-drugs, cosmetics, medical devices and regenerative medicine products (GVP ordinance) as a license requirement for MAHs effective from April, 2005, it states that collection and examination of safety management information, drafting and conducting of safety assurance measures and preparation of standard operating procedures (SOPs) for postmarketing safety management are obligatory.

Also, in the revised GVP ordinance that will come into force in October 2014, the preparation of "written procedures for drug risk management" in cases performing drug risk management and the preparation of "written procedures for mutual collaboration with the Post-marketing studies manager" are obligatory (see Chapter 2).

8.1 Basic Product Information

8.1.1 Company Core Data Sheet (CCDS)

MAHs generally prepare one Company Core Data Sheet (CCDS) for each drug globally in accordance with recommendations in the ICH E2C (R1). A CCDS provides the safety, approved indications, dosage and administration, pharmacology and other information on a drug. Core safety information contained in the CCDS is referred to as the Company Core Safety Information (CCSI).

The CCDS is prepared as an internal document and is not directly regulated by regulatory authorities or disclosed to the general public; thus, it has a different nature from that of "basic product information". However, under current circumstances where drugs are used globally, the CCDS is used as a fundamental document presenting the

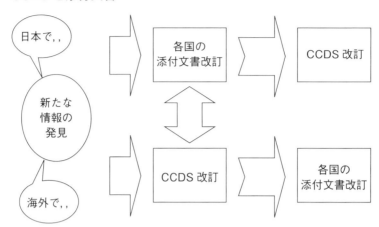

図 8.1　CCDS と添付文書

性格を異にするものである．しかしながら，医薬品がグローバルな状況下で使用される現在においては，企業の当該医薬品に対する世界共通の基本的なポジションを示した文書として，製品基本情報作成の際，基礎となるものであり，近年，グローバル企業においてはCCDSの作成に日本法人が関与する事例も出てきている．

　企業はCCDSに基づいて，製品基本情報を作成するべきであるとともに，新たな情報や各国規制当局からの指示等により各国の製品基本情報が変更された場合等には，CCDSの改訂の要否を検討する必要がある．日本においても，CCDSが改訂された場合には，製品基本情報（特に添付文書）の記載内容の改訂についてGVP手順書に基づき検討することになる（図8.1参照）．

8.1.2　添付文書

　わが国の添付文書は，医師，歯科医師，薬剤師等の医療関係者向けの製品基本情報であり，適正使用情報の中核をなし，医療用医薬品については，医薬品医療機器等法で表8.1のとおりに定められており，生物由来製品についてはさらに，表8.2に示した事項が追加される．また，添付文書は医薬品に添付される公的文書で，医療訴訟においての法的根拠となりうる．

　なお，現行の添付文書への記載事項（表8.3）と記載要領は1997年4月25日付の以下の3通知により定められていた．

- 「医療用医薬品添付文書記載要領について」(薬発第606号厚生省薬務局長通知)
- 「医療用医薬品の使用上の注意記載要領について」(薬発第607号薬務局長通知)
- 「医療用医薬品添付文書の記載要領について」(薬安第59号薬務局安全課長通知)

　その後，医薬品をめぐる環境の変化と添付文書をめぐる状況の変化により記載要領の改正についての検討が行われ，2017年6月8日付の2通知，1)「医療用医薬

CCDS and package inserts

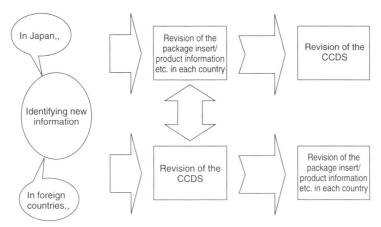

Fig.8.1 CCDS and package inserts

universal core position on the drug taken by a company when preparing product information. In recent years, there are cases where a Japanese corporation is involved in the preparation of a CCDS in a global company.

Companies should prepare basic product information based on the CCDS, and when changes in the basic product information in each country are made based on new information or upon instructions of regulatory authorities, whether or not the CCDS should be revised needs to be considered. In Japan, when a CCDS is revised, revision of the contents of basic product information (particularly the package insert) should be considered based on GVP (see **Fig.8.1**).

8.1.2 Package Inserts

Package inserts in Japan are the basic product information aimed at healthcare professionals such as physicians, dentists and pharmacists. They also constitute the core of information on proper use, and package inserts for ethical drugs are specified in the PMD Act as shown in **Table 8.1**. Items added for biological products are shown in **Table 8.2**. In addition, package inserts are official documents attached to drugs and may be legal evidence in medical lawsuits.

Items to be presented in and guidelines for current package inserts (**Table 8.3**) are stipulated in the following three notifications dated April 25, 1997:
- "Guidelines for descriptions in package inserts of ethical drugs" (PAB/MHW Notification No. 606)
- "Guidelines for descriptions in precautions for use of ethical drugs" (PAB Notification No. 607)
- "Guidelines for descriptions in package inserts of ethical drugs" (PAB/SD Notification No. 59)

Thereafter, a revision of the guide to drafting was considered due to changes in the environment surrounding drugs and the circumstances around package inserts. As a

196   第 8 章　製品基本情報と適正使用情報（の内容と伝達）

表 8.1　医療用医薬品の添付文書に関する医薬品医療機器等法上の規定 [1, 2]

条文番号　条名	規　定
第 52 条　添付文書等の記載事項	当該医薬品に関する最新の論文その他により得られた知見に基づき，以下の事項が記載されていなければならない。 ・用法，用量その他使用および取り扱い上の必要な注意 ・日本薬局方収載医薬品については，日本薬局方で添付文書等に記載するよう定められた事項 ・保健衛生上特別の注意を要する医薬品等で添付文書に記載するよう定められた事項 ・その他，厚生労働省令で定める事項
第 52 条の 2　添付文書等の記載事項の届出等	・製造販売業者は，厚生労働大臣が指定する医薬品の製造販売をするときは，あらかじめ，厚生労働省令で定めるところにより当該医薬品の添付文書等記載事項のうち使用および取り扱い上の必要な注意等について厚生労働大臣に届け出なければならない。変更しようとするときも同様とする。 ・製造販売業者は，上記届出をしたときは，直ちに当該医薬品の添付文書等記載事項について，電子情報処理組織を使用する方法等であって，厚生労働省令で定めるもの（PMDA Web サイト等）により公表しなければならない。
第 52 条の 3　機構(PMDA)による添付文書等記載事項の届出の受理	厚生労働大臣が機構（PMDA）に届出の受理に係る事務を行わせることとしたときは厚生労働大臣が指定する医薬品についての第 52 条の 2 第 1 項の規定による届出をしようとするものは，厚生労働省令で定めるところにより機構（PMDA）に届け出なければならない。
第 53 条　記載方法	・毒薬，劇薬又は第 50 条から第 52 条までに規定する事項（直接の容器等，添付文書等の記載事項）の記載は他の文字，記事，図画又は図案に比較して見やすい場所に記載 ・医薬品を一般に購入し，又は使用するものが読みやすく，理解しやすい用語により正確に記載しなければならない。
第 54 条　記載禁止事項	・当該医薬品に関し虚偽又は誤解を招くおそれのある事項 ・承認を受けていない効能，効果又は性能 ・保健衛生上，危険がある用法，用量又は使用期間

表 8.2　生物由来製品の添付文書に関する医薬品医療機器等法上の規定 [3]

条文番号　条名	規　定
第 68 条の 18　添付文書等の記載事項	生物由来製品は，第 52 条第 1 項各号又は第 63 条の 2 第 1 項各号に掲げる事項のほか，以下の事項が記載されていなければならない。 ・生物由来製品の特性に関して注意を促すための厚生労働省令で定める事項 ・生物由来製品の基準において記載するように定められた事項 ・その他，厚生労働省令で定める事項
第 63 条の 2　添付文書等の記載事項	医療機器は，添付文書等に，当該医療機器に関する最新の論文その他により得られた知見に基づき，次の事項が記載されていなければならない。 ・使用方法その他使用及び取扱い上の必要な注意 ・厚生労働大臣の指定する医療機器にあつては，その保守点検に関する事項 ・厚生労働大臣が性状，品質及び性能の適正を図るために設けた基準において，添付文書等に記載する事項 ・厚生労働大臣がその製法，性状，品質，貯法等に関して設けた基準において添付文書等に記載するように定められた事項 ・その他，厚生労働省令で定める事項

Chapter 8 (The Contents and Communication of) Basic Product Information and Information on Proper Use   197

Table 8.1   Specifications in the PMD Act related to package inserts of ethical drugs[1, 2]

Article No./Article name	Specification
Article 52 Matters to be indicated in package inserts etc.	Based on knowledge obtained from latest research papers, etc. related to the drug, the following matters must be described. • Dosage and administration and other necessary precautions for use and handling • For drugs listed on the Japanese Pharmacopoeia, matters specified in the Japanese Pharmacopoeia • Items specified for entry in package inserts for drugs which require special attention from public health • Other items specified by MHLW ordinance
Article 52-2: Notification, etc. of matters to be indicated in package inserts, etc.	• When intending to market a drug designated by the Minister of Health, Labour and Welfare, MAHs shall notify the Minister of Health, Labour and Welfare of necessary precautions for use and handling of the drug among matters indicated in the package insert, etc. of the drug according to the items specified by MHLW ordinance. The same rule applies when making a change. • When having made the above notification, MAHs shall promptly release the matters indicated in the package insert, etc. of the drug by a method using an electronic information processing organization among those specified in the MHLW Ordinance (PMDA's website).
Article 52-3: PMDA's acceptance of notification of matters indicated in package inserts, etc.	When the Minister of Health, Labour and Welfare decides to have the PMDA conduct clerical work related to the acceptance of notifications, parties who intend to make a notification pursuant to the provisions of Article 52-2, Paragraph 1 regarding drugs designated by the Minister of Health, Labour and Welfare must notify the PMDA as specified in the MHLW Ordinance.
Article 53 way of entries	• Entries for poisonous and powerful drugs and matters specified in Articles 50 to 52 (matters to be indicated on direct containers and package inserts, etc.) must be shown more prominently than other words, articles, drawings or designs • Entries for drugs must be accurate, easy to read and in language easy to understand for those who generally purchase and use them
Article 54 Prohibited entries	• Entries that are false or might lead to misunderstandings concerning the drug • Indications or efficacy for which approval has not been obtained • Dosage and administration or duration of use that might jeopardize public health

Table 8.2   Specifications in the PMD Act related to package inserts of biological products[3]

Article No./Article name	Specification
Article 68-18: Matters to be indicated in package inserts, etc.	In addition to the items in Article 52 Paragraph 1, and Article 63-2 Paragraph 1, the following items must be entered for biological products. • Precautions based on characteristics of biological products specified by MHLW ordinance • Items specified in Standards for Biological Products • Other items as specified by MHLW ordinance
Article 63-2: Matters to be indicated in package inserts, etc.	For medical devices, the following matters must be described in package inserts, etc. based on knowledge obtained from latest research papers, etc. related to the medical device. • Instructions for use and precautions necessary for use and handling • For medical devices designated by the Minister of Health, Labour and Welfare , matters related to maintenance and inspection • Matters to be indicated in package inserts, etc. based on the standards established by the Minister of Health, Labour and Welfare regarding appropriate properties, quality and performance • Matters to be indicated in package inserts, etc. based on the standards established by the Minister of Health, Labour and Welfare in relation to the manufacturing method, properties, quality and storage conditions of the medical device • Other items specified by MHLW ordinance

198 　第8章　製品基本情報と適正使用情報（の内容と伝達）

表 8.3 　添付文書の構成 [1, 2, 4]

①作成または改訂年月
②日本標準商品分類番号等
　日本標準商品分類番号, 承認番号, 薬価基準収載年月, 販売開始年月, 再審査結果公表年月（最新の期日）,
　再評価結果公表年月（最新の期日）, 効能又は効果追加承認年月（最新の期日）, 貯法等
③薬効分類名
④規制区分
⑤名称
◆本文冒頭
⑥警告
⑦禁忌
⑧組成・性状
⑨効能または効果
　効能または効果に関連する使用上の注意
⑩用法および用量
　用法および用量に関連する使用上の注意
⑪使用上の注意
⑫薬物動態
⑬臨床成績
⑭薬効薬理
⑮有効成分に関する理化学的知見
⑯取り扱い上の注意
⑰承認条件
⑱包装
⑲主要文献および文献請求先
　投薬期間制限医薬品に関する情報
⑳製造販売業者の氏名または名称および住所

品の添付文書等の記載要領について」（薬生発 0608 第 1 号厚生労働省医薬・生活衛生局長通知）, 2)「医療用医薬品の添付文書等の記載要領の留意事項について」（薬生安発 0608 第 1 号厚生労働省医薬・生活衛生局安全対策課長通知）により, 2019年 4 月 1 日から 2024 年 3 月 31 日までの 5 年間で, 以下のように記載要領が変更される（図 8.2 参照）.

　① 　項目の通し番号の設定
　　「警告」以降の全ての項目に番号を付与, 記載すべき内容がない項目は欠番.
　② 　「原則禁忌」,「慎重投与」の廃止
　　「原則禁忌」,「慎重投与」は廃止し,「特定の背景を有する患者に関する注意」など, その他の適切な項へ記載する.
　③ 　「特定の背景を有する患者に関する注意」の新設
　　「高齢者への投与」,「妊婦, 産婦, 授乳婦等への投与」,「小児等への投与」を廃止し,「特定の背景を有する患者に関する注意」を新設し,「妊婦」,「生殖能を有する者」,「授乳婦」,「小児等」,「高齢者」,「腎機能障害患者」,「肝

Chapter 8 (The Contents and Communication of) Basic Product Information and Information on Proper Use

Table 8.3 Contents of package inserts[1, 2, 4]

[1] Preparation and revision dates

[2] Standard Commodity Classification No. of Japan, etc. Standard Commodity Classification No. of Japan, Approval No., Date of entry in Health Insurance Price List, Date of marketing, Date of publication of Reexamination results*, Date of publication of Reevaluation results*, Date of approval of extended indications*, Storage conditions, etc.(* latest date)

[3] Therapeutic category

[4] Regulatory classification

[5] Name

◆ Beginning of text

[6] Warnings

[7] Contraindications

[8] Composition, Properties

[9] Indications (Precautions related to indications)

[10] Dosage and administration (Precautions related to dosage and administration)

[11] Precautions

[12] Pharmacokinetics

[13] Clinical studies

[14] Pharmacology

[15] Physicochemistry

[16] Precautions for handling

[17] Approval conditions

[18] Packaging

[19] Main references and requests for literature
      Information on restrictions to duration of administration

[20] Name and address of MAH

result, the guide to drafting will be changed as described below over a period of 5 years from April 1, 2019 to March 31, 2024 pursuant to two notifications dated June 8, 2017: 1) "Guide to Drafting Package Inserts of Ethical Drugs" (PSEHB Notification No. 0608-1, MHLW); and 2) "Points to Consider for Guide to Drafting Package Inserts of Ethical Drugs" (PSEHB/SD Notification No. 0608-1, MHLW) (see **Fig. 8.2**).

[1]   Establishment of serial numbers of sections
       Numbers will be assigned to all sections after the "WARNINGS" section. For sections without information to be recorded, the numbers will be unused.

[2]   Abolition of "Relative Contraindications" and "Careful Administration"
       The Sections "Relative Contraindications" and "Careful Administration" will be abolished and provided in other appropriate sections such as "PRECAUTIONS CONCERNING PATIENTS WITH SPECIFIC BACKGROUNDS."

[3]   New establishment of the Section "PRECAUTIONS CONCERNING PATIENTS WITH SPECIFIC BACKGROUNDS"
       The Sections "Use in the Elderly," "Use during Pregnancy, Delivery or Lactation" and "Pediatric Use" will be abolished, and the Section

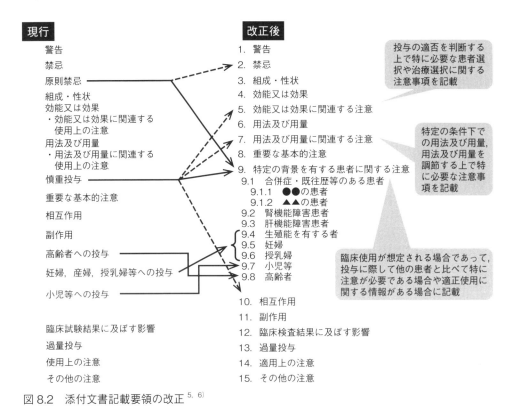

図8.2 添付文書記載要領の改正 [5, 6)]

機能障害患者」等の項目に分けて記載する。

④ 後発医薬品，バイオ後続品の情報提供の充実

後発医薬品およびバイオ後続品の「使用上の注意」および「取扱い上の注意」の記載は，原則として，それぞれの先発医薬品および先行バイオ医薬品と同一とする。

8.1.3 患者向医薬品ガイド

2014年11月に施行された医薬品医療機器等法の第1条の6（国民の役割）として「国民は，医薬品等を適正に使用するとともに，これらの有効性及び安全性に関する知識と理解を深めるように努めなければならない。」と記載されたが，患者向医薬品ガイドは，すべての医療用医薬品において作成するものではなく，重篤な副作用の早期発見等を促すために，特に患者へ注意喚起すべき適正使用に関する情報等を有する以下の医療用医薬品において，作成が望まれている（2005年6月30日付「患者向医薬品ガイドの作成要領」について（薬食発第0630001号厚生労働省医薬食品局長通知)[7)]。

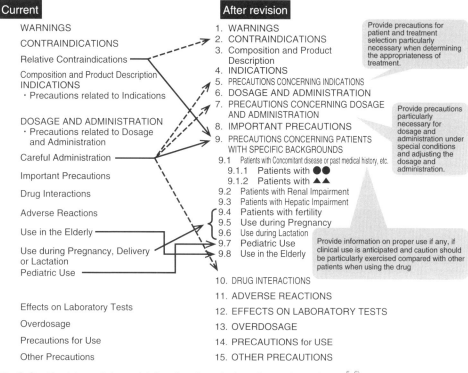

Fig.8.2 Revision of the guideline for descriptions in package insert[5, 6]

"PRECAUTIONS CONCERNING PATIENTS WITH SPECIFIC BACKGROUNDS" will be newly set out to present information by classifying it into sections such as "Use during Pregnancy," "Patients with fertility," "Use during Lactation," "Pediatric Use," "Use in the Elderly," "Patients with Renal Impairment" and "Patients with Hepatic Impairment."

[4] Enhancement of provision of information on generic drugs and biosimilars

Information to be provided in the Section "PRECAUTIONS" and "PRECAUTIONS FOR HANDLING" for generic drugs and biosimilars should be, in principle, the same as that for each of their original drugs and original biological drugs.

8.1.3 Drug Guides for Patients

As stated in Article 1-6 (Roles of the Public) of the PMD Act which came into force in November 2014, "The public must make efforts to properly use drugs, etc. and also to deepen the knowledge and understanding of their efficacy and safety." However drug guides for patients are not prepared for all ethical drugs. It is hoped that such guides will be prepared for the following ethical drugs for which there is information, etc. on proper use that requires attention particularly among patients to promote activities such as early detection of serious ADRs. ("Guide to the Preparation of Drug Guides for Patients;" PFSB Notification No. 0630001, MHLW dated June 30, 2005)[7].

- Drugs with a "Warning" section in the package insert. However, selection of patients for administration, careful reading of the package insert, and warnings to

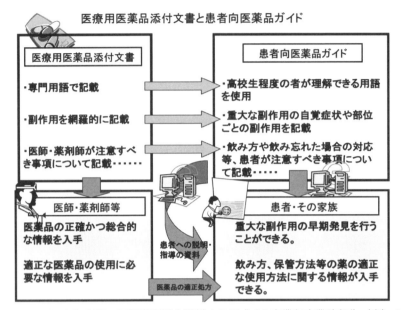

図 8.3　PMDA 2018 年度第 1 回運営評議会資料 1-3 平成 29 事業年度業務報告（案）より引用

- 添付文書に警告欄が設けられているもの。ただし，投与に際しての患者の選択，添付文書を熟読すること，治療経験等の医師等への警告は除く。
- 添付文書の「効能・効果に関連する使用上の注意」，「用法・用量に関連する使用上の注意」，または「重要な基本的注意」の項に，重篤な副作用回避等のために「患者に説明する」旨が記載されているもので，かつ「重大な副作用」の記載のあるもの。
- 患者に対して，特別に適正使用に関する情報提供が行われているもの。なお，診断や処置目的で病院や診療所のみで使用されるものは除く。

なお，医療用医薬品添付文書と患者向医薬品ガイドの位置付けについては図 8.3 を参照。

また，2006 年 1 月以降，患者向医薬品ガイドそのもの，ならびに関連通知が PMDA ホームページに掲載されている。

8.2　製品基本情報補完媒体（適正使用情報）

8.2.1　新医薬品の「使用上の注意」の解説

新医薬品の「使用上の注意」の解説は，製薬企業が市販開始直後の安全性確保を目的に，「使用上の注意」について設定理由や根拠となった副作用症例をあげて，わかりやすく解説した資料である。新発売後 1 年間を目安に新規納入先に集中して配布され，市販直後調査のツールとしても利用されている。

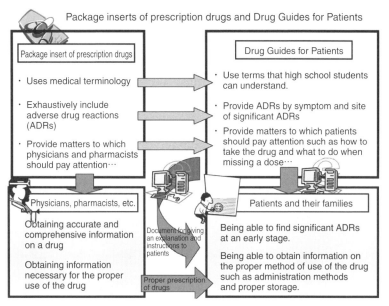

Fig.8-3 Cited from Documents 1 to 3 at the FY 2018 first Governing Council, PMDA: FY 2017 business report (draft)

  physicians, etc. in terms of treatment experience, etc. are excluded.
- Drugs with the statement "to be explained to patients" and "significant ADRs" to avoid serious ADRs in the "Precautions related to indications", "Precautions related to dosage and administration" or "important precautions" sections of the package insert.
- Drugs for which information on proper use is specially provided to patients. Those used only at hospitals or clinics for the purposes of diagnosis or treatment are excluded.

For the positioning of package inserts of prescription drugs and drug guides for patients, see **Fig. 8.3**.

In addition, since January 2006, Drug Guides for Patients and related notifications have been posted on the PMDA website.

8.2 Supplementary Materials to Basic Product Information (Information on Proper Use)

8.2.1 Explanation on the "Precautions" of a new drug

The explanation on the "Precautions" of a new drug is material prepared by an MAH to ensure safety during early post-marketing phase in which cases of ADRs that were the basis for setting "Precautions" are listed to facilitate understanding. Around one year after the launch of a new drug, these materials are distributed mainly to new sites to which the drug is delivered, and also are utilized as a tool of EPPV.

8.2.2　インタビューフォーム

インタビューフォーム（IF）[8]は，薬剤師などが日常業務上必要となる医薬品の適正使用や評価，医薬品管理のための情報，薬剤情報提供の裏付けとなる情報などが集約された総合的な個別の医薬品解説書として，日本病院薬剤師会が記載要領を策定し，その作成の手引きを日本製薬工業協会が作成している。従来はMRによる紙媒体情報提供物であったが，2009年5月からPMDAのホームページの「医療用医薬品情報検索→検索結果一覧で表示する文書を選ぶ」で，IFを選択すると該当製品のIFにたどりつける。

8.2.3　医療用医薬品製品情報概要

医療用医薬品製品情報概要とは，「個々の医療用医薬品に関する正確な情報を医薬関係者に伝達し，その製品の適正な使用を推進することを目的として作成される資材である。」と，日本製薬工業協会（以下，製薬協）医療用医薬品製品情報概要審査会で定めた「医療用医薬品製品情報概要等に関する作成要領（作成要領）」に規定されている。記載内容は添付文書の記載範囲内であるが，広告宣伝媒体であるので，医薬品医療機器等法第66条（誇大広告等），第67条（特定疾病用の医薬品等の広告の制限），第68条（承認前の医薬品等の広告の禁止）を遵守することはもとより，医薬品等適正広告基準，医療用医薬品の販売情報提供活動に関するガイドラインや製薬協コード・オブ・プラクティス，製薬協通知に留意して作成するよう求められている。

8.2.4　くすりのしおり

製薬企業が作成して，くすりの適正使用協議会が取りまとめている患者を対象とした服薬説明書で，従来はくすりの適正使用協議会（https://www.rad-ar.or.jp/）や製薬企業のホームページのみに掲載されていた。2007年3月からはPMDAホームページにも掲載され，現時点ではPMDAのホームページの「医療用医薬品情報検索→検索結果一覧で表示する文書を選ぶ」で，くすりのしおりを選択すると該当製品のくすりのしおりにたどりつける。参考までに，患者向医薬品ガイドとくすりのしおりの対比表を表8.4に示す。

8.3　添付文書の改訂等適正使用情報の重要度に応じた情報提供

死亡，障害もしくはこれらにつながるおそれのある症例または治療の困難な症例の発生を防止するため，厚労省からの命令，指示，製造販売業者の自主的な決定などにより，国民（患者），医療関係者に対して緊急な安全対策上の措置を講じる必

Chapter 8 (The Contents and Communication of) Basic Product Information and Information on Proper Use   205

8.2.2 Interview Form

The Interview Form (IF)[8] is a comprehensive explanatory document for individual drugs summarizing the information on proper use and evaluation, information for management of the drug, and information for substantiating the drug information that is required by pharmacists in their routine activities. The Japanese Association of Hospital Pharmacists developed guidelines for description in Interview Forms and JPMA prepares the guide to drafting based on these guidelines. It has been distributed in paper format by MRs but it has become accessible on the PMDA website since May 2009. By selecting the IF on the screen "prescription drug information search → select a document on a list of search results" in the PMDA's website, the IF of an applicable product can be obtained.

8.2.3 Ethical Drug Product Information Brochure

The ethical drug Product Information Brochure is stipulated in the guidelines for entries specified by the Review Board for product information brochures of the Japan Pharmaceutical Manufacturers Association (hereinafter, JPMA) as "the material prepared to communicate accurate information on individual ethical drugs to HCPs for the purpose of promoting proper use." The contents are within the scope of the package insert but since it is advertising material, it should be prepared in compliance with Article 66 (exaggerated advertisement), Article 67 (restriction of the advertisement of drugs for designated diseases), Article 68 (prohibition of advertisement of drugs prior to approval) of the PMD Act and by heeding the appropriate advertising standards for drugs, guidelines for activities to provide marketing information on prescription drugs, the JPMA Code of Practice and JPMA notifications.

8.2.4 Drug Information Sheet

Drug Information Sheets are patient medication information prepared by each MAH and are handled by the Risk/ Benefit Assessment of Drugs-Analysis and Response (RAD-AR) Council, Japan (https://www.rad-ar.or.jp/). They have been accessible on the website of RAD-AR and MAHs but they have also become accessible on the PMDA website since March 2007 and by selecting the Drug Information Sheet on the screen "prescription drug information search → select a document on a list of search results" in the PMDA website, the Drug Information Sheet of an applicable product can now be obtained. For reference, a comparison table of Drug Guides for Patients and the Drug Information Sheet is shown in **Table 8.4**.

8.3 Provision of Information According to the Degree of Importance of Information on Proper Use Such as a Revision of a Package Insert

To prevent deaths, disabilities, events that may result in death or disability, or untreatable diseases, when it is judged necessary for the general public (patients) and healthcare professionals (HCPs) to take urgent safety measures under orders and instructions from the MHLW, voluntary decision of the MAH, and others, Emergent/

206　第8章　製品基本情報と適正使用情報（の内容と伝達）

表8.4　患者向医薬品ガイドとくすりのしおりの対比表

患者向医薬品ガイド（経口剤）		くすりのしおり（経口剤）	
添付文書と対応して作成，おおむね数ページ。		剤形ごとに作成，おおむね1ページ。	
表題	対応する添付文書の内容	表題	対応する添付文書の内容
この薬は？	販売名，一般名，含有量	商品名	販売名，一般名，含有量，剤形写真
この薬の効果は？	薬効薬理，効能・効果，効能・効果に関連する使用上の注意	この薬の作用と効果について	薬効薬理，効能・効果
この薬を使う前に，確認すべきことは？	警告，禁忌・原則禁忌，効能・効果に関連する使用上の注意，用法・用量に関連する使用上の注意，慎重投与，重要な基本的注意，相互作用	次のような方は使う前に必ず担当の医師と薬剤師に伝えてください。	警告，禁忌・原則禁忌，相互作用，妊婦・産婦・授乳婦への投与
この薬の使い方は？ ・使用量及び回数 ・どのように飲むか？ ・飲み忘れた場合の対応 ・多く使用した時（過量使用時)の対応	用法・用量 過量投与	用法・用量 （この薬の使い方）	用法・用量，用法・用量に関連する使用上の注意，過量投与
この薬の使用中に気をつけなければならないことは？	重要な基本的注意，相互作用，妊婦・産婦・授乳婦への投与	生活上の注意	相互作用，その他の関連する使用上の注意
副作用は？	重大な副作用	この薬を使ったあと気をつけていただくこと(副作用)	重大な副作用，その他の副作用
この薬の形は？	剤形，識別コード		
この薬に含まれているのは？	主成分及び添加物の名称		
その他 ・この薬の保管方法は？ ・薬が残ってしまったら？	貯法	保管方法その他	貯法
この薬についてのお問い合わせ先は？			
		医療担当者記入欄	

Chapter 8 (The Contents and Communication of) Basic Product Information and Information on Proper Use   207

Table 8.4   Comparison of Drug Guide for Patients and Drug Information Sheet

Drug Guide for Patients (oral medications)		Drug Information Sheet (oral medications)	
Prepared based on package inserts, several pages		Prepared for each dose form, about 1 page	
Title	Corresponding contents of package insert	Title	Corresponding contents of package insert
What is this drug?	Brand name, non-proprietary name, content	Brand name	Brand name, non-proprietary name, content, photograph of dosage form
What are the effects of this drug?	Pharmacology, indications, precautions related to indications	Actions and effects of the drug	Pharmacology, indications
What should be checked before using the drug?	Warnings, contraindications, relative contraindications, precautions related to indications, precautions related to dosage and administration, careful administration, important precautions, drug interactions	Those to whom the following applies should consult with the attending physician and pharmacist before use.	Warnings, contraindications, relative contraindications, drug interactions, use during pregnancy or lactation
How is the drug used? • Dose and number of doses • How is it taken? • Measures when forgetting to take drug • Measures when taking too much (overdosage)	Dosage and administration overdosage	Dosage and administration (method of use of the drug)	Dosage and administration, precautions related to dosage and administration, overdosage
What should be watched for during use of the drug?	Important precautions, drug interactions, use during pregnancy or lactation	Precautions in daily life	Drug interactions, other related precautions
Adverse reactions?	Clinically significant ADRs	What should be watched for during use of the drug? (ADRs)	Clinically significant ADRs, other ADRs
Dosage form of the drug?	Dosage form, ID code		
What does the drug include?	Names of main ingredients and excipients		
Others • How should the drug be stored? • What should be done with left-over drug?	Storage conditions	Storage conditions etc.	Storage conditions
Person to contact concerning drug			
		For use by attending healthcare provider	

208　第8章　製品基本情報と適正使用情報（の内容と伝達）

表 8.5　緊急安全性情報等の提供に関する指針について（2014 年（平成 26 年）10 月 31 日付薬食安発 1031 第 1 号）[9]

1．緊急安全性情報等の作成基準

◇医薬品等について，（ア）に掲げるいずれかの状況からみて，国民（患者），医薬関係者に対して緊急かつ重大な注意喚起や使用制限に係る対策が必要な状況にある場合に，（イ）に掲げる措置を実施するに当たって，厚生労働省からの命令，指示，製造販売業者の自主的な決定その他により作成する。

（ア）項
　①法第 68 条の 10 に基づく副作用・不具合等の報告における死亡，障害若しくはこれらにつながるおそれのある症例又は治療の困難な症例の発生状況
　②未知重篤な副作用・不具合等の発現など安全性上の問題が有効性に比して顕著である等の新たな知見
　③外国における緊急かつ重大な安全性に関する行政措置の実施
　④緊急安全性情報又は安全性速報等による対策によってもなお効果が十分でないと評価された安全性上の問題

（イ）項
　①警告欄の新設又は警告事項の追加
　②禁忌事項若しくは禁忌・禁止事項の新設又は追加
　③新たな安全対策の実施（検査の実施等）を伴う使用上の注意の改訂
　④安全性上の理由による効能効果，使用目的，性能，用法用量，使用方法等の変更
　⑤安全性上の理由により，回収を伴った行政措置（販売中止，販売停止，承認取り消し）
　⑥その他，当該副作用・不具合等の発現防止，早期発見等のための具体的な対策

2．緊急安全性情報等の提供方法

①　医薬食品局安全対策課は，緊急安全性情報又は安全性速報の作成及び配布について，製造販売業者等に対し，命令，指示を行う場合は，その理由等を記した書面により通知する。

②　製造販売業者は，厚生労働省及び PMDA と協議し，緊急安全性情報又は安全性速報を作成する。

③　製造販売業者及び医薬食品局安全対策課は，国民（患者），医薬関係者への周知のため，緊急安全性情配布開始後，速やかに報道発表を行う。また，製造販売業者は，回収等の国民（患者）が直接の対応を行う必要がある事案においては，新聞の社告等の媒体への情報の掲載を考慮する。なお，緊急安全性情報には，広告宣伝に関連する内容や緊急性を伴わない他の製品に関連する内容（代替となる製品に関するものを除く。）を含んではならないものとする。

④　製造販売業者は，医薬関係者向けのみならず，国民（患者）向けの緊急安全性情報を報道発表にも活用する。

⑤　PMDA は，①の通知，緊急安全性情報又は安全性速報及び添付文書の改訂内容を，緊急安全性情報又は安全性速報の配布開始後，速やかに PMDA のホームページに掲載し，PMDA による PMDA メディナビにて速やかに配信する。また，製造販売業者においても同様の情報を速やかに自社等のホームページ（特定の利用者のみ対象としたものではない場所をいう。）に掲載する。なお，法第 52 条の 2 第 1 項，法第 63 条の 3 第 1 項又は法第 65 条の 4 第 1 項の規定により添付文書等記載事項の届出の対象となる医薬品等については，製造販売業者は添付文書の改訂内容を自社等のホームページに掲載する前に PMDA に届け出る。

⑥　製造販売業者は，直接配布を原則とするが，⑦の配布計画に従い，医療機関，薬局等に対し，緊急安全性情報又は安全性速報及び改訂添付文書（添付文書情報）等について，迅速性及び網羅性を考慮し，直接配布，ダイレクトメール，ファックス，電子メール等を活用し，効果的に組み合わせる等により情報提供を実施する。また，当該製品の納入が確認されている医療機関の適切な部署（医療安全管理者，医薬品安全管理責任者，医療機器安全管理責任者，又は医療機関の製品情報担当者等の所属する部署），薬局等に，①の通知日又は製造販売業者が自主的に配布を行うと決定した日から 1 か月以内に情報が到達していることを確認する。

⑦　製造販売業者は，PMDA 安全部門（医薬品は安全第二部，医療機器及び再生医療等製品は安全第一部をいう。）と緊急安全性情報又は安全性速報の配布計画について事前に協議し，配布（等）計画書を提出する。医療機関，薬局等への訪問等による配布については，配布計画に従い実施し，その結果を PMDA 安全部門に提出する。

⑧　製造販売業者は，緊急安全性情報の場合は，医学，薬学等の関係団体に対して情報提供を行い，会員等への情報提供の協力及び関係団体のホームページ等への掲載等の効果的な広報手段での周知を依頼する。また，当該製品を使用する患者団体を把握している場合には，当該団体に対しても情報提供を行うことも考慮する。なお，安全性速報の場合は，必要に応じて上記対応を行う。

⑨　製造販売業者は，厚生労働省からの命令，指示，社内各部門での連絡等に関する文書，訪問記録及び配布記録を，当該製品の安全性情報に関する記録を利用しなくなった日から 5 年間保存する。（ただし，生物由来製品:10 年，特定生物由来製品:30 年，特定保守管理医療機器及び設置管理医療機器:15 年，再生医療等製品 10 年，指定再生医療製品 30 年）

Chapter 8 (The Contents and Communication of) Basic Product Information and Information on Proper Use   **209**

Table 8.5 The Guidelines on Provision of Emergency/Rapid Safety Communication DHPLs (dated October 31, 2014, PFSB Notification No. 1031-1) [9]

---

1. Criteria for preparation of Emergent Safety Communication DHPL, etc.

For drugs, etc., Emergent Safety Communication DHPL, etc. are prepared when emergency or critical warnings for the general public (patients) and HCPs or measures related to restriction of use are required based on situations listed in (A), in order to implement actions listed in (B) based on orders and instructions from the MHLW or voluntary decision of the MAH.

Section (A)

[1] Occurrence of deaths, impairment, or cases that may result in death or impairment, or cases that are difficult to treat in reports of adverse reactions/defects, etc. based on Article 68-10 of the PMD Act

[2] New findings, such as a prominent safety issue compared to efficacy, including the occurrence of unknown serious adverse reactions/defects, etc.

[3] Implementation of emergency and critical administrative actions related to safety in foreign countries

[4] Safety issue for which the efficacy is assessed to be insufficient despite measures with Emergency/Rapid Safety Communications, etc.

Section (B)

[1] New establishment of a warning column or addition of warnings

[2] New establishment or addition of contraindications or contraindications/prohibition

[3] Revision of precautions for use accompanied by implementation of a new safety measure (implementation of a test, etc.)

[4] Changes in indication, intended use, performance, dosage and administration, and methods for use, etc., for safety reasons

[5] Administrative actions accompanied by recall (discontinuation, suspension, withdrawal of the approval) for safety reasons

[6] Other specific measures for prevention and/or early detection of the relevant adverse reactions/defect, etc.

---

2. Methods for providing Emergent Safety Communication DHPL, etc.

[1]   The Safety Division of the Pharmaceutical and Food Safety Bureau (PFSB) orders or instructs the MAH, etc. in writing with reasons, etc. to prepare and distribute Emergent/Rapid Safety Communication DHPLs.

[2]   The MAH prepares Emergent/Rapid Safety Communication DHPLs upon discussion with the MHLW and the PMDA.

[3]   The MAH and Safety Division of the PFSB issue a press release immediately after the start of distribution of Emergent Safety Communication DHPL to disseminate the information to the general public (patients) and HCPs. Also, the MAH considers posting the information in media including newspaper announcements (press release) for issues such as recall for which the general public (patients) are required to take direct actions. In addition, Emergent Safety Communication DHPL must not include information related to advertisement or other products that do not require emergency actions (excluding information on alternative products).

[4]   The MAH utilizes Emergent Safety Communication DHPL for the general public (patients) for a press release, in addition to those for HCPs.

[5]   The PMDA posts the notification in [1], Emergent/Rapid Safety Communication DHPLs, and contents of revision of package inserts on the PMDA website immediately after the start of distribution of Emergent/Rapid Safety Communication DHPLs, in addition to promptly sending them via PMDA medi-navi. The MAH also promptly posts the same information on the website of the company, etc. (which are not restricted to specific users). For drugs, etc. that require submission of matters to be indicated in package inserts, etc. based on the regulations in Article 52-2 Paragraph 1, Article 63-3 Paragraph 1, or Article 65-4 Paragraph 1, the MAHs must submit the contents of a revision of package inserts to the PMDA before posting them on the website of the company, etc.

[6]   In principle, the MAH distributes the information directly. However, in accordance with the distribution plan in [7], Emergent/Rapid Safety Communication DHPLs and revised package inserts (package insert information), etc. are provided to medical institutions and pharmacies utilizing and efficiently combining direct distribution, direct mail, fax and e-mail, etc. taking account of rapidity and comprehensiveness. In addition, the MAH confirms that the information is delivered to appropriate departments of medical institutions and pharmacies, etc. to which the relevant product is confirmed to be delivered (departments to which medical safety manager, pharmaceutical safety control manager, medical device safety control manager, or product information manager belongs) within one month of the day of notification in [1] or the day when the MAH decides to perform voluntary distribution.

[7]   The MAH discusses a plan for distribution of Emergent/Rapid Safety Communication DHPLs with the Safety Division of the PMDA (Office of Safety II for drugs and Office of Safety I for medical devices and regenerative medicine products) in advance, and submits a plan for distribution (etc.). The information is distributed to medical institutions and pharmacies, etc. by visiting them in accordance with the distribution plan, and the results are submitted to the Safety Division of the PMDA.

[8]   For Emergent Safety Communication DHPL, the MAH provides the information to the relevant medical and pharmaceutical parties, and asks their members, etc. to cooperate in information provision and dissemination by effective means such as posting on their websites, etc. In addition, in case associations of patients who use the relevant product are known, consideration should be given to provide the information to such associations. The above actions should also be taken for Rapid Safety Communication DHPL as required.

[9]   The MAH retains documents and records of visits and distributions related to orders or instructions from the MHLW and communications among departments of the company for 5 years after the day when the records related to the safety information of the relevant product are no longer used. (However, the retention periods shall be as follows: biological products, 10 years; specified biological products, 30 years; controlled medical devices requiring special maintenance and installation controlled medical devices, 15 years; regenerative medicine products, 10 years; designated regenerative medicine products, 30 years).

表 8.6　医療用医薬品添付文書使用上の注意及び取扱い上の注意の改訂に伴う改訂添付文書等の情報対応について（2015年〔平成27年〕2月26日付 日薬連発第129号）

1. 緊急安全性情報（イエローレター），安全性速報（ブルーレター）
   製造販売業者は，緊急安全性情報又は安全性速報に係る薬食安通知に際し，「添付文書の改訂内容」についてPMDAへの届出及び掲載手続を行い，原則として薬食安通知発出及び届出の受理を確認後に情報提供を開始する。また，自社等のホームページ（特定の利用者のみを対象としたものではない場所）に，速やか（原則として緊急安全性情報又は安全性速報に係る薬食安通知受理後，3日以内，遅くとも1週間以内）に「緊急安全性情報」又は「安全性速報」及び「改訂添付文書情報」等を掲載する。

2. 使用上の注意事項等を改訂した場合
   1) 薬食安通知による使用上の注意等の改訂
      製造販売業者は，薬食安通知に際し，「添付文書の改訂内容」についてPMDAへの届出及び掲載手続を行い，原則として薬食安通知発出及び届出の受理を確認後に情報提供を開始する。また，「改訂添付文書情報」等を自社等のホームページに薬食安通知受理後，原則として2週間以内に掲載する。なお，改訂内容は「医薬品安全対策情報」（以下，DSU）に掲載される。
   2) 薬食安通知によらない使用上の注意等の改訂
      製造販売業者は，「添付文書の改訂内容」についてPMDAへの届出及び掲載手続を行い，原則として届出が受理された後，情報提供を開始する。また，「改訂添付文書情報」等を自社等のホームページに改訂後，原則として2週間以内に掲載する。PMDA相談企業は，必要に応じて改訂内容をDSUに掲載依頼する。
      なお，DSUとは別に「改訂内容を明らかにした文書」を作成した場合は，その文書も原則として薬食安通知発出及び届出の受理を確認後に（薬食安通知によらない場合は改訂後），自社等のホームページに掲載する。

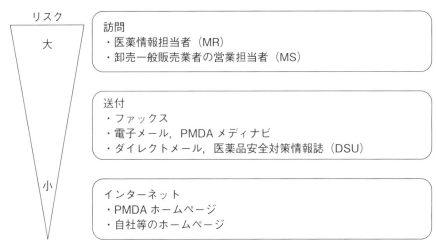

図 8.4　わが国における適正使用情報の提供・伝達の特徴

要があると判断された場合は，「緊急安全性情報等の提供に関する指針について」に基づき，緊急安全性情報等を配布する（表 8.5）。緊急安全性情報等は製造販売業者の自主的な決定であっても，厚労省およびPMDAと協議し作成する。また，原則として国民（患者）向け情報も併せて作成する。なお，日本製薬団体連合会（以下，日薬連）の自主基準により，表 8.6 の情報対応が実施されている。緊急安全性情報等以外の使用上の注意の改訂案内は，「改訂のお知らせ」などを用いてMR等を通じて，厚労省 医薬・生活衛生局安全対策課からの指示書受理後1か月以内に，医療関係者に伝達が行われる（図 8.4）。その他自主改訂等の場合においても，で

Table 8.6 Handling of information such as revised package inserts, etc. associated with revision of precautions for use and handling in package inserts of ethical drugs (FPMAJ Notification No. 129 dated March 26, 2015)

---

1. **"Emergent Safety Communication DHPL" (yellow letter) and "Rapid Safety Communication DHPL" (blue letter)**
   The MAH submits "contents of revision of package insert" to the PMDA and performs procedures for posting based on the PFSB notification on Emergent/Rapid Safety Communication DHPLs. In principle, information provision is started after the confirmation of issuance of the PFSB notification and receipt of the notification. In addition, the MAH posts "Emergent/Rapid Safety Communication DHPLs" and "revised package insert information", etc. on the website of the company, etc. (which are not restricted to specific users) promptly (within 3 days after the receipt of the PFSB notification on the Emergent/Rapid Safety Communication DHPLs in principle, within one week at the latest).

2. **In case precautions for use, etc. are revised**
   1) Revision of precautions for use, etc. based on the PFSB notification
   The MAH submits "contents of revision of package insert" to the PMDA and performs procedures for posting based on the PFSB notification, and starts providing information after the confirmation of issuance of the PFSB notification and receipt of the notification in principle. In addition, the MAH posts "revised package insert information", etc. on the website of the company, etc. within 2 weeks after the receipt of the PFSB notification in principle. Also, the contents of revision are posted on "Drug Safety Update" (DSU).
   2) Revision of precautions for use, etc. independent of the PFSB notification
   The MAH submits "contents of revision of package insert" to the PMDA and performs procedures for posting, and starts providing information after the notification is accepted in principle. In addition, the MAH posts "revised package insert information", etc. on the company website, etc. within 2 weeks after the revision in principle. Also, the MAH asks the PMDA to post the contents of revision on DSU as required.
   In addition, in case a "document in which contents of revision are specified" is prepared separately from the DSU, it is also posted on the company website, etc. after the confirmation of issuance of the PFSB notification and receipt of the application in principle.

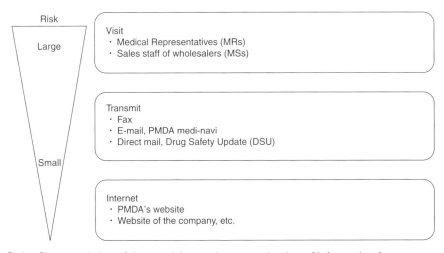

Fig.8-4 Characteristics of the provision and communication of information for proper use in Japan

Rapid Safety Communication DHPLs are distributed based on the "Guidelines for Preparation of Emergent/Rapid Safety Communication DHPLs" (**Table 8.5**). In addition, Emergent/Rapid Safety Communication DHPLs are prepared by the MAH after consulting with the MHLW and PMDA, even if it is a voluntary decision by the MAH. Furthermore, in principle the information is to be prepared not only for

表 8.7 緊急安全性情報・安全性速報以外の使用上の注意の改訂

薬生安	医薬・生活衛生局安全対策課長通知
自主改訂	企業自主

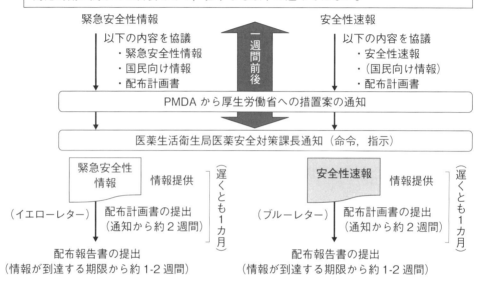

製薬協「医療用医薬品添付文書」情報提供の手引き（平成28年4月版）
図 8.5 緊急安全性情報，安全性速報による情報提供対応の流れ

きるだけ1か月以内を目安に医療関係者に伝達される（表8.6, 8.7）。

なお、「緊急安全性情報」は、黄色系の紙に赤枠で囲む（最大4ページとする）ことから「イエローレター」と呼ばれている。また、「安全性速報」は、緊急安全性情報に準じ、一般的な「使用上の注意」の改訂情報よりも迅速な安全対策措置をとる場合に発出され、青色系の紙に赤枠で囲むことから「ブルーレター」と呼ばれる。医療関係者向けならびに患者向けの緊急安全性情報・安全性速報はPMDAホームページに掲載されている（安全対策業務→情報提供業務→医薬品→注意喚起情報→緊急安全性情報・安全性速報）。

〈医薬品安全対策情報〉

医薬品安全対策情報（日本版 Drug Safety Update、略称：DSU）は、使用上の注意改訂時の情報伝達を徹底するため、日薬連が編集発行、厚労省が監修する情報誌で、1992年11月に第1号が発刊され、通常年10回発行されている。DSUは、通常、通知後3週間以内に病院、診療所、保険薬局等の約24万施設に直接郵送される。また、2004年3月から、郵送のみでなく、PMDAホームページにも掲載されている（安全対策業務→情報提供業務→医薬品→注意喚起情報→DSU（日本製薬団体

Table 8.7 Revision of precautions other than Emergent/Rapid Safety Communication DHPLs

PSEHB/SD	Notification by Safety Division, Pharmaceutical Safety and Environmental Health Bureau
Voluntary revision	Voluntary revision by an MAH

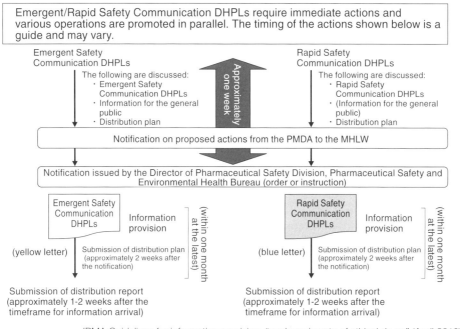

JPMA Guidelines for information provision, "package inserts of ethical drugs" (April 2016)

Fig.8-5 Flow of information provision via Emergent/Rapid Safety Communication DHPLs

healthcare professionals but also for the general public (patients). The methods of dealing with information shown in **Table 8.6** have been implemented according to the voluntary standards of the Federation of Pharmaceutical Manufacturers Association of Japan (FPMAJ). Information on Revision of Precautions other than DHPLs of Emergent/Rapid Safety Communications are communicated within one month after receipt of instructions from the Safety Division, Pharmaceuticals and Food Safety Bureau, MHLW via MRs, etc, using "Revision notices" (**Fig. 8.4**). For other voluntary revisions by the MAH, HCPs should be notified within one month whenever possible (**Table 8.6**, **8.7**).

"Emergent Safety Communication DHPL" are provided in (up to four) yellow pages with a red frame, and therefore is called a "Yellow Letter." A "Rapid Safety Communication DHPL" are issued when a safety measure is taken more promptly than modified information of general "precautions for use" in accordance with Emergent Safety Communication DHPL in blue paper with a red frame, and therefore is called a "Blue Letter." Emergent/Rapid Safety Communication DHPLs for healthcare professionals and patients are presented on the PMDA website (Post-marketing Safety Measures → Information Services → Drugs → Information Calling attention → The Yellow Letter / Blue Letter).

連合会発行))。

さらに，2018年6月発行のWeb版のDSUから，商標名をクリックすると各社のお知らせ文書の閲覧が可能となっている。

8.4 わが国における適正使用情報の提供・伝達の特徴

わが国における適正使用情報の提供・伝達の特徴は，図8.4に示すように，医師・薬剤師等医薬関係者へのMR/MSの直接訪問による伝達を中心として，郵便等による送付，インターネットでの情報提供の3種の方法により行われていることである。特に重要な使用上の注意の改訂等では，同時に3種の方法により情報が提供・伝達される。

その他，添付文書改訂を伴わない場合においても，PMDA，学会，企業の判断により，添付文書情報のリマインド等の重要な適正使用情報が医療関係者や患者に情報提供される場合がある。これらはいずれもPMDAのホームページに掲載され公表されるとともに，企業の判断により行われるものについては，企業のMRによっても医療機関等に伝達されている。

また，医療用医薬品の添付文書は，1999年5月以降，新規作成，改訂に際し製造販売業者等がSGMLデータおよびPDFデータとしてPMDAホームページに掲載

表8.8 PMDAメディナビ[12]

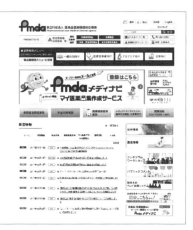

＜主な配信内容＞
- 緊急安全性情報・安全性速報
- 使用上の注意の改訂指示通知
- 回収情報（クラスI，クラスII）
- 承認情報
- 医薬品リスク管理計画（RMP）
- 適正使用等に関するお知らせ
- 医薬品に関する評価中のリスク等情報
- 副作用救済給付の決定のお知らせ　等

<Drug Safety Update>

Drug Safety Update (DSU, Japanese version) is an information journal edited and issued by the FPMAJ and supervised by the MHLW to adequately communicate information at the time of revision of precautions. The first issue was published in November 1992 and it is usually published 10 times a year. DSU is usually mailed directly to about 240,000 institutions such as hospitals, clinics, health insurance pharmacies, etc. within 3 weeks of notification. It has also become accessible on the PMDA website since March 2004 in addition to direct mail. (Post-marketing Safety Measures → Information Services → Drugs → Information Calling attention → DSU [issued by the Federation of Pharmaceutical Manufacturers Association of Japan]).

Furthermore, from the Web version of DSUs issued in June 2018, clicking on a brand name enables access to written notices by each company.

8.4 Characteristics of the Provision and Communication of Information for Proper Use in Japan

The characteristics of provision and communication of information for proper use are shown in **Fig. 8.4**. There are three methods of communication. The main method consists of direct visits to HCPs such as physicians and pharmacists by MRs/MSs etc. The other two methods are sending by direct mail, etc. and provision of information via the Internet. Especially in cases of revision of important precautions, information is provided and communicated by all three methods simultaneously.

In addition, even if no revision of a package insert is included, important information on proper use such as a reminder of package insert information may be provided to healthcare professionals and patients at the discretion of the PMDA, academic societies or companies. Each of these is presented on the PMDA website, and for those implemented at the discretion of companies, the information is also transmitted to medical institution and other relevant institutions by the companies' MRs.

Package inserts for ethical drugs newly prepared or revised after May 1999 must be placed on the PMDA's website which provides information on pharmaceuticals and medical devices as SGML data or PDF data by the MAHs. With enforcement of the

Fig.8.8   PMDA medi-navi[12)]

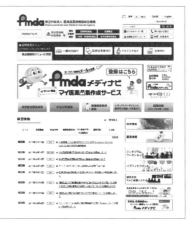

<Main information delivered>
- Emergent/Rapid Safety Communication DHPLs (The Yellow Letter / Blue Letter)
- Notifications for instructions on revision of precautions for use
- Recall information (Classes I and II)
- Approval information
- Risk Management Plan (RMP)
- Alert for proper use, etc.
- Information on risks, etc. under evaluation regarding drugs
- Notices of determination of ADR relief/benefits, etc.

216   第 8 章　製品基本情報と適正使用情報（の内容と伝達）

するよう指導されていたが，2014 年 11 月医薬品医療機器等法の施行により届出が
義務付けられた。

　なお，2005 年 8 月 1 日からは PMDA メディナビが開始され，ユーザー登録者（無
料で登録ができる）には表 8.8 にあげた内容の新着情報が自動的に配信されるよう
になっている（2018 年 3 月 30 日時点のユーザー登録件数は 16 万 4,821 件と報告さ
れている）。

8.5　PMDA ホームページ

　本書第 8 章中でも繰り返し参照している PMDA ホームページ [11] は，当初医薬品
医療機器情報提供ホームページとして，医薬品の安全な使用を推進するため，医師，
歯科医師，薬剤師を対象として，旧医薬品副作用被害救済・研究振興調査機構が日
本製薬団体連合会（通称，日薬連）とともに 1999 年 5 月に医薬品情報提供システ
ム事業を発足したことによるものである。なお，2006 年 1 月以降から「患者向医
薬品ガイド」を掲載することに伴い，2007 年 3 月にはユーザー別に必要な情報を
得やすくするために，「一般の皆様」向けの情報と「医療関係者」向けの情報に分
けて掲載することになった。その後，数回の改訂が行われ，2018 年 10 月時点では，
訪問別ナビゲーションとして，「一般の方向け」，「医療従事者向け」，「アカデミア
向け」，「企業向け」と構成されている。

　掲載情報は表 8.9 のとおりである。

　なお，厚労省では 2017 年以降，新規作用機序を有する革新的な医薬品については，
最新の科学的見地に基づく最適な使用を推進する観点から，当該医薬品の使用に係

表 8.9　PMDA ホームページに掲載されている主な医薬品関連情報（2018 年 10 月時点）

1）添付文書情報
2）患者向医薬品ガイド
3）ワクチン接種を受ける人へのガイド
4）厚生労働省発出の安全性情報；

- 医療用医薬品
- 医療機器
- 再生医療等製品
- 一般用医薬品
- 要指導医薬品
- 体外診断薬

- 使用上の注意の改訂指示通知
- 安全対策に関する通知
- 自主点検通知
- 医薬品・医療機器等安全性情報
- 厚生労働省発表資料

5）緊急安全性情報・安全性速報
6）医薬品リスク管理計画（RMP）
7）Drug Safety Update（日薬連）
8）OTC 版 Drug Safety Update（一般薬連）
9）症例報告に関する情報
10）医療安全対策に関連する通知等
11）PMDA 医療安全情報
12）重篤副作用疾患別対応マニュアル
13）新薬の承認に関する情報
14）回収情報
　　（医薬品，医薬部外品，化粧品，
　　医療機器）

- 副作用が疑われる症例報告に関する情報
- 不具合が疑われる症例報告に関する情報
- 再生医療等製品の不具合が疑われる症例報告に関する情報
- コンビネーション医薬品の機械器具部分の不具合等が疑われる症例報告に関する情報

PMD Act in November 2014, the notification of package inserts is obligatory.

On August 1, 2005, PMDA medi-navi was started. Newly arriving information listed in **Table 8.8** are automatically distributed to registered users (can register without charge) (As of March 30, 2018, 164,821 users are reportedly registered.).

8.5 PMDA Website

PMDA website[11] which provides information on pharmaceuticals and medical devices, which is repeatedly referred to in Chapter 8 of this book, was originally created following the inauguration of the drug information provision system project by the former Organization for Pharmaceutical Safety and Research and the FPMAJ in May 1999 for physicians, dentists and pharmacists to promote safe use of drugs. With the publication of "Drug Guide for Patients" in January 2006, information for the "general public" and for "healthcare professionals" was listed separately from March 2007 so that the necessary information can be easily obtained for each user. Thereafter, several revisions were made. As of October 2018, navigation by visit is composed of "for General public," "for Healthcare professionals" "for Academia" and "for Business."

The information listed as of October 2018 is shown in **Table 8.9**.

For innovative drugs with novel mechanisms of actions, the MHLW has specified to prepare "Guidelines for Promotion of Optimal Use" providing requirements for patients and healthcare professionals, concepts and points to note for the use of the concerned drug from the viewpoint of promoting optimal use based on the latest scientific evidence, and prepared Guidelines for Promotion of Optimal Use have been presented on the said

Table 8.9 Main drug-related information presented on the PMDA website (as of October 2018)

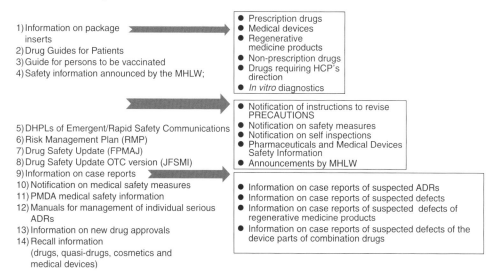

る患者および医療機関等の要件，考え方および留意事項を示す「最適使用推進ガイドライン」を作成することとし，作成された最適使用推進ガイドラインを当該ホームページに掲載している。

文　　献

1) 厚生省薬務局長通知，1997 年（平成 9 年）4 月 25 日付 薬発第 606 号（医療用医薬品添付文書の記載要領について）
2) 厚生省薬務局安全課長通知，1997 年（平成 9 年）4 月 25 日付 薬安第 59 号（医療用医薬品添付文書記載要領について）
3) 厚生省薬務局長通知，1997 年（平成 9 年）4 月 25 日付 薬発第 607 号（医療用医薬品の使用上の注意記載要領について）
4) 厚生労働省医薬局長通知, 2003 年（平成 15 年）5 月 15 日付 医薬発第 0515005 号（生物由来製品の添付文書に記載すべき事項について）
5) 厚労省医薬・生活衛生局長通知，2017 年（平成 29 年）6 月 8 日付 薬生発第 0608 第 1 号（医療用医薬品の添付文書の記載要領について）
6) 厚労省医薬・生活衛生局安全対策課課長通知，2017 年（平成 29 年）6 月 8 日付 薬生安発 0608 第 1 号（医療用医薬品の添付文書等の記載要領の留意事項について）
7) 厚生労働省医薬局長通知, 2005 年（平成 17 年）6 月 30 日付 薬食発第 0630001 号（患者向医薬品ガイドの作成要領）
8) 医薬品インタビューフォーム記載要領 2018 —日本病院薬剤師会—
（https://www.jshp.or.jp/cont/18/1108-2-3.pdf）
9) 医療用医薬品製品情報概要等に関する作成要領，2017 年 10 月
（http://www.jpma.or.jp/about/basis/drug_info/pdf/drug_info05.pdf）
10) 日本製薬工業協会医薬品評価委員会 PMS 部会，「医療用医薬品添付文書」情報提供の手引き—平成 28 年 4 月版—，2016 年
11) PMDA ホームページ：https://www.pmda.go.jp
12) 医薬品医療機器情報配信サービス（PMDA メディナビ）：
http://www.pmda.go.jp/safety/info-services/medi-navi/0007.html

website since 2017.

References

1) PAB Notification No. 607 MHW dated April 25, 1997 (Guide to Drafting Package Inserts of Ethical Drugs)

2) PAB/SD Notification No. 59 MHLW, dated April 25, 1997 (Guidelines for descriptions in package inserts of ethical drugs)

3) PFSB Notification No. 0515005 MHLW, dated May 15, 2003 (Items to be described in package inserts of biological products)

4) PAB Notification No. 607 MHLW, dated April 25, 1997 (Guidelines for descriptions in precautions for use of ethical drugs)

5) PSEHB Notification No. 0608-1, MHLW dated June 8, 2017 (Guidelines for descriptions in precautions for use of ethical drugs)

6) PSEHB Notification No. 0608-1, MHLW dated June 8, 2017 (Points to Consider for guidelines for descriptions in precautions for use of ethical drugs)

7) PFSB Notification No. 6030001 MHLW, dated June 30, 2005 (Guidelines for preparation of drug guides for patients)

8) Guidelines for descriptions in Drug Interview Forms - Japanese Society of Hospital Pharmacists (JSHP) - (https://www.jshp.or.jp/cont/18/1108-2-3.pdf)

9) Guidelines for preparation of ethical drug product information brochure, October 2017 (http://www.jpma.or.jp/about/basis/drug_info/pdf/drug_info05.pdf)

10) PMS Subcommittee, Drug Evaluation Committee, Japan Pharmaceutical Manufacturers Association, "Package Inserts of Ethical Drugs", Guidelines for information provision –April 2016-, 2016

11) PMDA's website: https://www.pmda.go.jp

12) Pharmaceuticals and Medical Devices Information E-mail Alert Service (PMDA medinavi): http://www.pmda.go.jp/safety/info-services/medi-navi/0007.html

和 文 索 引

※ 本書偶数ページ（左側）に掲載しているものを，アルファベットを含めて，すべてこの和文
索引にまとめた。当該分野では略称など，日本語でもアルファベットのままで使用されるも
のが多くあるためである。

アルファベット

AESI　　78

Aggregate Data　　76

AI・機械学習　　36

AMED　　4, 26

BSE　　102

CAPA　　142

CCDS　　164, 192, 194

CCSI　　192

CIOMS VI　　180

CIOMS　　78

Core RMP　　124

CSV 形式　　28

CTD　　124

DCSI　　78

DHPL　　164

DPC 調査　　188

DSU　　212

DSUR　　74

EPPV　　4

EU GVP　　138, 172

EU RMP　　124

European Union　　138

GCP renovation　　6

GCP　　54

GCTP　　42

Global RMP　　124

GMP　　42, 58

GPMSP　　12

GPSP (Good Post-marketing Study Practice)　　12, 14, 22, 54, 66

GQP (Good Quality Practice)　　58, 64

GVP (Good Vigilance Practice)　　12, 54, 58, 136

GVP モジュール I　　138

GVP モジュール II　　142

GVP モジュール IV　　138

HIV (Human Immunodeficiency Virus)　　84

ICH E17　　8

ICH E19　　36

ICH E2A　　70

ICH E2C　　112

ICH E2C (R2)　　112

ICH E2E　　108, 120

ICH E2F　　74

ICH E6　　6, 54

ICH E8　　6

ICH E2B (R3)　　26, 72

Identified/Potential Risk　76

JADER (Japanese Adverse Drug Event Report database)　28

MAH (Marketing Authorisation Holder)　140

Managing the Risks from Medical Product Use　94

MID-NET　4, 16, 18, 22, 28, 34, 182

MID-NET 運用開始記念シンポジウム　28

MIHARI Archive　186

MIHARI Communication　186

MIHARI Project　186

MIHARI (Medical Information for Risk Assessment Initiative)　22

MIHARI プロジェクト　22, 24

MTS 調査　188

PACMP　44

PASS　172

PBRER (Periodic Benefit-Risk Evaluation Report)　108, 110, 112, 114, 124

PMDA 信頼性保証部　132

PMDA 第 3 期 5 か年計画　26

PMDA 第 4 期中期計画　34

PMDA ホームページ　172, 184, 202, 204, 212, 214, 216

PMDA メディナビ　22, 30, 32, 214, 216

Pragmatic clinical trials　6

PSMF (Pharmacovigilance System Master File)　140, 142

PSUR (Periodic Safety Update Report)　108, 110

PV 監査　132, 140, 142

PV 契約　138, 142

PV システム　138

QR コード　46

Quality Management　56

Quality Management System：QMS　56

Real World Data　6

Reference RMP　124

REMS (Risk Evaluation and Mitigation Strategy)　124

RMP　4, 14, 22, 32, 78, 82, 106, 120

RMP 掲載のお知らせ　30

RMP マーク　34

SAE　76

SMT (Safety Management Team)　78

solicited　160

TERMS　186

unsolicited　158

vCJD (変異型クロイツフェルト・ヤコブ病)　102

WHO モニタリング制度　90

あ行

安全確保措置　62, 66

安全管理情報の評価・分析・検討　62

安全管理責任者　58

安全管理統括部門　62, 160

安全性確保の措置　82

安全性監視　8

安全性監視活動　82

和文索引　223

安全性監視計画策定の検討の進め方
　14, 16, 108

安全性管理チーム　78

安全性検討事項　124

安全性速報　128, 182, 212

安全性定期報告　108

安全性データの評価　78

イエローレター　128, 212

異常行動　34

遺族一時金　148

遺族年金　148

委託　66

一般医療機器　60

一般使用成績調査　66, 166

一般用医薬品　62

遺伝子組換え製品　104

イベントの性質　180

医薬品安全性情報の入手・伝達・活用状況
　等に関する調査　32

医薬品安全対策情報　212

医薬品医療機器情報配信サービス（PMDA
　メディナビ）　30

医薬品・医療機器等の品質，有効性及び安
　全性の確保等に関する法律　4

医薬品医療機器等法改正　38, 40, 160,
　196

医薬品等適正広告基準　204

医薬品の安全管理審査に関する調査事業
　186

医薬品の市販後調査の基準に関する省令の
　一部を改正する省令　100

医薬品の臨床試験の実施基準　54

医薬品副作用救済基金　144

医薬品副作用被害救済基金法　144

医薬品リスク管理計画　4, 14, 22, 32, 82,
　124

医薬品リスク管理計画指針について
　122

医薬品リスク管理計画書の概要の作成及び
　公表について　110

医薬部外品　60

依頼に基づかない情報源　158

依頼に基づく情報源　160

医療関係者へのお知らせ　164

医療機関からの副作用等報告制度　12,
　20

医療機関における安全性情報の伝達・活用
　状況に関する調査　186

医療機関報告制度　86

医療機関モニター報告制度　86

医療情報データベース　4, 16, 18, 22, 28,
　34, 182

医療情報データベース基盤整備事業
　186

医療手当　148

医療費　148

医療用医薬品製品情報概要　204

医療用医薬品製品情報概要等に関する作成
　要領　204

医療用医薬品の製造販売後調査等の実施方
　法に関するガイドラインについて
　166, 174

医療用医薬品の販売情報提供活動に関する
　ガイドライン　26, 52, 204

因果関係の評価　180

インタビューフォーム　204

牛海綿状脳症（BSE）　102

疫学調査相談　4

オセルタミビル　34

オンサイトセンター研修　28

か行

回収処理　64

改正 GPSP　4, 58

改正 GVP　58

改善措置　134

介入研究　164

開発中止届出　76

各対処方法の関連法令下における位置づけ
の整理　14

カテゴリー 1　112, 118

カテゴリー 2　112, 118

カテゴリー 3　112, 118

観察研究　6, 164

患者からの副作用報告制度　14, 90

患者登録システム（レジストリ）　28

患者向医薬品ガイド　30, 200, 206

患者向医薬品ガイドの作成要領について
200

感染症定期報告制度　12, 102

感染等被害救済制度　144

管理医療機器　60

企業中核データシート　164, 192

企業報告制度　84, 88

希少疾病用医薬品　166

休薬中止基準　76

教育訓練　62, 64

行政指導による再評価（第一次）　116

許可区分　62

緊急安全性情報　128, 182, 208, 212

緊急安全性情報等の提供に関する指針につ
いて　208

くすりのしおり　204, 206

化粧品　62

健康被害事件　2

研究報告　158, 162

抗がん剤併用療法実態把握調査　188

抗体医薬品　104

高度管理医療機器　62

後発医薬品の RMP　128

国際共同治験　8, 80

国際共同治験の計画及びデザインに関する
一般原則　8

国際誕生日　76, 110

国内販売提携先　136

国民への情報提供　30

国立研究開発法人 日本医療研究開発機構
4

国立成育医療研究センター　188

コンプライアンス　136

さ行

再審査期間　104

再審査結果の判定　112

再審査・再評価申請資料　56

再審査終了後の RMP 定期報告　128

再審査制度　12, 82, 104

再生医療等製品　6

再評価制度　82, 112

先駆け審査指定制度　6, 8, 12, 38

サリドマイド薬害　82, 144, 158

時間的関連性　180

シグナル　176

シグナル検出　176

シグナル評価　176

自己点検　62, 64, 134, 136

システム調査（プロセス調査）　134

事前評価　6

疾患登録レジストリ　48, 172

実践的臨床試験　6

実地調査　136

自発報告制度　82, 158

市販後安全対策　14

市販後リスク管理　82

市販直後調査　22, 94, 100

市販直後調査計画書　102

市販直後調査実施報告書　102

市販直後調査制度　4

市販直後の定点観測　188

社内規則　136

集積情報　180

重篤性　178

重篤度分類基準　180

重篤副作用疾患別対応マニュアル　178

重要な潜在的リスク　108, 122

重要な特定されたリスク　122

出荷時の品質管理　58

障害児養育年金　148

障害年金　148

条件及び期限付承認制度　8, 10

条件付き承認制度　4, 8

条件付き早期承認制度　8, 10, 38, 42

使用上の注意　88, 182, 202

使用成績調査　16, 66, 168

使用成績比較調査　66, 166, 168

承認後変更管理計画書（PACMP）　44

承認取得日　76

承認条件　8

承認申請資料（CTD）　124

情報伝達　92

症例登録方法　174

初回治験計画届出日　76

処方実態調査　22

処方せん医薬品　62

処方せん医薬品以外の医療用医薬品　62

書面調査　134

新再評価　116

審査ラグ　2

申請資料の信頼性の基準　132, 134

申請ラグ　8

診断書　146

真のエンドポイント　170

信頼性保証部（PMDA）　132

診療データベース　182

スモン事件　144

製造管理及び品質管理基準　58

製造出荷判定　58

製造販売業三役　58

製造販売業の許可　58

製造販売業の許可区分　60

製造販売後安全管理基準　12, 54

製造販売後安全管理業務手順書　60

製造販売後調査及び試験の実施基準　12, 54

製造販売後調査等基本計画書　106, 172

製造販売後調査等実施計画書　66

製造販売後データベース調査　16, 22, 66, 164, 170

製造販売後の医薬品安全性監視における医療情報データベースの利用に関する基本的考え方について　170

製造販売後の有効性の検討　14

製造販売後臨床試験　8, 16, 164, 168

製品回収　64

製品基本情報　192, 202

生物由来製品　64, 196

生物由来製品感染症等被害救済制度
　144, 152
是正措置及び予防措置　**142**
説明的臨床試験　**6**
選択除外基準　**76**
全例調査方式　**166, 174**

総括製造販売業者　**132**
総括製造販売責任者　**48, 50, 58, 62**
葬祭料　**148**
措置報告　**158, 164**
ソリブジン　**84**

た行

第一次再評価　**116**
第1種製造販売業者　**62**
体外診断用医薬品　**60**
大規模臨床試験　**170**
第3種製造販売業者　**62**
対照群　**170**
代替のエンドポイント　**170**
第二次再評価　**116**
第2種製造販売業者　**62**

チェックリスト　**136**
治験安全性最新報告（DSUR）　**74**
治験安全性最新報告概要　**74**
治験依頼者　**72, 74**
治験計画届　**72**
治験実施計画書　**72, 78**
治験実施施設　**70, 76**
治験責任医師　**76**
治験中核安全性情報（DCSI）　**78**
治験薬概要書　**70, 76**
治験薬副作用等緊急報告制度　**70**

中央登録方式　**166, 174**
注目すべき AE（AESI）　**78**
貯蔵等の管理　**64**

追加の医薬品安全性監視活動　**124**
追加の安全性監視方法　**16, 124**
追加のリスク最小化計画　**32, 122, 126**
追跡（詳細）調査　**160**
通常のリスク最小化活動　**126**

ディオバン　**24**
定期的安全性最新報告（PSUR）　**110,
112**
定期的ベネフィット・リスク評価報告
（PBRER）　**112, 114**
定期の予防接種　**92**
定期の予防接種等による副反応の報告等の
取扱いについて　**92**
データベース分析手法高度化事業　**186**
データマイニング　**176**
適合性調査（信頼性保証査察）　**42**
適合性評価　**132**
適正使用情報　**214**
電子保存された診療録等を用いた医薬品の
安全性に関する調査　**188**
電送化率　**28**
添付文書情報　**44, 46, 194, 198, 200**

同意文書　**76**
投薬証明書　**146**
特定使用成績調査　**66, 164**
特定臨床研究　**6**
ドラッグ・ラグ　**2, 8**
トレーサビリティー　**46, 50**

な行

日本医療研究開発機構　4, 26
日本版 Drug Safety Update　212
妊娠と薬情報センター　188

年次報告（治験薬）　72

は行

バーコード　46
バイオ後続品　122
バリデーション研究　172
販売部門　62

ヒト免疫不全ウイルス　84
病院情報システムデータ　172
非臨床データ　76, 78
品質管理業務手順書　60
品質管理統括部門　64
品質再評価　116, 118
品質システム　138
品質不良　64
品質保証責任者　58
品質保証部門　64

フィジビリティー調査　172
フォローアップ監査　138
不具合報告　86
副作用・感染救済給付　146
副作用・感染症報告制度　12, 82, 158
副作用等報告制度　92
副作用症例データセット　28
副作用被害判定部会　148
副作用・不具合情報収集　26
副作用用語集　30

副反応検討部会　94
副反応報告制度　90, 92
ブルーレター　128, 212
プロスペクティブな調査　176
プロセス調査　134
プロモーションコード　136

別の要因　156, 180
変異型クロイツフェルト・ヤコブ病　102

補遺（ICH E6 ガイドライン）　56
ホライゾン・スキャンニング　36

ま行

未承認薬審査迅速化のためのリスク管理体制構築に資する調査事業　186

尤もらしさ　180
モニター病院　86

や行

薬害肝炎事件の検証及び再発防止のための医薬品行政のあり方検討委員会　18, 52, 56
薬害肝炎訴訟　56
薬害再発防止のための医薬品行政等の見直し　18
薬害事件　2
薬剤師　48, 62, 64
薬事・食品衛生審議会（副作用被害判定部会）　92, 148
薬価制度改革　4

優先審査　6

優先相談　6

溶出試験　116, 118
予測性　178
予防接種健康被害救済制度　146, 154
予防接種法　90, 92, 154

ら行

利活用開始前研修　28
利活用申出前研修　28
リサーチ・クエスチョン　172
リスク管理計画（RMP）　78
リスクコミュニケーション　24, 32
リスク最小化策　14, 78
リスクマネジメント　70

臨時の再評価　116
臨床研究　6
臨床データ　76
臨床評価ガイドライン　168

類薬情報　78
類薬データ　76

レジストリ　28
レセプトデータベース　182
レトロスペクティブな調査　176
連続調査方式　166, 174

わ行

ワクチン　90, 92, 104

Alphabetical Index

* For readers in English, the following index listed terms only in right-hand pages of this book.

abnormal behavior   35

acquisition,transmission and utilization of pharmaceutical safety information   33

Ad Hoc Reevaluation   117

additional pharmacovigilance activities   127

additional risk minimization   33

additional risk minization activities   123, 127

aditional pharmacovigilance methods   17

administrative database   183

Adverse drug reactions and infections reporting system   83

ADRs reported directly from medical institutions   21

Advanced Database Analysis Method Project   187

Adverse Drug Reaction Relief Service Fund   145

Adverse Drug Reaction Relief Service System   145

Adverse Events of Special Interest (AESI)   79

Adverse drug reaction (ADR) and infection reporting system   13

aggregate data   77

AI and machine learning   37

all-patient investigations   167

all-patient investigation system   167,

175

Alternative cases   181

analysis safety assurance measures   63

Annual reporting   73

antibody drug   105

application lag   9

approval conditions   9

appropriate advertising standards for drugs   205

assessment   177

barcodes   47

Basic plan for implementation of post-marketing studies   107

Basic Product Information   193

Biological plausibility   181

biological products   65, 123

biosimilar products   123

Blue Letter   213

bovine spongiform encephalopathy (BSE)   103

CAPA (Corrective Action and Preventive Action)   141

Category 1   113, 119

Category 2   113, 119

Category 3   113, 119

Causality assessment   181

CCDS (Company Core Data Sheet)

165, 193, 195

central registration system   167, 175

CIOMS VI   181

CIOMS (Council for International
Organization of Medical Science)
79

claim database   183

clinical evaluation guidelines   169

clinical studies   7

clinical trial in the protocol   73

clinical trial plan   73

clinical trial safety updated report (DSUR)
75

collection of ADR/defect information
27

Commemorative Symposium for Initiation
of MID-NET   29

Committee on judgement of Sufferers from
Adverse Drug Reactions   149

Common Technical documents (CTD)
125

Company Core Data Sheet (CCDS)
165, 193, 195

Company Core Safety Information (CCSI)
193

compliance evaluation   133

compliance inspection   43

conditional and fixed-term approval system
9, 11

conditional approval system   5, 7, 9

Conditional Early Approval System   9,
11, 39, 43

consultation service for epidemiological
studies   5

continuous investigation system   167,
175

Core RMP   125

cosmetics   63

CSV format   29

data-mining   177

dependent on a request (solicited)   161

Development Core Safety Information
(DCSI)   79

Development Safety Update Report
(DSUR)   75

Dear Healthcare Professional Letters
(DHPL)   165

DHPL of Emergent Safety Communication
183

DHPL of Rapid Safety Communication
183

Diovan   27

Disability pension   149

disabled child support pension   149

disease registry   49

DPC Survey   189

Drug Guides for Patients   31, 201, 207

drug-induced hepatitis   57

Drug Information Sheet   205, 207

drug lag   3, 9

Drug Safety Update   215

drug-induced hepatitis   57

DSU, Japanese version   215

DSUR   75

Early post-marketing phase risk
minimization and vigilance   95, 101

Early Post-marketing Phase Risk
Minimization and Vigilance (EPPV)
5

education and training   63, 65

electronic healthcare database   183

electronic transmission rate   29

Emergency Safety Communication DHPL
129, 209

Emergent Safety Communication DHPL
(Yellow Letter)   129, 183

Emergent/Rapid Safety Communiation DHPLs 205, 209, 213

Eropean Union (EU) 139

Ethical Drug Product Information Brochure 205

ethical drugs 197

EU GVP 139

EU RMP 125

Expectedness 179

explanatory clinical trials 6, 7

First Reevaluation 117

Fixed-point observations of pharmacovigilance activities in medical institutions at an early post-marketing stage 189

funeral expenses 149

GCP (Good Clinical Practice) 55

GCP renovation 7

General Drug Use Investigations 167

General Principles for planning and Design of Multi-Regional Clinical Trials 9

General Safety Management Division 63, 161

global clinical trials 9, 81

Global RMP 125

Glossary of Adverse Drug Reaction 31

GMP (Good Manufacturing Practice) 59

GMP/GCTP 43

GPMSP 13

GPSP (Good Post-marketing Study Practice) 13, 15, 55, 67

GPSP Ordinance 23

GQP 59, 65

Guide to the Preparation of Drug Guides for Patients 201

guidelines for activities to provide marketing information on prescription drugs 205

Guideline for Promotion Information Provision Activities of Prescription Drugs 27, 53

GVP (Good Vigilance Practice) 13, 55, 59

GVP Modulu I 139

GVP Modulu II 141

highly controlled medical devices 63

horizon scanning 39

hospital-information system data 173

How to develop pharmacovigilance planning 15, 17

human immunodeficiency virus (HIV) 87

ICH E17 9

ICH E19 37

ICH E2A 71

ICH E2B (R3) 27, 73

ICH E2C 113

ICH E2C (R2) 113

ICH E2E 109, 121

ICH E2F 75

ICH E6 7, 55

ICH E8 7

Identified/Potential Risk 77

imprementation plan 103

incidence of thalidomide 83

incidents of health damage caused by adverse drug reaction (ADRs) 3

Information for Proper Use 215

information on other drugs in the same class 79

information provision to the public 31

Information source of measures-taken reports   165

information source of research reports   163

Infrastructure Development Project for Medical Information Database   187

international birth date   111

interventional studies   165

interview form   205

Introduction of the Periodic Reporting System for Infections   13

Investigation and Prevention of Recurrence of Drug-induced Hepatitis Cases   19

investigation of actual prescription practice   25

Investigation of Post-marketing Efficacy   15

Investigations regarding pharmaceutical safety using electronic medical records   187

investigators   77

investigator's brochure   71

Japan Agency for Medical Research and Development (AMED)   5, 27

Japanese Adverse Drug Event Report database (JADER)   29

Law for Adverse Drug Reaction Relief Service Fund   145

license category   63

MAH reporting system   85, 89

Managing the Risks from Medical Product Use   95

Mandatory ADR Reporting Medical Institutions   13

Manuals for management of individual serious ADRs   179

marketing division   63

material prepared to communicate accurate information on individual ethical drugs to HCPs for the purpose of promoting proper use   205

measures-taken report   159

medical allowances   149

medical evaluation for the safety   79

Medical expenses   149

medical information database   5, 17, 19, 23, 29, 37

Medical Information for Risk Management Initiative (MIHARI)   23

Medical Informations System (MIS) survey   189

medical institution monitoring report system   87

Method of provision of package insert information   47

MID-NET   5, 17, 19, 23, 29, 35, 183

MIHARI Communication   187

MIHARI Archive   187

MIHARI Project   25, 185

Modulu IV   139

monitoring hospitals   87

multiple cases   181

National Center of Child Health and Development   189

Nature of event   181

New Reevaluation   117

non-clinical data   79

not dependent on a request (unsolicited)   159

Notice of posting of RMP   31

notification of discontinuation of development   77

observational studies   165

Organization of the Position of Each Measure under the Relevant Laws and Regulations   15

office of conformity Audit   133

On-site center training   29

orphan drugs   167

oseltamivir   35

other factors   157

package insert information   45

Package Inserts   195, 199

PACMP (post-approval change management plan)   45

PASS (Post-authorisation Safety Studies)   173

Patient Adverse Drug Reaction Reporting System   15, 91

Patient enrollment methods   175

patient registration system (registry)   29

PBRER   111, 113

Periodic Benefit-Risk Evaluation Report (PERER)   112, 115, 125

Periodic reporting on RMP following Reexamination period   129

Periodic reporting system for infections   103

periodic safety reports   109

Pharmaceutical Affairs and Food Sanitation Council   149

pharmaceutical and medical devices information e-mail service (PMDA Medi-navi)   31

Pharmaceuticals and Medical Devices Agency (PMDA)   133, 161

Pharmaceutical Officer   49, 51, 59, 63, 65

pharmacist   49

Pharmacovigilance System Master File (PSMF)   141

pharmacovigilance activities   83

pharmacovigilance planning   109

Pharmacovigilance system Master File   141

Pharmacovigilance (PV)   9, 133

patient ADR reporting system   91

PMDA Medi-navi   23, 31, 33, 215, 217

PMDA's third-term five-year plan   27

PMDA's fourth medium-term plan   35

PMDA website   29, 33, 173, 185, 203, 205, 213, 215, 217

Post-marketing clinical trials   9, 17, 165, 169

post-marketing database studies   67, 171

post-marketing database study   17, 167

Post-marketing database survey   23

post-marketing safety management and quality management   61

pre-application evaluation   7

Precautions   203

pregmatic clinical trials   6, 7

Pregnancy and Medicine Information Center   189

prescription drug   63

Preventive Vaccination Act   155

Preventive Vaccination Law   91, 93

priority consultation   7

priority review   7

promotion code   137

prospective investigations   177

protocol   79

PSNF   141

PSUR (Periodic Safety Update Report)   111

PSUR/PBRER   109

PV audits   141

PV contracts   139, 143

PV system   139

QR code   47

Quality Assurance Officer   59

quality defects   65

Quality Management   57

quality management division   65

Quality Management System (QMS)   57

Quality Revaluation   117, 119

Rapid Safety Communication DHPL (Blue Letter)   129, 183

real world data   7

recalls   65

Reevaluation system   13, 83, 113, 117

Reexamination period   105

Reexamination results   113

Reexamination system   13, 83, 105

Reference RMP   125

reformation of the drug pricing system in Japan   5

regenerative medicine products   7

Relief Service for Infections derived from Biological Products   153

Relief Service System for Adverse Health Effects following Vaccination   155

relief service system for infections   145

relief service system for infections derived from biological products   145

Relief Services System for Adverse Health Effects with Vaccination   147

REMS (Risk Evaluation and Mitigation Strategy)   125

reporting system for ADRs   93, 159

research questions   173, 175

research reports   159

Retrospective investigations   177

Review Committee on Drug Administration for Investigation and Prevention of Recurrence of Drug-induced Hepatitis Cases   53

review lag   3

Review of drug administration, etc. for prevention of recurrence of incidents of drug-induced suffering   19

revised GPSP Ordinance   5

revised package inserts   211

revision of package inserts   183

revision of Pharmaceutical and Medical Device Act   41

risk communication   25, 33

Risk Management Plan (RMP)   5, 15, 23, 79, 83, 125

risk minimization plan   15, 33, 79, 83

RMP   33, 79, 83, 107, 121, 129

RMP for generic medicines   129

RMP mark   35

routine risk minimization activities   127

SAE   77

safety assurance measures   67, 83

Safety Management Officer   59

Safety Management Team (SMT)   79

Safety Specification   125

safety assurance measures   63, 83

SAKIGAKE Designation System   7, 9, 13, 39

Second Reevaluation   117

self inspections   63, 65, 135, 137

Seriousness   179

Seriousness classification criteria   179

signal   177

single detection   177

single genetically-modified product

105

SMON   145

solicited   161

sorivudine   85

Specified clinical studies   7

Specified use-results survey   67, 167

sponsor   73, 77

spontaneous reporting system   83, 159

standard operating procedures (SOP)
61

Standards for the Reliability of Application
Data   135

studies performed for Reexamination and
Reevaluation applications   57

study sites   71, 77

summary of the clinical trial safety updated
report   75

Survey project for drug safety management
review   187

Survey project to help establish a risk
management system to promote a
shorter-review period for unapproved
drugs   187

Surveys for communication/utilization
status of safety information at medical
institutions   187

survivor lump sum payments   149

Survivor pensions   149

system for expedited reporting of Adverse
Drug Reaction (ADRs)   71

system inspections (process inspectoins)
135

Temporal relationship   181

TERMS   187

thalidomide   145, 159

Thalidomide Education and Risk
Management System   187

the Act Securing Quality,Efficacy and

Safety of Pharmaceuticals,Medical
Devices, Regenerative and Cellular
Therapy Products and Cosmetics   7

The Blue Letter   183, 213

the Good Post-marketing Study Practice
13

the Japan Agency for Medical Research and
Development (AMED)   5

the Pharmaceutical and Medical Device Act
(PMD Act)   39

the Pharmaceutical Officer   49, 51

the PMD Act   7, 39, 197

the post-marketing studies implementation
plan   67

the SAKIGAKE Designattion System
7, 9

the survey on the current status of
combination therapy with anticancer
agents   189

The Yellow Letter   183, 213

Three Officers in Marketing Authorization
Holders   59

traceability   47, 53

Training before applying for utilization of
MID-NET   29

Training before utilizing MID-NET   29

type 1 marketing business   63

type 2 marketing businesses   63

type 3 marketing businesses   63

unsolicited   159

Use-results surveys   17, 67

Use-results survey with comparative group
67, 167, 169

vaccine   105

Vaccine adverse Reactions reporting system
91, 93

Vaccine Adverse Reaction Review

Committee   95

vCJD (variant Creutzfeldt-Jakob disease)
    103

WHO monitoring system   91

Yellow Letter   213

日英対訳

日本における医薬品のリスクマネジメント 第3版

－新たな改正GPSP省令への対応と医薬品医療機器等法の改正に向けて－

定価　本体14,000円（税別）

2010年 3 月19日	初版発行
2014年 10月30日	第2版発行
2019年 5 月20日	第3版発行

企画・編集　　一般財団法人 医薬品医療機器レギュラトリーサイエンス財団

発 行 人　　武田 正一郎

発 行 所　　株式会社 じ ほ う

　　　　　101-8421　東京都千代田区神田猿楽町1-5-15（猿楽町SSビル）
　　　　　電話　編集　03-3233-6361　販売　03-3233-6333
　　　　　振替　00190-0-900481
　　　　　＜大阪支局＞
　　　　　541-0044　大阪市中央区伏見町2-1-1（三井住友銀行高麗橋ビル）
　　　　　電話　06-6231-7061

©2019　　　　　　　　　　　　　　　組版・印刷　（株）日本制作センター
Printed in Japan

本書の複写にかかる複製，上映，譲渡，公衆送信（送信可能化を含む）の各権利は
株式会社じほうが管理の委託を受けています。

JCOPY ＜出版者著作権管理機構 委託出版物＞

本書の無断複製は著作権法上での例外を除き禁じられています。
複製される場合は，そのつど事前に，出版者著作権管理機構（電話 03-5244-5088，
FAX 03-5244-5089，e-mail：info@jcopy.or.jp）の許諾を得てください。

万一落丁，乱丁の場合は，お取替えいたします。

ISBN 978-4-8407-5170-4